PSYCHIATRIC SYMPTOMS AND COGNITIVE LOSS IN THE ELDERLY

Evaluation and Assessment Techniques

EDITED BY

Allen Raskin

NATIONAL INSTITUTE OF MENTAL HEALTH

Lissy F. Jarvik

BRENTWOOD VETERANS ADMINISTRATION HOSPITAL
AND
UNIVERSITY OF CALIFORNIA, LOS ANGELES

HEMISPHERE PUBLISHING CORPORATION

Washington New York London

A HALSTED PRESS BOOK

JOHN WILEY & SONS

New York Chichester Brisbane Toronto

Hemisphere Publishing Corporation
1025 Vermont Ave., N.W., Washington, D.C. 20005

Distributed solely by Halsted Press, a Division of John Wiley & Sons, Inc., New York.

1 2 3 4 5 6 7 8 9 0 L I L I 7 8 3 2 1 0 9

Library of Congress Cataloging in Publication Data

Main entry under title:

Psychiatric symptoms and cognitive loss in the elderly.

Includes indexes.
1. Geriatric psychiatry. 2. Cognitive disorders–Testing. 3. Mental illness–Diagnosis. I. Raskin, Allen, date II. Jarvik, Lissy. [DNLM: 1. Cognition disorders–In old age–Congresses. 2. Psychiatric status rating scales–In old age–Congresses. 3. Evaluation studies–Congresses. 4. Depression–In old age–Congresses. 5. Psychopathology–In old age–Congresses. 5. Psychopathology–In old age–Congresses. WT150 P967]
RC451.4.A5P76 618.9'76'89075 78-23705
ISBN 0-470-26579-5

Printed in the United States of America

Contents

Contributors

Bertram S. Brown, MD, Assistant Surgeon General, U.S. Public Health Service, National Institute of Mental Health, Rockville, Maryland

Donna Cohen, PhD, Assistant Professor and Chief, Behavioral Biology Unit, Department of Psychiatry and Behavioral Sciences, University of Washington School of Medicine, Seattle, Washington

Thomas H. Crook, PhD, Research Psychologist, Psychopharmacology Research Branch, National Institute of Mental Health, Rockville, Maryland

Carl Eisdorfer, MD, PhD, Professor and Chairman, Department of Psychiatry and Behavioral Sciences, University of Washington School of Medicine, Seattle, Washington

Lissy F. Jarvik, MD, PhD, Chief, Psychogenetics Unit, Brentwood VA Hospital, and Professor, Department of Psychiatry and Biobehavioral Sciences, University of California at Los Angeles, Los Angeles, California

Gerald E. Kochansky, PhD, Assistant Professor of Psychiatry (Psychology), Massachusetts Mental Health Center, Boston, Massachusetts

Nanette A. Kramer, PhD, Clinical/Aging Psychology Program, University of Southern California, Los Angeles, California

Margaret W. Linn, PhD, Director, Social Science Research, Veterans Administration Hospital, and Associate Professor of Psychiatry, University of Miami School of Medicine, Miami, Florida

Douglas M. McNair, PhD, Professor of Psychiatry (Psychology), Boston University School of Medicine, Boston, Massachusetts

Henry J. Michalewski, PhD, Postdoctoral Fellow, Ethel Percy Andrus Gerontology Center, University of Southern California, Los Angeles, California

Julie V. Patterson, MA, Research Assistant, Department of Psychology, Ethel Percy Andrus Gerontology Center, University of Southern California, Los Angeles, California

Robert Plutchik, PhD, Associate Professor, Department of Psychiatry, Albert Einstein College of Medicine, Bronx, New York

Allen Raskin, PhD, Research Psychologist, Psychopharmacology Research Branch, National Institute of Mental Health, Rockville, Maryland

Carl Salzman, MD, Assistant Professor of Psychiatry, Harvard Medical School, Massachusetts Mental Health Center, Boston, Massachusetts

Richard I. Shader, MD, Associate Professor of Psychiatry, Harvard Medical School, Massachusetts Mental Health Center, Boston, Massachusetts

James M. Smith, PhD, Harlem Valley Psychiatric Center, Wingdale, New York

Larry W. Thompson, PhD, Professor of Psychology, Ethel Percy Andrus Gerontology Center, University of Southern California, Los Angeles, California

Foreword

While the overall population of the United States more than doubled in the years 1900 to 1960, one subgroup—comprised of persons over 65 years of age—increased fivefold, from 3.1 million to 16.7 million. Further, according to current projections, by 1980 the number of people age 65 and over will exceed 24 million.

This increase in the proportion of older people has been associated with a parallel increase in the use of psychiatric services by this age group. However, the available services have fallen far short of the need, qualifying the elderly as undeservedly underserved. Thus, during my tenure as director of the National Institute of Mental Health (NIMH), I was pleased to have the opportunity to authorize establishment of an NIMH Center for Studies of the Mental Health of the Aging as the focal point of our activities responsive to the emerging public health issues. Simultaneously, I encouraged other components of the institute to expand existing programs and develop new initiatives pertinent to the mental health needs of the elderly. We clearly needed more advocacy for and knowledge of older citizens.

As part of the institute's response to my request for new initiatives, an aging program was established within the Psychopharmacology Research Branch. Staff responsible for the program were concerned primarily with the use of psychoactive drugs among this age group. However, as Drs. Raskin and Jarvik note in the Preface, the fact readily became apparent that instruments currently available for assessing psychiatric symptoms and cognitive loss among the elderly suffer from serious shortcomings. A workshop was convened on this particular issue, and this volume is one outcome of that workshop.

I was pleased to learn that the workshop also had other effects. Many of the participants were encouraged to take a more active role in refining existing assessment instruments and in developing more meaningful instruments for measuring psychopathology in the elderly. I hope that these efforts, aimed at an increased sensitivity in measuring treatment effects, will rebound ultimately in the discovery of new and more effective methods for treating mental illness in the elderly.

Bertram S. Brown, MD
Assistant Surgeon General
U.S. Public Health Service

Preface

A major stumbling block in research with the elderly has been the lack of valid and reliable instruments for assessing both cognitive functioning and psychiatric symptoms in these individuals. Tests designed for use with a general psychiatric population are not always appropriate when applied to the elderly. For example, clinicians who have worked with the elderly have long felt that depression and anxiety often take somewhat different forms in older than in younger depressed and anxious patients. The syndrome known as depressive pseudodementia is a good illustration of this phenomenon. The term refers to memory loss and other signs of cognitive disturbance that superficially resemble an organic brain syndrome but where the symptoms are, in fact, concomitants of depression. This syndrome is not uncommon in the aged but is often misdiagnosed and hence improperly treated.

The past decade has also witnessed an increase in research with the elderly, especially treatment-oriented research. As a result, more investigators have become aware of the failings and shortcomings of existing assessment instruments in this field and of the need for more meaningful assessment devices.

With this background in mind we decided to bring together experts in this field to critically review the present state of the art with regard to the diagnosis and evaluation of psychopathology in the elderly. A workshop on this topic was subsequently held on April 8–9, 1977 under the joint sponsorship of the National Institute of Mental Health and the University of California at Los Angeles. Prior to the workshop each participant was asked to prepare a review paper evaluating existing rating scales in his or her field and to include recommendations for improving existing scales or for the development of new scales. The workshop provided an opportunity to bring into focus the most critical needs in this field, such as the need for more meaningful measures of memory loss, and to discuss techniques and approaches for meeting these needs.

For the most part, the chapters in this book represent an amalgam of the critical reviews that were prepared prior to the workshop and new information the authors added based on comments and suggestions of their colleagues at the workshop. This book also contains a number of chapters solicited after the workshop to fill gaps that were not closed in the papers prepared by the workshop participants.

This book deals with the assessment of psychopathology and the assessment of cognitive disturbances in the elderly. The chapters by Drs. Robert Plutchik and Thomas Crook discuss both conceptual and practical issues relating to assessment in these areas. Dr. Plutchik raises a number of fundamental questions about the goals of assessment in the elderly and the appropriate criteria for evaluating strengths and weaknesses of existing measurement instruments. Dr. Crook focuses on the special problems associated with efforts to measure memory loss and other aspects of cognitive dysfunction in the elderly. He discusses such issues as the need to make cognitive tests meaningful by relating them to cognitive tasks that aged individuals face in their daily lives.

Chapters 5 through 8 are devoted to critical reviews of instruments that have been used to assess psychopathology in the elderly. There are separate chapters on psychiatric rating scales, self-rating scales, nurse and psychiatric aide rating scales, and community adjustment scales. These chapters provide the reader with an opportunity to weigh the advantages and disadvantages of the major measures of psychopathology currently being used with the aged and to decide which of these instruments best meet his or her own needs. Chapter 10 by Drs. Nanette A. Kramer and Lissy F. Jarvik provides a similar service to the reader interested in tests presently in use to measure cognitive performance in the elderly. Drs. Donna Cohen and Carl Eisdorfer (chapter 11) take the reader one step further. They discuss recent developments in the area of cognitive testing with an emphasis on tests that have evolved from cognitive theories.

This book also offers the reader an understanding of the genesis and development of psychopathology in the elderly and why certain forms of psychopathology occur with greater frequency in older than in younger patients. These issues are discussed in chapter 1 by Dr. Allen Raskin and in chapter 3 by Drs. Carl Salzman and Richard I. Shader. Chapter 3, in particular, describes how both psychological and somatic factors, such as endocrine disturbances, can lead to depression in the elderly.

From the prior description it should be evident that this book was designed to be more than a compendium of geriatric rating scales. First, it provides a conceptual framework for understanding some of the psychosocial and biological bases for mental illness in the elderly. Second, broad issues such as the purpose of testing in this age group and the special problems of assessing psychopathology and cognitive dysfunction in elderly subjects are discussed. Finally, the heart of the book is devoted to detailed critical analyses of the major assessment instruments in this field with specific recommendations included for improving existing scales, or where necessary, developing new assessment devices.

The book should have obvious appeal to researchers and others who need assessment instruments to evaluate the clinical status of elderly patients and the effects of various therapeutic modalities such as drug treatment or hospital milieu effects. However, we hope this book will also appeal to other mental health professionals who either desire a better understanding of the symptomatic behaviors they are likely to encounter in elderly psychiatric patients or possible biological as well as psychosocial bases for this behavior. This book can also assist the clinician by providing information on quantitative techniques for establishing the presence and degree of psychopathology in elderly patients as an aid to both differential diagnosis and treatment.

We wish to acknowledge the efforts of the various contributors who made this book possible. It is a very time-consuming, thought-provoking, and often tedious task to prepare critical literature reviews, especially reviews of rating scales, and we are grateful to all authors for a job well done. As we have noted elsewhere the impetus for this book grew out of a workshop on geriatric assessment measures that was jointly sponsored by the National Institute of Mental Health and the University of California at Los Angeles. Many individuals from both institutions generously permitted us to call upon their special expertise and experience to make that meeting a success. However, we would like to single out for special mention Drs. Jerome Levine and Louis A. Wienckowski of the National Institute of Mental Health for their consultation, encouragement, and support in all stages of this endeavor. Ms. Sue Dohan of the University of California at Los Angeles assumed major responsibility for coordinating the myriad administrative details associated with organizing and running the workshop in Los Angeles for which we are most appreciative. Last, but certainly not least, Diane Cheslosky of the National Institute of Mental Health prepared correspondence, proofed and retyped manuscripts, and performed many other functions essential to the preparation of this book.

Allen Raskin
Lissy F. Jarvik

I

ASSESSING PSYCHOPATHOLOGY

1

Signs and Symptoms of Psychopathology in the Elderly

Allen Raskin
National Institute of Mental Health

This chapter focuses on the unique expressions and forms of psychopathology in elderly persons. In particular, attention is directed to the following issues: Do depression and anxiety manifest themselves in somewhat different form in older as compared to younger patients? What signs and symptoms distinguish depressive pseudodementia from true dementia? What are the characteristics of the schizophrenias noted in later life? What similarities and differences exist in the sleep disturbances of young and old adults? Do some symptoms have different meaning when they occur in older as compared to younger patients?

DEPRESSION

General

Affective disorders, and depression in particular, constitute a serious mental health problem for persons 65 years of age and older. Epstein (1976) has reported the incidence of affective disorders in older persons in communities as well as in hospitals as 10–65%. Roth (1955) has estimated that approximately 50% of older persons admitted to mental hospitals have depression. Essen-Möller and Hagnell (1961) have reported lifetime risks of depression to be 17.7% for men and 8.5% for women who were followed to age 80. In the latter study most of the subjects were examined by a psychiatrist to establish the diagnosis of depression. The sex differences noted by Essen-Möller and Hagnell are consistent with the results of a study by Gurland (1976) who reported a higher incidence of depression in women than in men prior to age 45 and a tendency for this difference to equalize at age 45 and then to reverse after age 65.

The wide disparity in the incidence and prevalence of depression noted above is related to two factors. First, the rates drop if one uses psychiatric diagnosis rather than symptom pattern for classifying patients as depressed. Gurland (1976) has cited data from the U.S.-U.K. Cross National Project indicating that only 5% of patients over age 60 were diagnosed as depressed by the study psychiatrists but that many more patients were given high depression ratings on a symptom checklist. The psychiatrists had an apparent bias toward diagnosing patients age 60 and over as chronic organic brain syndrome rather than depression and overassigning depression diagnoses to patients 35-59 years of age. The second factor is the high incidence of transient depressive episodes in older individuals, episodes lasting a few hours to a few days and precipitated by external events. Psychiatrists and other mental health professionals differ on whether to label these transient attacks as true depressive episodes.

In order to understand why there would be a high incidence of transient depressive attacks in older persons and also why these individuals might present with somewhat different symptoms than younger depressed patients, one needs to consider the stresses and pressures that are unique to the older age group. First, there are significant sensory losses and health problems associated with aging. It has been estimated that 29% of individuals 65 and older have significantly impaired hearing (Butler, 1975), many may have decreased visual acuity, and many experience crippling arthritis and losses from vascular disease that restrict physical movement and impair speech. Even among the healthy elderly, psychomotor responses are slowed (Schaie & Strother, 1968), and recent memory is often impaired (Kahn, Zarit, Hilbert, & Niederehe, 1975; Whitehead, 1973). The consequences of these losses are more isolation and withdrawal among the elderly than among the young.

The elderly are also host to a variety of psychosocial factors that can precipitate depression. Advancing age often leads to forced retirement, decreased financial resources, and loss of emotional support by the death of friends or relatives. Consequently, it is not remarkable that pessimism has been noted as a common characteristic in this age group (Zung & Green, 1972, pp. 213-224). An empirical study by Beckman and Brody (1973) has confirmed the relationship between role loss and depression in the elderly. These authors have found a statistically significant correlation between a Role Loss Index derived from Dean's Powerless Scale and The Beck Depression Inventory in 167 older men and women. Unfortunately, the age range in this study is not specified.

Even if one acknowledges that the elderly are especially vulnerable to physical and psychosocial factors that can lead to depression and that depression is epidemic in this age group, it does not necessarily follow that depression manifests itself differently in older than in younger individuals. There remains the need to document differences in the frequency, quality, and intensity of depressive attacks in younger and older adults. Unfortunately, hard evidence of this kind is hard to come by. For example, no studies have specifically examined differences between younger and older adults in the frequency of depressive attacks or in the duration of these attacks.

Some data do exist on differences in presenting symptoms between young and old depressed patients and signs of depression in depressed and normal elderly persons.

Differences between Normal and Depressed Elderly

In two separate studies young and old normal adults were compared on the Zung Self-Rating Depression Scale (SDS). Zung and Green (1972, pp. 213-224) reported high total SDS scores in two groups of normals, those under 19 years of age and those 65 years of age and older. Zung offered no explanation for these differences, but Blumenthal (1975) stated that the somatic items on the SDS, such as constipation, weight loss, fatigue, and heart racing, may have resulted in spuriously high total scores for those over 65. It is her contention that somatic complaints in persons 65 and older often reflect true physical problems rather than depression. In other words, these items have different meaning for older than for younger adults (cf. chapters 2, 5, and 6 for further discussion of the SDS).

An analysis of the rank ordering of the 20 SDS items for those age 65 and older revealed that these normal individuals tended to rate the somatic items high and the depression items low. Specifically, items reflecting decreased libido, psychomotor retardation, anorexia, diurnal variation, constipation, and confusion were ranked high, whereas depression and crying spells were ranked low (Zung, 1967).

Zung (1967) also performed a factor analysis of the SDS on a sample of 169 normal geriatric subjects 65 and older and labeled the first principal component Loss of Self-Esteem. His Depressed Affect item loaded .43 on this factor compared to loadings of .68 for Personal Devaluation, .65 for Emptiness, and .62 for Indecisiveness. However, when a normal varimax rotation was performed, the first rotated factor continued to have high factor loadings for the items Personal Devaluation, Emptiness, and Indecisiveness, but Depressed Affect now had a loading of .73 on this factor. The somatic complaint items had high loadings on the second factor indicating they were relatively independent of the depression and self-esteem items. This would be consistent with Blumenthal's (1975) comments about the meaning of somatic complaint items in elderly persons. In commenting on these results, Zung (1967) referred to statements by other authors that depression in the elderly tends to take a form different from that usually found in younger individuals. He noted that elderly depressed patients are often characterized by apathy, disinterest in their surroundings, lack of drive, inertia, and gloominess.

Blumenthal (1975) performed a cluster analysis of the SDS on a sample of 160 normal married couples, including 72 individuals 58 years of age or older. She extracted four clusters that she labeled Well-Being, Depressed Mood, Somatic Symptoms, and Optimism. Her Well-Being cluster included many of the items with high loadings on Zung's Loss of Self-Esteem factor. She ran separate correlations among these clusters for those over 57 years of age and found the correlations with the Somatic Symptoms cluster were particularly low. This finding led her to comment that the somatic symptom items may have different meaning in older individuals than in younger ones and may be primarily a measure of the reduced physical endurance and cardiovascular problems that often occur in older age groups rather than a measure of depressive symptomatology. Blumenthal also noted that the Optimism cluster for those over 57 years of age had low correlations with the other clusters. This cluster contains the items, "My mind is as clear as it used to be" and "I feel hopeful about the future." Here too she stated that these items may have different meaning for older than for younger adults. She commented on the increasing memory problems in older individuals, which may have a physical basis, and on the lack of optimism about the future, which is not unusual in older individuals with significant physical infirmities and health problems.

Salzman and Shader (1972, pp. 159–168) compared two separate samples of normal individuals, 60 years of age and older, with a sample of young volunteers, (21–35 years of age, on the depression factor from the Profile of Mood States (POMS) (McNair & Lorr, 1964), the D60 depression scale of the Minnesota Multiphasic Personality Inventory (MMPI), and the shortened Dempsey modification of the D60. These results ran counter to Zung and Green's (1972, pp. 213–224) findings as the two samples of elderly subjects rated themselves lower on depression than the young volunteers, especially on the Depression factor from the POMS. The POMS is a self-rated adjective checklist. One explanation for these disparate findings could be the presence of somatic complaint items on Zung's SDS and the absence of these items on the Depression factor from the POMS. As noted previously, it has been suggested that the inclusion of somatic complaint items on a depression scale designed for use with elderly subjects with significant health problems may result in spuriously high depression ratings (Blumenthal, 1975).

Although Blumenthal's comments about the differences in meaning of somatic complaint items in young and old persons have obvious merit, one has to be cautious not to label all somatic concerns, complaints of body slowness, and expressions of fatigue and apathy as normal for elderly subjects. Gurland, Fleiss, Goldberg, Sharpe, Copeland, Kelleher, and Kellett (1976) extracted a rather large Depression factor from the Geriatric Mental State Schedule, which had been administered to 100 elderly subjects 65 years of age and older. This factor included complaints of memory impairment, a loss of interest in social activities, a lack of energy and listlessness, and sleep and vegetative disturbances. As a result these authors concluded that one has to be careful to disengage behaviors that can legitimately be ascribed to the aging process from those associated with depression.

Differences between Elderly and Nonelderly Depressed Patients

Studies in this area have generally focused on two issues, the preponderance of somatic complaints in elderly depressed patients and the state of apathy and withdrawal that characterizes many elderly depressed patients (cf. chapters 2, 3, and 5).

Birkmayer, Neumayer, and Riederer (1973, pp. 158–166) studied symptomatology of depression using a self-devised rating scale in 105 patients below age 65 and in 53 patients above age 65. The symptom profile was similar in both groups, but the geriatric patients showed an increased incidence of insomnia, loss of appetite and weight, headaches, and dizziness. There was no difference between the groups in feelings of guilt. This latter finding is interesting because other authors have reported that expressions or feelings of guilt occur less frequently in elderly than in young depressed patients (Busse, 1961, pp. 274–284; Busse & Reckless, 1961).

On the basis of clinical observation, a number of authors noted that somatic complaints tend to be emphasized and may be the predominant complaints in elderly depressed patients (Busse & Pfeiffer, 1973, pp. 109-144; de Alarcon, 1964). Using data from the U.S.-U.K. Cross National Project, Gurland (1976) compared a group of 32 patients 65 years of age and older with a group of 173 patients 20–59 years of age on scores derived from the Geriatric Mental Status examination. Both groups were diagnosed by project psychiatrists as suffering from depressive disorders. He found that somatic concerns were more evident in the older than in the younger depressed patients. Similarly, Salzman, Van der Kolk, and Shader (1975) reported that of 152 consecutive admissions with depression in patients over age 60, 64% were found to have "physically unjustified bodily complaints." The most frequent complaints (32%) were gastrointestinal disorders, 19% were head symptoms, and 8% were cardiovascular symptoms.

The distinction between justified and unjustified physical complaints is not always easy to make. It has been reported, for example, that about 80% of people 64–74 years of age have some form of chronic medical disorder and that this figure rises to 87% for those over age 74 (Bell, 1973; Shanas, 1974).

There is a frequent reference in the literature to the observation that depressed elderly patients appear apathetic, seem disinterested in their surroundings, and lack drive (Epstein, 1976; Fann, Wheless, & Richman, 1976; Levin, 1963; Zung & Green, 1972, pp. 213–224). Smith, Bright, and McCloskey (1977) rated 370 ambulatory geriatric patients on the 28-item Geriatric Rating Scale. Of the three factors that emerged, the first and largest factor consisted of 11 items and was labeled Withdrawal-Apathy. However, this study was performed on a heterogeneous sample of ambulatory geriatric patients with a variety of psychiatric disorders. Hence, one has to be careful to separate the apathy and withdrawal that is often seen in older persons from the apathy specific to depression in this age group. One also needs to be careful to distinguish the apathy seen in depressed elderly persons from the motor retardation and emotional withdrawal that occurs in other psychiatric conditions, such as schizophrenia.

The observation has also been made that elderly depressed patients are often reluctant to admit feelings of dysphoric mood and sadness (Davies, 1965; Salzman & Shader, 1972, pp. 159–168). As a result, many clinicians base their diagnosis of depression on what they feel are unjustified somatic complaints and on the appearance of apathy and withdrawal. One is reminded in this context of a similar problem with young children and adolescents where depression is often masked or not readily observable but still central to much of the acting out and antisocial behavior displayed by disturbed youngsters. However, the efforts by Spitzer, Endicott, and Robins (1975) and Feighner, Robins, Guze, Woodruff, Winokur, and Munoz (1972) to operationalize psychiatric diagnosis require the presence of dysphoric mood as a necessary precondition to the diagnosis of depression. It may be, particularly with older individuals, that diagnosis will have to depend more on observation of the patient's behavior than on the patient's verbal comments to establish the presence of dysphoric mood. Does the patient look sad or cry easily? It is also possible the patient may be more willing to admit feeling sad and blue on an instrument (such as a self-report adjective checklist that can be completed with no one else present) than to a psychiatrist, psychologist, or other mental health professional.

Changes in Depressive Symptomatology as Patients Get Older

Long-term studies of elderly depressed patients do not exist. Consequently, there is no evidence to indicate whether the symptom pattern changes over time. The concept of the "burnt out" schizophrenic seems to have no direct counterpart in the depression literature. In a review article of depression in the elderly, Epstein (1976) reported that depressive symptomatology in senescence was found to improve. However, senescence was not defined and this observation was apparently based on clinical impression rather than evidence from longitudinal or follow-up studies. Post (1972) did conduct a 3-year follow-up of 92 depressed inpatients over age 60. He reported only 26% had lasting recoveries, 37% had further attacks, 25% showed some residual depressive invalidism, and 12% remained clinically depressed throughout the follow-up period. Lest one become overly pessimistic about the prognosis of depressive illness in the elderly, it now appears prognosis is equally guarded for younger depressed patients. Weissman and Kasl (1976) recently reported the results of a 1-year follow-up of 150 depressed women, 24–60 years of age, treated initially as outpatients. In the year following 8 months of maintenance treatment with amitriptyline, 21% of these women had a new, documented episode of depression, 60% experienced some recurrences of symptoms, and 15% were as symptomatic at 1 year as they had been when they received acute treatment.

Table 1 lists the major signs and symptoms of depression in the elderly as gleaned from the literature in this area. Because there is so little empirical

TABLE 1 Signs and Symptoms of Depression in the Elderly

Dysphoric mood
- Looks sad; mournful or depressed
- Cries easily; eyes moist or tearful
- Reports feeling depressed or blue
- Speaks in a sad, gloomy, or mournful voice

Suicidal behavior and ideation
- Reports recurrent thoughts of death, dying, or suicide
- Expresses wish to be dead
- Says life is not worth living
- Has made suicide attempts

Pessimism and inadequacy
- Reports future seems bleak, dark, or unbearable
- Reports feeling hopeless
- Is preoccupied with feelings of inadequacy
- Has clinging dependency
- Worries continually about something
- Reports feeling indecisive

Guilt, shame, or worthlessness
- Blames self for things done or not done
- Feels worthless and no good to anyone
- Reports feeling inferior to others
- Suffers from troubled conscience

Anergia or fatigue
- Feels everything is an effort
- Feels tired, worn-out, lacking in energy
- Looks tired and lacking in energy
- Reports waking up feeling tired
- Sits or lies around because of lack of energy

Apathy and social withdrawal
- Lacks interest in hobbies previously enjoyed
- Does not enjoy being with others
- Is alone most of the time
- Spends little free time at recreational activities
- Has lost interest in TV or radio

Retardation in speech or behavior
- Speaks slowly
- Moves slowly and deliberately
- Subjectively feels slowed down in movements

Memory
- Has trouble remembering recent events
- Has trouble remembering past events such as those from childhood
- Has good memory one day, bad the next

Attention or concentration
- Has difficulty in attending or concentrating
- Checks and double-checks every action

Confusion or perplexity
- Reports feeling confused
- Appears bewildered by events
- Rambles or drifts off topic being discussed

Sleep disturbances
- *See text discussion*

Vegetative disturbances
- Loss of appetite
- Recent weight loss of 10 pounds or more

Sex difficulties
- No longer shows interest in sex
- Derives little pleasure from sexual activities previously enjoyed

Somatic complaints
- Headaches
- Constipation
- Dry mouth
- Pains in stomach
- Pressure in the head
- Nausea or upset stomach

data on this topic, no attempt was made to assess the validity of these specific behaviors as measures of depression in the elderly. For that purpose, better criteria for diagnosing elderly individuals as depressed are needed. Also needed are large representative samples of young and old normal subjects and young and old depressed patients to determine which items characterize depression in general, which are idiosyncratic to older depressed patients, and which are related to age rather than depression (i.e., characterize both the old depressed and the old normal subjects and distinguish them from the two younger groups).

A number of points were previously raised about scale construction. Reference was made to the fact that somatic complaints may have different meaning for an older than for a younger depressed patient. In persons 65 years of age and older, chronic physical illness is the rule rather than the exception. Physical complaints may be tapping real health problems rather than be concomitants of depression. Consequently, in rating these somatic complaints it may be worthwhile to include a separate column for indicating whether the rater feels that a given complaint represents a real health problem or a hypochondriacal complaint. Items so rated would be treated separately in the scoring and in subsequent data analysis.

It may also be necessary to provide more detailed definitions and guidance to raters for distinguishing behaviors, such as apathy, fatigue, motor retardation, and emotional withdrawal, that tap different aspects of behavior and can have important diagnostic and treatment implications. In this context Overall and Gorham's (1962) manual for the Brief Psychiatric Rating Scale is recommended. It provides guidelines for distinguishing between tension and anxiety and between motor retardation and emotional withdrawal.

One solution that has been suggested for getting elderly individuals to admit they feel depressed is the use of a self-report scale. The individuals can complete the scale in private without having to admit openly to a psychiatrist or psychologist that they have been feeling sad or blue. Another possibility is to develop scale items that measure the tendency to deny mental health problems, the converse of a problem encountered in some young neurotic patients, labeled the "sick set," who openly admit to any and all deviant or psychopathological behaviors.

SLEEP DISTURBANCES

Although sleep disturbances are considered among the major symptoms of depression, they are discussed separately because of their common occurrence (50% or higher) in persons 60 years of age or older (Feinberg & Carlson, 1968; Kahn & Fisher, 1969; Kahn, Fisher, & Lieberman, 1970). The symptoms commonly noted in elderly individuals experiencing sleep difficulties include: increased latency or time to fall asleep (initial insomnia), frequent awakening during the night (middle insomnia), increased frequency of dreaming, lighter sleep, and an increase in total time spent in bed with a decrease in total amount of sleep (Amin, 1976). An especially serious problem in older individuals is early awakening and an inability to fall asleep again (late insomnia), one of the characteristics of endogenous depression.

Electroencephalographic (EEG) recordings indicate an increase in arousals and a decline in rapid eye movement (REM) latency and in deep (stage IV) sleep with advancing age. Stage IV sleep at age 60 is about 55% of that at age 20 (Agnew, Webb, & Williams, 1967; Kales, Wilson, Kales et al., 1967; Karacan, Williams, Littell, & Salis, 1973, pp. 120-132). It has also been reported that the amount of REM sleep in elderly adults may be related to the general vigor and health of the individual (Kahn & Fisher, 1968).

In using assessment instruments it may be worthwhile to include items that tap the range of sleep disturbances rather than one all-inclusive item that asks if the patient has difficulty in sleeping. In addition to items on initial, middle, and late insomnia, information about the depth of the patient's sleep and about the frequency of dreaming should also be obtained. It would also be worthwhile to consider other ways of increasing the accuracy of this information, which is notoriously unreliable when based solely on reports from the patients themselves, but without doing intensive sleep studies with EEG recordings.

Distinguishing Depressive Pseudodementia from True Dementia

The term *depressive pseudodementia* has been applied to elderly individuals who complain both of depression and of memory and other cognitive problems, but for whom there is no clear evidence of organic brain damage. Post (1976, pp. 205-234) estimated the incidence of these reversible dementias, or pseudodementias, to be between 7 and 19%. It is often difficult to know whether the memory problems reported are concomitants of depression and/or anxiety, or if anxiety and depression are the natural accompaniments of memory loss in the early stages of senile dementia or other forms of organic brain damage. The ability to distinguish depressive pseudodementia from true dementia may be of more than academic interest. It is conceivable that in both groups the anxiety and depression would respond to treatment with an antidepressant. It is also conceivable that the true dementia group might have a higher susceptibility to the adverse effects of these drugs, especially their anticholinergic effects. At present, we do not have answers to these questions, but an obvious first step would be to distinguish true dementias from the pseudodementias. Psychiatric symptoms may provide clues for distinguishing these groups and may aid in the differential diagnosis, as may differential test patterns on psychological tests such as the Wechsler Adult Intelligence Scale (WAIS) (Crookes, 1974).

Nevertheless, the differential diagnosis is difficult to make. Zung and Green

(1972, pp. 213–224), for example, noted that psychomotor slowing or agitation, labile affect, decreased libido, constipation, and paranoid ideation may be features common to both depression and organic brain syndrome. The depressive pseudodementias may also mimic, at times, the progressive deterioration that is the hallmark of senile dementia. In severe depressions one often sees a loss of concentration and attention that may affect not only recent memory but also orientation. A progressive deterioration in personal habits may also exist. Poor appetite, weight loss, and other physical changes may add to the impression of a progressive deterioration (Kiloh, 1961). Differentiating these two groups can be further complicated by the effects of poor nutritional intake or the discontinuation of therapeutic drugs for certain physical illnesses. These actions can lead to metabolic disturbances that may, in turn, result in states of delirium.

Despite these problems in diagnosis, differences in symptoms have been noted in these two groups of patients. Studies have shown (Roth, 1955; Roth & Morrissey, 1952) that in 150 patients over age 60, those with affective psychoses had symptoms of depression, retardation, self-reproach, and nihilistic, somatic, or paranoid delusions that occurred with a clearly defined onset and without evidence of progressive deterioration in adjustment prior to the presenting illness. Patients with senile psychosis, on the other hand, were characterized by an insidious onset with progressive failure at work, in routine activities, or both. The principal symptoms in these latter patients were confusion with disorientation, intellectual deterioration, impairment of memory, restlessness, and hallucinations.

Roth's results suggest that patients with senile psychosis or organic brain disease (OBD) generally do not report feeling blue or depressed. A similar finding has been noted by Gurland et al. (1976) who compared a group of 32 depressed patients with a group of 39 OBD patients on factors derived from the Geriatric Mental State Schedule. These authors have reported that the depressive group showed more depression, anxiety, somatic concerns, and depersonalization than the OBD group but showed less impairment on the dimensions of cognitive function such as impaired memory, cortical dysfunction, and disorientation. They also have noted that the OBD group was best separated from the depressive group on disorientation. This latter finding suggests that the OBD subjects in the study by Gurland et al. (1976) were probably a chronic group of fairly deteriorated patients. The absence of depression in these patients by no means rules out the possibility of patients in the early stages of senile dementia becoming depressed and anxious when memory and other cognitive problems first become apparent. A recent study by Kahn, Zarit, Hilbert and Niederehe (1975) has given some credence to this view. These authors found that in a group of depressed elderly subjects and a group of organically impaired elderly subjects memory complaints were more prevalent in those with high scores on the Hamilton Depression Scale (Hamilton, 1967). However, the group of organically impaired subjects who did not have memory complaints and were also rated low on the Hamilton Depression Scale showed significantly greater impairment on performance tests that tapped cognitive function than the organically impaired patients with high memory complaints and high scores on the Hamilton Depression Scale. Consequently, it appears that there is a lessening of both depression and verbalized complaints of memory loss in individuals as they become more cognitively impaired as a result of chronic OBD (cf. chapters 3 and 9 for further reference to depressive pseudodementia).

ANXIETY

There is a more substantial literature on depression in the elderly than there is on anxiety in this age group. However, it is generally accepted that anxiety is also a serious problem in the elderly. Clinical practitioners in this field have reported that, as is true of depression, anxiety in the elderly generally does not take the same form as anxiety in younger persons. Kral and Papetropoulus (1965, pp. 775-786) noted, for example, that only a small number of elderly patients have phobic anxiety reactions or obsessive compulsive neuroses. Lehmann and Ban (1969) have indicated that intrapsychic conflicts are rarely central to the anxiety seen in the elderly. Instead, anxiety, agitation, and restless tension in the elderly are said to be most often associated with some physical disorder and to take the forms of sleeplessness, hypochondriacal fears regarding the heart, lung, or other organ systems, loss of appetite, and, in some cases, obsessive eating.

Again, as was true of depression, the major psychosocial factors associated with anxiety in the elderly are reported to be fear of getting old, losing one's role in society, and becoming isolated and rejected. The occurrence of both anxiety and depression in the same elderly persons is also a common phenomenon. Finally, the tendency noted for normal elderly subjects to deny feelings of depression, as compared to younger adults, is also apparent for feelings of anxiety and tension. Specifically, Salzman and Shader (1972, pp. 159-168) found that two samples of normal elderly subjects 60 years of age and older scored significantly lower on the Tension factor of the POMS, a self-administered adjective checklist, and on the Taylor Manifest Anxiety Scale than a sample of normal volunteers 21-35 years of age.

Many of the prior comments on the paucity of empirical data and the need for additional research on depression in the elderly have equal validity for anxiety in the elderly and will not be repeated. Further, much of the research proposed for dealing with problems of assessing depression in the elderly may also be applied to assessing anxiety in the elderly.

SCHIZOPHRENIA AND PARANOID DISORDERS

Friedel and Raskind (1976) have proposed five meanings or definitions of schizophreniform psychosis as applied to the elderly. These include: (1)

patients with no cognitive impairment who develop acute schizophreniform illness with hallucinations and delusions; (2) patients with chronic progressive organic brain syndrome with memory loss, disorientation, and general intellectual impairment; (3) patients who have suffered from chronic schizophrenia since early adulthood; (4) patients with chronic brain syndrome who have also developed schizophreniform symptoms such as delusions and hallucinations; and (5) patients with chronic organic brain syndrome whose behavioral symptoms (agitation, irritability, assaultiveness) have become severe enough to cause distress to themselves or to their environment.

Because the condition is both serious and unique to elderly individuals, attention is focused on the first group of patients described by Friedel and Raskind (1976) and identified earlier (Roth, 1955) as suffering from late paraphrenia. These patients are generally characterized by a closely knit paranoid delusional system, a late onset of hallucinations, and a deterioration of the schizophrenic type occurring relatively late in life. Although some authors refer to this condition as a form of schizophrenia, most prefer to skirt the issue by regarding the late paraphrenias as a schizophreniform illness. These late paraphrenias make their first appearance during the fifth or sixth decade of life and sometimes later. They account for about 10% of the patients of an inhospital population (Roth, 1955) and about 7% of the patients in a geriatric clinic (Kral, 1961).

Factors that contribute to the development of paranoid reactions at any age tend to be more frequent in old age and include social isolation, solitary living, general insecurity, and sensory deficits, particularly visual and auditory loss (Busse & Pfeiffer, 1969, pp. 183–235). Individuals with schizoid dispositions may become overtly psychotic or develop late paraphrenia when senile degeneration or cerebral arteriosclerosis occurs (Bromley, 1966). Post (1973) also suggested that many of these patients have always been regarded as eccentric and may have, in fact, been borderline schizophrenics all of their lives.

To some extent there is also a uniqueness to the kinds of paranoid reactions and hallucinations that predominate in the elderly and that are often extensions of the physical and psychological losses they have undergone. For example, patients who believe that talk is being directed at them from next door or from the next floor often have significant hearing loss (Post, 1973). Post regards this as the most common form of paranoid symptomatology in the elderly. Feelings of being unwanted or of being subjected to annoyances may also become more intense in the elderly. Interference with one's property, such as theft of belongings or rearrangement of drawers, is also a common complaint in the elderly and may reflect some paranoid thinking.

It is worth noting that many of the scales that have been developed for use with a general psychiatric population or for assessing schizophrenic symptoms, including paranoid reactions, often fail to sample the kinds of paranoid reactions and hallucinations seen in elderly patients. Consequently, if a scale were devised that included these behaviors, we might see a significant rise in the recorded incidence of paranoid reactions in the elderly, a matter of practical importance since these elderly patients tend to show a good response to the major tranquilizers (Post, 1973).

DISCUSSION

The original intent of this chapter was to present a critical review and analysis of the bases for many of the widely held and reported beliefs regarding the occurrence of psychopathology in the elderly. Of special interest were the comments that the symptoms of depression, anxiety, and schizophrenia often differ in older as compared to younger persons. As we have seen, a good deal has been written on these topics, but, for the most part, what has been reported are clinical impressions and case histories rather than data from empirical studies. Consequently, as outlined in the review on the depression literature, we do not know, for example, which signs and symptoms of depression are unique to elderly depressed patients, which signs characterize depression in general, and which signs are found in all elderly persons, normal as well as depressed, and are therefore not pathognomonic of depression in this age group. Data on these questions are also lacking with regard to anxiety in the elderly.

Even in those studies that did make comparisons between indexes of depression in normal young and normal old adults or between young and old depressed patients, the authors seldom spelled out the criteria used for calling an individual depressed or, for that matter, for saying someone was normal and not depressed. One wonders, for example, how many of the elderly subjects would have been categorized as depressed had the authors used the Spitzer et al. (1975) or Feighner et al. (1972) criteria for the diagnosis of depressive disorders. This is an important point as so much of the depression reported in the elderly is transient and may last no more than a few days. To be diagnosed as depressed, using the Feighner et al. criteria, the depression must have lasted at least 1 month. Spitzer et al. have a category called episodic minor depressive disorder that requires a duration of symptoms for 1 week for a probable diagnosis and for 2 weeks for a definite diagnosis. It may be that in the elderly there is a transient form of depression, lasting no more than a few days, and Spitzer and associates may need to consider incorporating it in their Research Diagnostic Criteria (RDC). However, at the present time, when an author has examined a group of elderly depressed patients and does not list the criteria used for labeling these patients as depressed, we have no way of knowing whether these were primarily transient depressions or one of the 11 forms of major depressive disorders in the second edition of the RDC. Greater diagnostic clarity is obviously needed in this field if we are to sort out possible differences in the presenting symptoms of young and old depressed and/or anxious patients. Late paraphrenia also does not appear as a separate diagnostic entity in the RDC, although patients with this disorder would probably meet the diagnostic criteria specified for schizophrenia.

This review has highlighted some of the special problems one is likely to encounter in testing elderly subjects. Reference has been made to the fact that certain symptoms, such as somatic complaints, may have different meaning in older persons than in younger persons. Some elderly individuals are reluctant to admit having psychological problems, and it may be necessary to develop more subtle techniques for probing for signs of mental illness in this age group. In sum, it should be possible to develop scales that will sample the major signs and symptoms of psychopathology in the elderly and to devise techniques to handle the special problems encountered in testing these patients. Development of these scales will enable us to accurately document the major presenting symptoms of an elderly patient. Unfortunately, it is doubtful that these scales will be of much value in clarifying the diagnostic heterogeneity that now exists in this field. Perhaps an approach that combines psychiatric rating scales, cognitive test measures, and some of the newer neurophysiological and vascular techniques, such as computerized axial tomography and the xenon inhalation technique, may prove useful for this purpose.

REFERENCES

Agnew, H. W., Webb, W. B., & Williams, R. L. Sleep patterns in late middle-aged males: An EEG study. *Electroencephalography and Clinical Neurophysiology*, 1967, *23*, 168–171.

Amin, M. M. Drug treatment of insomnia in old age. *Psychopharmacology Bulletin*, 1976, *12*, 52–55.

Beckman, A. C., & Brody, G. F. Role loss, powerlessness and depression among older men and women. *Gerontologist*, 1973, *13*, 100.

Bell, W. G. Community care for the elderly: An alternative to institutionalization. *Gerontologist*, 1973, *13*, 349–354.

Birkmayer, W., Neumayer, E., & Riederer, P. In P. Keilholz (Ed.), *Masked depression*. Bern: Hans Huber, 1973.

Blumenthal, M. D. Measuring depressive symptomatology in a general population. *Archives of General Psychiatry*, 1975, *32*, 971–978.

Bromley, D. B. *The psychology of human aging*. Baltimore: Penguin, 1966.

Busse, E. W. Psychoneurotic reactions and defense mechanisms in the aged. In P. H. Hoch & J. Zubin (Eds.), *Psychopathology of aging*. New York: Grune & Stratton, 1961.

Busse, E. W., & Pfeiffer, E. Functional psychiatric disorders in old age. In E. W. Busse & E. Pfeiffer (Eds.), *Behavior and adaptation*. Boston: Little Brown, 1969.

Busse, E. W., & Pfeiffer, E. Mental disorders in later life–Affective disorders, paranoid, neurotic and situational reactions. In E. W. Busse & E. Pfeiffer (Eds.), *Mental illness in later life*. Washington, D.C.: American Psychiatric Association, 1973.

Busse, E. W., & Reckless, J. B. Psychiatric management of the aged. *Journal of the American Medical Association*, 1961, *175*, 645–648.

Butler, R. M. *Why survive? Being old in America*. New York: Harper & Row, 1975.

Crookes, T. G. Indices of early dementia on the WAIS. *Psychological Reports*, 1974, *34*, 734.

Davies, B. M. Depressive illness in the elderly patient. *Postgraduate Medicine,* 1965, *38,* 314–320.

de Alarcon, R. Hypochondrias and depression in the aged. *Gerontologia Clinica,* 1964, *6,* 266–277.

Epstein, L. J. Depression in the elderly. *Journal of Gerontology,* 1976, *3,* 278–282.

Essen-Möller, E., & Hagnell, O. The frequency and risk of depression within a rural population in Scania. *Acta Psychiatrica Scandinavica,* 1961, *162,* 28–32. (Suppl.)

Fann, W. E., Wheless, J. C., & Richman, B. W. Treating the aged with psychotropic drugs. *Gerontologist,* 1976, *16,* 322–328.

Feighner, J. P., Robins, E., Guze, S. B., Woodruff, R. A., Winokur, G., & Munoz, R. Diagnostic criteria for use in psychiatric research. *Archives of General Psychiatry,* 1972, *26,* 57–63.

Feinberg, I., & Carlson, V. R. Sleep variables as a function of age in man. *Archives of General Psychiatry,* 1968, *18,* 239–250.

Friedel, R. O., & Raskind, M. A. Psychopharmacology of aging. In M. S. Elias, B. E. Ellefpheriou, & P. K. Elias (Eds.), *Special review of experimental aging research: Progress in biology.* Bar Harbor: EAR, Inc., 1976.

Gurland, B. J. The comparative frequency of depression in various adult age groups. *Journal of Gerontology,* 1976, *31,* 283–292.

Gurland, B. J., Fleiss, J. L., Goldberg, K., Sharpe, L., Copeland, J. R. M., Kelleher, M. J., & Kellett, J. M. A semi-structured clinical interview for the assessment of diagnosis and mental state in the elderly: The Geriatric Mental State Schedule II: A factor analysis. *Psychological Medicine,* 1976, *6,* 451–460.

Hamilton, M. Development of a rating scale for primary depressive illness. *British Journal of Social and Clinical Psychology,* 1967, *6,* 278–296.

Kahn, E., & Fisher, C. Individual differences and amount of rapid eye movement sleep in aged adulthood. *Psychophysiology,* 1968, *3,* 393.

Kahn, E., & Fisher, C. The sleep characteristics of the normal aged male. *Journal of Nervous and Mental Disease,* 1969, *148,* 477–494.

Kahn, E., Fisher, C., & Lieberman, L. Sleep characteristics of the human aged female. *Comprehensive Psychiatry,* 1970, *11,* 274–278.

Kahn, R. L., Zarit, S. H., Hilbert, N. M., & Niederehe, G. Memory complaint and impairment in the aged. *Archives of General Psychiatry,* 1975, *32,* 1569–1573.

Kales, A., Wilson, T., Kales, J. D. Measurement of all-night sleep in normal elderly persons: Effects of aging. *Journal of the American Geriatric Society,* 1967, *15,* 405–414.

Karacan, I., Williams, R. L., Littell, R. C., & Salis, P. J. Insomniacs: Unpredictable and idiosyncratic sleepers. In W. P. Koella & P. Levin (Eds.), *Sleep: Physiology, biochemistry, psychology, pharmacology,–clinical implications.* Basel: Karger, 1973.

Kiloh, L. G. Pseudo-dementia. *Acta Psychiatrica Scandinavica,* 1961, *37,* 336–351.

Kral, V. A. Recent research in prevention of mental disorders at later age levels. *Proceedings of the Third Institute on Preventative Psychiatry.* Iowa City: University of Iowa Press, 1961.

Kral, V. A., & Papetropoulos, D. Treatment of geriatric patients. In N. S. Kline & H. E. Lehmann (Eds.), *International psychiatry clinics, psychopharmacology.* Boston: Little Brown, 1965.

Lehmann, H. E., & Ban, T. A. Chemotherapy in aged psychiatric patients. *Canadian Psychiatric Association Journal,* 1969, *14,* 361–369.

Levin, S. Depression in the aged: A study of the salient external factors. *Geriatrics,* 1963, *18,* 302–307.

McNair, D. M., & Lorr, M. An analysis of mood in neurotics. *Journal of Abnormal and Social Psychology,* 1964, *69,* 620–627.

Overall, J. E., & Gorham, D. R. The brief psychiatric rating scale. *Psychological Reports,* 1962, *10,* 799–812.

Post, F. The management and nature of depressive illnesses in late life: A follow-through study. *British Journal of Psychiatry,* 1972, *121,* 393–404.

Post, F. Paranoid disorders in the elderly. *Postgraduate Medicine,* 1973, *53,* 52–56.

Post, F. Diagnosis of depression in geriatric patients and treatment modalities appropriate for the population. In D. M. Gallant & G. M. Simpson (Eds.), *Depression: Behavioral, biochemical, diagnostic and treatment concepts.* New York: Spectrum Publications, 1976.

Roth, M. The natural history of mental disorders in old age. *Journal of Mental Science,* 1955, *101,* 281–301.

Roth, M., & Morrissey, J. D. Problems in the diagnosis and classification of mental disorder in old age. With a study of case material. *Journal of Mental Science,* 1952, *98,* 66–80.

Salzman, C., & Shader, R. I. Responses to psychotropic drugs in the normal elderly. In C. Eisdorfer & W. E. Fann (Eds.), *Psychopharmacology and aging.* New York: Plenum Press, 1972.

Salzman, C., Van der Kolk, B., & Shader, R. I. Psychopharmacology and the geriatric patient. In R. I. Shader (Ed.), *Manual of psychiatric therapeutics.* Boston: Little Brown, 1975.

Schaie, K. W., & Strother, C. R. Limits of optimal functioning in superior old adults. *Interdisciplinary Topics in Gerontology,* 1968, *1,* 132–150.

Shanas, E. Health status of older people. *American Journal of Public Health,* 1974, *64,* 261–264.

Smith, J. M., Bright, B., & McCloskey, J. Factor analytic composition of the Geriatric Rating Scale (GRS). *Journal of Gerontology,* 1977, *32,* 58–62.

Spitzer, R. L., Endicott, J., & Robins, E. *Research diagnostic criteria (RDC)* (2nd ed.). New York: Biometric Research, New York State Department of Mental Hygiene, 1975.

Weissman, M. M., & Kasl, S. V. Help-seeking in depressed out-patients following maintenance therapy. *British Journal of Psychiatry,* 1976, *129,* 252–260.

Whitehead, A. Verbal learning and memory in elderly depressives. *British Journal of Psychiatry,* 1973, *123,* 203–208.

Zung, W. W. K. Depression in the normal aged. *Psychosomatics,* 1967, *8,* 287–292.

Zung, W. W. K., & Green, R. L. Detection of affective disorders in the aged. In C. Eisdorfer & W. E. Fann (Eds.), *Psychopharmacology and aging.* New York: Plenum Press, 1972.

2

Conceptual and Practical Issues in the Assessment of the Elderly

Robert Plutchik
Albert Einstein College of Medicine

INTRODUCTION

This chapter is concerned with a number of critical issues regarding the problem of assessing the elderly. Some of these issues deal with the question of goals; that is, assessment for what? Some deal with scale construction and evaluation. Others relate to specifying criteria for evaluating measurement instruments currently available. In examining these issues, both rating and self-report scales are considered.

The chapter is organized in the following way. An initial section reviews statistics about changes in age distribution in the world population and considers some of the problems resulting from this change. A second section examines the goals of assessing the elderly. The third section considers some problems of research with the elderly. The last section discusses criteria for evaluating measurement instruments, with examples of various scales in current use and critical evaluations of these instruments.

THE STATISTICS OF AGING

It is ironic that U.S. culture is referred to as youth-oriented when the population as a whole is growing older. The aging of the population reflects a decrease in fertility associated with an increase in longevity. This process has been going on for a long time. In the years between 1900 and 1960, the American population more than doubled, while the population of persons over age 65 increased 5 times, from 3.1 million to 16.7 million. This means that older persons increased from 4.1% of the population to over 10%. By 1980, it is expected that there will be 24 million Americans over the age of 65 (Pollack, Locke, & Kramer, 1961).

These changes in the age of the population have been paralleled by changes in the psychiatric status of the elderly as well as in their use of services and facilities. For example, it has been estimated that 277,000 persons over 65 received care in a psychiatric facility in 1964. In that year 70% of all psychiatric patients were served in public mental hospitals, 5% were served in private mental hospitals, 17% in general hospitals, and 8% in outpatient psychiatric clinics (Rosen, Anderson, & Bahn, 1968). The nationwide survey of Rosen et al. also revealed that 80% of the elderly who entered public mental hospitals were diagnosed as having senile brain disease or cerebral arteriosclerosis, although this figure was considerably lower for private facilities. Psychoneurotic depressive reactions were reported for 14% of those between 65 and 74 years of age, while 20% of this same group were reported as showing affective and schizophrenic psychotic reactions. Only about 8% of the elderly were served on an outpatient basis.

In an updating of their 1969 nursing home survey, the National Center for Health Statistics reported that about 800,000 persons were residents of 18,000 nursing and personal care homes (1973). About 90% of these residents were over the age of 65, an increase of 47% over the number of residents in 1964. About 95% were white. The number of female residents increased faster than the number of male residents, and by 1969, almost 70% of the residents were female. The median age for all females was 81.9 years and for all males was 78.7 years. In terms of mental status, 45% had a partial or complete disability.

Although the increase in the aged population has been well documented, the distribution of the aged into various care facilities is not as well known. For example, Kramer, Taube, and Starr (1968) reviewed a number of epidemiological studies dealing with this issue. They pointed out that the number of patients entering state and county mental hospitals decreased during the 10-year period from 1955 to 1965, while the number entering VA hospitals increased.

One reason for the decline of patients in mental hospitals was that more and more psychiatric patients went to the general hospitals that provided psychiatric services. Kramer et al. (1968) reported that "the number of admissions to general hospitals with psychiatric services exceeds that to mental hospitals by a considerable amount" (p. 122). They concluded: "If current trends are maintained, a 50 percent reduction in both the numbers of these patients and the corresponding rates in these groups of patients will be achieved in considerably less than 20 years" (p. 124). These reductions were due to increased use of general hospi*als, mental health centers, nursing homes, and home health care agencies.

Among the many problems of the elderly is drug misuse. Precise data are lacking but one survey reported that 198 million prescriptions were given to 19 million older Americans in 1968 (HEW Task Force, 1971). Older people are more prone to make medication errors (e.g., misread labels) and are more likely to develop adverse reactions to drugs (Smith, Seidl, & Cluff, 1966). In addition, alcohol abuse among the elderly is high. For example, 44% of elderly patients evaluated at a psychiatric screening clinic were found to have serious problems of alcohol abuse (Gaitz & Baer, 1971).

To get more detailed information on the problems of the elderly, Peak (Note 1) evaluated 100 referrals to an outpatient clinic in Durham, North Carolina. Most had severe impairments of both physical and mental health and had difficulty with activities of daily living. Organic brain syndromes and depression were the most common diagnoses.

In concluding this section about characteristics of the aged, it is important to note that similar population trends are occurring in all countries. In 1975 the United Nations reported that there were about 291 million people in the world over the age of 60. It was estimated that there will be a 100% increase in the elderly in 30 years.

IMPLICATIONS OF AN AGING POPULATION

According to Bozzetti and MacMurray (1977), the evidence clearly indicates that the aging population has certain sex, marital, and racial distributions and that the aged suffer from physical incapacities, memory defects, decline in intellectual capacities, depression, and isolation. Their ego defenses tend to be relatively primitive, their emotions muted, and their social roles limited.

It should be obvious that realistic assistance to aged persons must involve a multidimensional approach both in terms of assessment and in terms of services. For assessment, many parameters need to be considered. These include: the functional capacities of the elderly person; the person's diagnostic state; the nature of financial, social, or environmental supports the patient has; the social or environmental stress the patient is exposed to; and the quality of the services offered. For services, many disciplines must be involved. These include: general medicine, psychiatry, psychology, social work, nursing, rehabilitation, city planning, architecture, and even law enforcement.

Because the population of elderly patients in state mental hospitals is heavily weighted with never-married, separated, divorced, and widowed persons, when planning community placements for such patients, special attention must be given to living arrangements. Also, medical and psychiatric services for persons living in families may need to be different from those for persons living alone or in nonfamily settings.

Considerably more information is needed in various areas, including

> the incidence and prevalence of mental disorders in the non-institutionalized population; the needs of persons with mental disorders in both the non-institutionalized and institutionalized populations for specific types of preventive, curative, ameliorative, and rehabilitative services; the effectiveness of specific types of treatments and programs; the most effective ways of delivering services; the number of facilities and personnel needed to staff them; the most effective staffing patterns; and the quality of care. (Kramer et al., 1968, p. 146)

THE GOALS OF ASSESSMENT OF THE AGED

The previous section broadly stated some of the (largely) unmet needs regarding assessment and treatment of the elderly. In this section some of these goals are more fully considered.

From the standpoint of epidemiological systems, evaluation of a group of elderly people must involve an assessment not only of the people themselves, but also of the environment and the interactions among the various elements of each. Specifically this means that a complete evaluation should include the following classes of information:

1. How well can the person function?
2. Does the person have physical impairments that create service and support needs?
3. Does the person have psychological symptoms that create interpersonal difficulties?
4. What is the person's unique set of needs for socialization, recreation, sex, activity, and work?
5. How well are each person's needs being met?
6. What kinds of placement settings are most relevant to each person?
7. What kinds of living accommodations are most suitable for each person?
8. What kind of housing is productive of maximum satisfactions for which individuals?
9. What are the strengths and weaknesses of residence facilities in relation to the needs of the elderly?
10. What types of psychiatric, medical, drug, psychological, nursing, and rehabilitative treatments work best with the elderly?

These questions obviously reflect only some of the goals of assessment research. They emphasize the need to measure many different kinds of variables in order to develop a complete picture of elderly persons in their environment. However, it is impossible to measure everything. This is due, not to a lack of time, money, or effort, but to problems connected with the measurement tools. The following section deals with this latter issue.

SOME PROBLEMS OF ASSESSMENT RESEARCH WITH THE ELDERLY

The excellent review of rating scales for geriatric psychopharmacology by Salzman, Kochansky, and Shader (1972) also included some descriptions of research problems. They pointed out that the rating of cognitively and physically impaired elderly presents a greater problem than the rating of younger ambulatory persons. Older patients often can cooperate only to a slight degree; self-rating therefore becomes difficult and changes of function due to treatment are often minimal, at best. Salzman et al. concluded that rating scales must vary with the population being studied, but also noted that relatively few scales have been designed specifically for the geriatric patient. Even fewer have been designed to deal with the various subgroups among the aging population. This implies that the attainment of a general purpose, all-encompassing rating scale for all elderly people is probably an unattainable and untenable goal.

But these are only some of the problems of research with the aged. For example, psychological test performance is dependent on both functional and organic factors. If a patient does poorly on a block design test, this could reflect a cognitive deficit (i.e., not understanding the problem), a motivational deficit (i.e., not wanting to do the problem because of depression or apathy), a hearing or visual deficit (i.e., not being able to see the problem or hear the instructions), or a deficit in manipulative skills (i.e., not being able to do the problem). Without having other classes of information available it becomes very difficult to interpret the meaning of the poor performance.

Another problem that is occasionally debated concerns the issue of self-report versus observer ratings. The study by Kuriansky, Gurland, and Fleiss (1976) addressed this issue. Their research team evaluated 50 consecutive inpatient admissions of geriatric patients using the Performance Test of Activities of Daily Living. This test requires the patient to do a variety of simple tasks, e.g., pressing a light switch, combing one's hair, or drinking from a cup. The patient's degree of dependency is then estimated. These ratings of dependence were then compared with the patient's self-rating of capacity for personal care and functioning at home.

The degree of agreement between the test score and the self-assessment was zero. However, the performance test score correlated highly with physical health ratings made by a physician and discriminated organic patients from the nonorganics. The authors concluded that

> objective testing has the advantages of minimizing the interference on the measurement of functioning capacity of subjective aspects of a patient's condition, e.g., lack of insight into their disability, self-depreciation, and communication problems inherent in interviewing patients with impaired comprehension or who speak a foreign language (Kuriansky et al., 1976, p. 100)

Unfortunately, there are some considerations that question the implied generality of objective testing over self-report. For one thing, the test was concerned only with simple physical acts, and it is not at all certain that objective tests could even be devised for other types of functions such as interpersonal relations or emotional disturbances. Second, the tests were administered by one person, and no reliability data are given either for the test or for the administrator. Finally, one of the supposed advantages of testing, i.e., the use of scaled numerical data, was not considered in the study. Instead, the authors lost information by arbitrarily classifying the patients into one of three categories of dependency.

In addition, other studies found that self-report assessments are just as good as objective assessments. For example, Maddox and Douglass (1973) reported on 83 normal elderly who were examined by a physician for health status 6 times over a 15-year period. Each time the subjects rated their own health from poor to excellent. Results showed consistent, moderate, positive correlations between self-ratings and physician ratings of health. It was also found that self-ratings were better predictors of subsequent physicians' ratings than vice versa. Maddox and Douglass suggested that "the subjective belief that one is healthy or ill may be more important than actual medical status in predicting an individuals' general emotional state and behavior" (p. 88).

These reports imply that the issue of self-report or objective report is a moot question. There is no inherent reason to argue that one method is, in general, superior to the other. Both methods represent partial, limited ways of collecting information about individuals, and both are subject to various limitations or biases. No test score, be it self-report or objective, should ever be taken at face value; in all cases test scores require inferences to be made about hypothetical underlying variables of psychiatric interest, and many factors intervene to influence the adequacy (or validity) of such inferences. Multiple methods of data gathering are just as important as the gathering of data about many aspects of the individual and the individual's environment. Each test must be evaluated in detail for sources of bias, for psychometric properties, and for discriminative or predictive abilities. These points can be best illustrated by reference to studies that have attempted to evaluate some widely used measures.

A number of different types of indexes have been used to evaluate mental status in community studies of mental disorder. Among the best known is the Gurin Mental Status Index, a 20-item self-report measure, which has been reported to have both concurrent and discriminative validity. The use of this index has led to the often cited statement that there is a high prevalence of mental illness in the general community. In order to examine its properties, Schwartz, Myers, and Astrachan (1973) interviewed 132 ex-patients living in the community and obtained self-report data on the Gurin Mental Status Index as well as interviewer ratings on the Spitzer Psychiatric Evaluation form and on the New Haven Schizophrenia Index. Results of the survey showed that the Gurin Index systematically defined the sample as more impaired than did the other instruments. The authors interpreted these findings as indicating that the three measures of mental status tap different aspects of psychiatric symptomatology. Factor analysis of the items of all scales revealed that the Gurin Index measures neurotic symptoms almost exclusively, the Psychiatric Evaluation Form measures some neurotic symptoms and some schizophrenic symptoms, while the New Haven Index primarily measures the more extreme symptoms of schizophrenia.

One implication of these findings is that the Gurin Mental Status Index probably overestimates the need for psychiatric services by overestimating the prevalence of psychiatric disorders in the community. Although this study was carried out with the assistance of people in their middle years, the conclusion probably applies to studies of the elderly as well. Another implication of the findings is that each test instrument has its own built-in biases, which are often unknown, and it is only by various comparative analyses that these biases can be identified. Once known, each instrument can be used to answer the question for which it is most suitable.

Another illustration of these points may be found in the 22-item Langner Scale used by Srole, Langner, Michael, Opler, and Rennie (1962) in their Midtown Manhattan Study, and by many others in epidemiological studies. The content of their scale is very similar to that of Gurin's and it thus reflects neurotic symptoms (e.g., "Have you ever been bothered by nervousness, feeling fidgety and tense?") and psychophysiological reactions (e.g., "Are you ever troubled by headaches or pains in the head?"). The scale was not constructed to detect organic brain conditions, mental retardation, sociopathy, depression, or psychotic symptoms. Respondents who report more than four symptoms are considered sick; the others are well.

Validity for the scale has been claimed on the grounds that it discriminates between known ill and known well populations. However, in a critique of the scale, Seiler (1973) pointed out that college students get higher scores on it than predischarge ward patients do, outpatients get higher scores than inpatients on a psychiatric ward, and neurotics get higher scores than psychotics. Clearly, the summation of many mild symptoms of psychological disorder is not equivalent to a few symptoms of severe mental illness.

In addition, Seiler noted that although the cutoff of four symptoms identifies a large number of the mentally ill, it also produces a large number of false positives from the population of normals. In other words, even though patients in mental hospitals may have more symptoms, on the average, than community residents, this does not imply that community residents with many symptoms are mentally ill.

These ideas suggest that the content of the scale does not adequately reflect the universe of content related to mental illness; that is, it does not have content validity. This point is especially important in relation to scales used with geriatric patients. Relatively few scales have been designed specifically for use with the elderly; most have simply been borrowed from scales used for younger populations. In such cases, without appropriate norms, the meaning of the scores obtained is always in question.

Another important psychometric problem should be emphasized in relation to using tests or scales as selection or screening devices. The World Health

Organization developed a rating scale for identifying children in general medical settings who may require psychiatric consultation. Currently the recommended cutoff for referral is one symptom rated out of ten. When this criterion was applied to a population of children in Colombia, South America, over 70% of the children attending a general pediatric clinic were found to need psychiatric consultation (World Health Organization, Note 2). This finding was at variance with the referral rate (15%) found for adults in that community using a different scale for evaluation. It also would have been impossible to provide psychiatric services for such a huge number of referrals.

One other important research problem briefly mentioned before, bears elaboration. This concerns the question of norms and the meaning of scores. It can be best illustrated by a discussion of scales for the measurement of depression in the elderly.

The Zung Self-Rating Depression Scale (SDS) was originally developed as a simple, quick, self-report index of depression in adult psychiatric populations, but subsequently it has been used a good deal with elderly patients as well. Whether such use is appropriate and whether it provides a valid index of depression in the aged is questionable in light of a number of considerations (cf. chapters 1 and 5 for additional discussions of the SDS).

For one thing, cross-cultural studies of depression demonstrate that different groups or subgroups express depression somewhat differently. In one study, Marsella, Kinzie, and Gordon (1973) administered the Zung scale to over 500 Hawaiian college students of Japanese, Chinese, or Caucasian ancestry. Of these students, 196 (39%) had clinically significant depression as reflected in a score of 50 or more on the SDS, a surprisingly high number. A factor analysis of these and other depression items was then computed separately for each ethnic group. Although there were a number of overlapping symptoms, gastrointestinal complaints (e.g., poor appetite, gas belching) differentiated the depressed from the nondepressed in the two Oriental groups, but not in the Caucasian one. The authors suggested that in Oriental cultures there is embarrassment about the expression of loneliness and sadness but no problem with the expression of somatic complaints.

These ideas were further documented in an extensive review of cross-cultural studies of depression (Marsella, Note 3). Marsella cited reports indicating that some languages have no terms for depression as such, and that different investigators have reported widely varying prevalence rates for depression, depending upon their theoretical expectations as well as the specific test used. A factor analysis of semantic differential scales for depression in Japan and the United States shows different connotative meanings for the term in the two cultures. One investigator cited by Marsella claimed that the only elements that are fairly consistent as signs of depression across non-European cultures are: disturbances of sleep, libido, and appetite. Mood changes, guilt, suicidal feelings, and motor agitation or apathy are not found consistently in all cultures as indexes of depression.

These problems of identifying depression even arise in very similar cultures as evidenced by the U.S.-U.K. diagnostic studies. For example, it has been found that 12-16% of new admissions to mental hospitals are diagnosed by U.S. psychiatrists as depressed, while British psychiatrists diagnose 30-46% of a comparable sample of English hospital admissions as depressed (Cooper, Kendell, Gurland, Sharpe, Copeland, & Simon, 1972). When the SDS was tried in several countries, the correlations of symptom frequency with physicians' ratings of depression ranged from +.65 (England) to +.43 (Japan). The fact that the correlation was lowest in Japan (the only non-Western country that was sampled) suggests that the depressive pattern in Japan is not the same as it is in Western countries. It was also found that normal populations in some of these countries produced much higher depression scores than was true in the United States. Thus, "the use of American norms would suggest that many normal Czechs, Swedes and Germans are 'clinically' depressed" (Marsella, Note 3, p. 38).

Further light was thrown on this issue by a comparison of five different depression scales as applied to normal college populations of Japanese, Chinese, and Caucasian ancestry. The scales used were the SDS, the Beck Depression Inventory, the Multiple Affect Adjective Checklist, the Minnesota Multiphasic Personality Inventory (MMPI) Depression Scale, and the KAS-Hogarty Depression Scale. The SDS and KAS-Hogarty use symptom frequency, the Beck Depression Inventory uses symptom intensity, the Multiple Affect Adjective Checklist uses mood descriptors, and the MMPI-Depression Scale requires a yes or no to indicator items that have no face validity for depression. The results showed that college students from these countries had minimal levels of depression on the Beck Depression Inventory, the Multiple Affect Adjective Checklist, and the KAS-Hogarty, but approached borderline levels of clinical depression on the SDS and the MMPI-Depression Scale. Marsella (Note 3) concluded that the various studies cited

> point to the importance of defining the concept of depression in terms which are relevant to the culture under study. . . . Formats which emphasize the measurement of depression through the endorsement of mood descriptors may be inappropriate for cultures which do not label inner mood states. Similarly, the use of formats based on indicator items which are validated on specific cultural samples (e.g., MMPI) is also inappropriate since there is no basis for determining whether the indicator items (e.g., "I like mechanics magazines") are relevant to the culture under study. . . . The most useful approach may be to develop symptom norms for both depressed and normal populations in every culture. (p. 46)

The more Westernized a culture, the more one can expect a picture of depression which includes both vegetative and psychological components. In contrast, depression in less Westernized cultures often does

> not involve psychological components. . . . Some orientations emphasize the labeling of psychological experience while others do not. Suicide appears to be associated more with depressive disorders which include psychological dimensions. (p. 57)

These ideas are relevant to research with the elderly. It may be argued that the aged population in any given country is a special subgroup with cultural norms and expectations that differ from those of the younger population. Although there is almost no direct evidence available on this hypothesis, one recent survey does bear on it. Warheit, Holzer, and Schwab (1973) interviewed a random sample of 1645 adults in a southwestern county in the United States. The respondents' scores on an 18-item depression scale, developed by the authors, were analyzed in terms of age, race, sex, income, education, and socioeconomic status. Results showed that females had significantly higher depression scores than males; that blacks had higher scores than whites; and that depression scores were high in persons with low income, education, and socioeconomic status. There were no significant changes associated with age per se. When whites and blacks were matched for socioeconomic level, there were also no significant differences between them. The authors cautioned that the variables studied in the regression analyses accounted for only 12.6% of the total variance. It is thus evident that many untapped variables contribute to the presence of depression in the general population. The hypothesis that the elderly are a special cultural subgroup of the population clearly requires further research.

SOME PRACTICAL ISSUES ASSOCIATED WITH THE USE OF RATING OR SELF-REPORT SCALES

There is a great difference in what one can expect to accomplish in a research setting in contrast to a normally functioning institutional setting. In general, professional and subprofessional staffs have very little free time to do extra things (fill out forms, make ratings, test patients) for research. Consequently, forms or rating scales must be brief and clear and require a minimum of inference. For the most part, it is impractical to use tests or rating scales that contain more than 30 items or that take more than 10–15 minutes to complete. One way of getting around this is by developing several short forms each of which can be completed in 10 minutes or so and that can be completed on different days at the convenience of the rater.

It is unrealistic to develop a long, complex research form, administered with the assistance of graduate students, and to turn it over to nurses, aides, or psychiatrists expecting them to use the form routinely. Once in a while, an institutional staff will tolerate a tedious rating form if it is to be used for a specific, time-limited project. They will resist strongly if it is imposed on them as a permanent requirement.

There are many specific things one can say about the details of test or scale construction. Three examples are discussed here: the Zung Self-Rating Depression Scale (SDS) as a self-report index, the Missouri Geriatric Profile, and the Geriatric Rating Scale (GRS).

The Zung Self-Report Scale: A Critique

Reliability

Ten of the items are worded symptomatically positive for depression and ten are worded symptomatically negative for depression. Although this is designed to avoid yea-saying or nay-saying patterns of response, the frequent change of mental set confuses many patients who then check boxes that indicate the opposite of what they intend, or must repeatedly ask the interviewer for help in clearing up the confusion. The attempt to avoid response biases sometimes creates more problems than it solves. Kerlinger (1967) provided evidence to show that items should not be reversed and that the best items are written in the way that people naturally express themselves.

The printed format is visually difficult for many patients. The scale has been unnecessarily squeezed onto a 6-inch piece of paper and the place for patients to put checkmarks is a 4 X 20 cell grid. The result is that patients often erroneously put checks in the wrong box (e.g., mark responses for two successive items on the same line). Patients generally need to be observed as they take the test to call their attention to this type of error when it occurs.

Validity

Several of the items from this scale, when used with particular patient populations, are inappropriate or appear to be tapping something other than depression:

4. "I have trouble sleeping at night." It is unclear how a patient who routinely takes sleeping medication should answer this.
6. "I still enjoy sex." First, this question is felt by many patients to be unduly intrusive and the response is therefore likely to be defensive rather than honest. Second, since most geriatric patients or patients with medical illnesses respond in the negative to this item, it seems to have little validity for depression for these patients.
7. "I notice that I am losing weight." This has questionable validity for depression in patients who are on diets or who suffer from certain medical illnesses (e.g., cancer).
8. "I have trouble with constipation." This symptom is often the side effect of particular medications or diets.
11. "My mind is as clear as it used to be." This item has questionable validity among geriatric patients where mental confusion may very likely be due to organic deterioration rather than depressive mood.

12. "I find it easy to do the things I used to do." Again, validity of this item as a measure of depression is questionable among geriatric or medically ill patients.
19. "I feel that others would be better off if I were dead." This item was found to be anxiety provoking and inappropriate for patients with serious, and possibly terminal, medical illnesses.

Administration

Although the SDS is clearly intended to be a self-administered questionnaire, most patients require assistance while filling out the scale. It is often necessary to assist those patients who become confused by the mixture of positively and negatively worded items as well as those who find the printed format cumbersome and mark the form incorrectly. Also, it is often necessary to have an examiner present to answer questions frequently raised by many patients. Certain types of patients often ask for assistance in understanding how particular items apply to them (notably items 4, 5, 6, 7, 8, 19). The standardization of the test then suffers considerably as it is left to each individual examiner to interpret the applicability of the item to the patient.

The Missouri Geriatric Profile Scale (Evenson, Note 4): A Critique

This scale has the advantage of being designed specifically for geriatric inpatients. It is meant to be completed by nurses or aides on the basis of behavior observed during a preceding 2- or 3-day period. The instrument consists of 73 items rated on a 4-point scale of "Never observed," "Occasionally observed," "Often observed," or "Always observed." In addition, there are two global ratings of rate of progress and of readiness for discharge. The items are stated in such a way that a high rating on 49 of the items indicates poor functioning, while a high rating on the remaining 24 items indicates good functioning.

The scale is unnecessarily long for routine use. The redundancy is highlighted by the presence of a number of items that have a similar meaning and the ratings are probably highly correlated. For example, there does not seem to be any need for both the following items: "Is objectionable to other patients during night" and "Is objectionable to other patients during the day." Nor does it seem necessary to document depression with all the following items: "Cries," "Looks sad and unhappy," "Talks about death or suicide," "Attempts to kill or harm self," and "Talks about feeling blue or depressed." Some of these items are obviously more important than others from the viewpoint of hospital management or prognosis. Similarly, there are several items that tap delusions as well as several items that tap aggressive, acting-out behavior.

If we consider the 24 items that attempt to measure good functioning, there also appears to be considerable repetitiveness. For example, the items "Knows and responds to own name," "Understands what others communicate," "Knows where he is," and "Knows the time and date" all tap the implicit dimension of orientation and do it with unnecessary redundancy. Some items are not generally applicable, for example, "Handles own money or spending" and "Goes on weekend home visits." Some items are vague, for example, "Claims that things have special meanings." It thus appears that the extensive overlap of item connotations would justify a reduction in the length of the overall scale.

A second reason to reduce the scale length is that some items are of trivial significance in an inpatient setting. For example, it makes no difference for disposition, prognosis, or ward management if a patient "Hoards meaningless items," "Talks about influential friends or enemies," "Gets upset if something doesn't suit him," or "Requires a special diet." Items that are not centrally related to the patient's functional capacities can usefully be omitted.

The last 15 items are all concerned with physical symptoms. The list looks very much like a side effects symptom checklist. The purpose of the list is not clear, and here again some symptoms seem to be trivial (dry mouth or nasal congestion, rash or itchy skin), while some seem to have much greater medical significance (a seizure). Some items are puzzling. For example, a frequent request for additional medications is considered just as bad as a frequent refusal to take medications.

One of the global ratings asks the ward attendant to judge the patient's progress on a scale ranging from "Getting worse" to "Rapid progress." However, the instructions tell the rater to use the past 2 or 3 days as the basis for a judgment. This seems inconsistent with the well-known fact that geriatric inpatients do not usually show rapid changes over short periods of time.

It thus appears that the Missouri Geriatric Profile Scale is overly long, unnecessarily redundant, and not always clear in its goals. A thoughtful reduction in items would go a long way toward solving these problems.

The Geriatric Rating Scale: A Critique

The Geriatric Rating Scale (GRS) was developed as a brief, objective rating scale to be used by nonprofessional ward staff for rating hospitalized geriatric patients. The items consist of 31 incomplete sentence stems, each of which can be completed by three alternatives. The alternatives are indicative of varying degrees of impairment. The sum of the ratings on all items is used as a global measure of impairment. Studies reported high interjudge reliability (+.87) and evidence for validity (Plutchik, Conte, Lieberman, Bakur, Grossman, & Lehrman, 1970; Plutchik & Conte, 1972; Dastoor, Norton, Boillat, Minty, Papadopoulou, & Muller, 1975).

The scale is brief and easy to use. However, three items of the GRS were found difficult to rate. These dealt with the behavior of patients at night (e.g.,

"With regard to sleep, the patient: Sleeps most of the night; Is sometimes awake; Is often awake), and they were discarded because of the difficulty the day staff had in obtaining this information. Of the remaining 28 items, most deal with functional capacities (e.g., continence, hearing, vision, ambulation) and with social behavior. Little emphasis is given in the GRS to traditional psychiatric categories such as delusions, hallucinations, or depression. This focus may reflect the fact that it was developed in the context of a facility for the long-term care of chronic patients most of whom suffered from organic brain disease rather than from schizophrenia-spectrum illness. The issue remains, however, of the adequacy of the sample of items for all varieties of geriatric inpatients.

Another aspect of the sampling problem concerns the applicability of the scale to geriatric outpatients. Attempts to apply GRS to outpatients have shown that the items are too easy; that is, most patients who can function outside of a hospital get very good ratings on most items, and thus no discrimination is possible. It is therefore evident that quite different items are needed to discriminate among moderately functioning geriatric patients in the general community.

One drawback of the GRS is that it yields only a single global score as a measure of overall physical and social functioning. Thus the scale may lack precision in identifying special areas of dysfunction that may be affected by drugs or other therapies. Fortunately this drawback has been recently remedied. Smith, Bright, and McCloskey (1977) administered the GRS to 370 geriatric patients and factor analyzed the data. The scale was found to be composed of three factors: Withdrawal/Apathy (11 items), Antisocial Disruptive Behavior (6 items), and Deficits in Activities of Daily Living (7 items). Although the male and female patients did not differ significantly on overall scores, differences were found on two of the factor scales with women showing a greater degree of impairment. Females scored significantly higher than males on Antisocial Disruptive Behavior and Deficits in Activities of Daily Living. The use of factor scores, or subscales, thus seems to increase the sensitivity of the GRS. The use of subscales to obtain profiles is probably desirable for all scales.

Basic Questions for Evaluating Any Scale

For what specific subpopulation is the scale designed? Is it for regressed mental patients in a state hospital or for ambulatory senior citizens in a nursing home? The answer to this question will determine the general content and level of functioning that is tapped by the scale.

What is the purpose of making ratings of individuals? Usually, ratings are made to: determine a diagnosis, establish a level of functioning, select a group of people for admission to a service, decide on a disposition, make a prognosis, or determine the effectiveness of a drug or treatment. Ratings used for diagnostic purposes often differ from ratings for level of functioning. It is quite possible for two individuals to have the same diagnosis but markedly different functional capacities. Similarly, the decision to admit someone to a nursing home may require information different from that required in evaluating a drug.

Who is to make the ratings? A scale designed to be completed by psychiatrists and other professionals may involve more inference and may require finer discriminations than one that is to be completed by aides. Thus, some scales may have as many as seven or more rating categories, while others may have no more than two or three.

What is in it for the raters? In most settings where ratings and evaluations are to be made, well-trained research assistants are not available. Cooperation by the staff must be voluntary, and deliberate efforts must be made to justify the project in practical terms and to enlist the aid of the raters. The collection of data for the sake of science is seldom a source of motivation for the raters. Feedback of results helps but is not enough. Basically, the investigator must appear credible and concerned and should provide as much preliminary contact and explanation as possible.

How often are ratings to be made? The investigator should carefully consider how often ratings need to be repeated. Sometimes they need to be made only once, as in admission screening. Sometimes they need to be made every month or so to be able to identify changes in ill or debilitated patients. Cooperation is best insured if few ratings are required. In addition, if a specific research question can be answered in 3 months, there is no need to maintain the rating system beyond that time.

How much information is really needed? Cooperation by nonprofessional staff in completing long forms seems to decrease exponentially after the first page of questions. This issue relates to the understandable desire to cover everything for everyone in one form. If you have to rely on existing staff for data collection, long forms usually do not work out well.

How reliable is the scale? Interjudge reliabilities after minimum training should be better than +.80, or the scale is likely to be too unreliable for general use. Internal reliability should be checked for each scale or subscale separately.

How valid is the scale? In geriatric research, questions of discriminative and construct validity are more important than concurrent validity because there are so few standards against which to compare new scales. One problem that has come up in several studies is that discriminative validity is difficult to demonstrate though the use of various intact, age-related groups. For example, contrary to expectations, old people in nursing homes have no more death anxiety than do college students. Similarly, most measures of body image show no differences between normal old people and normal young people.

How can norms be established and false positives avoided? Some deficits are found in most older people on most tasks, relative to norms available on younger people. It is not easy to measure the relative degree of impairment in special subpopulations of the elderly unless very adequate norms are available on large elderly groups. Otherwise, there is a tendency to identify a large number of false positives as requiring services that may, in fact, not be necessary. A great deal more attention needs to be given to the establishment of age-appropriate norms on both new and old tests or scales.

Are the elderly a cultural subgroup? The possibility that people over 65 from various socioeconomic strata represent special cultural subgroups cannot be ignored. Questions used in tests and rating scales should be carefully examined for cross-cultural generality as well as for relevance to the population.

Should we distinguish between subjective and objective feelings of discomfort or distress? Many tests or scales ask patients how upset or troubled they are by various listed signs or symptoms. People sometimes report stomachaches, headaches, shyness, or compulsive behavior as characteristic of themselves, but at the same time, they report not feeling troubled by these things. In other words, people can recognize that they are shy and yet not feel troubled by their shyness.

In such cases, should the rater decide that the patient has a pathological problem, or should the rater take the patient's word at face value? In other words, is a problem a problem regardless of whether the patient thinks it is? It seems that here is a situation where diagnoses are less important than the functional living skills.

TWO MODELS FOR THE SELECTION OF TESTS

The point has already been emphasized that there is no single test, scale, or type of measurement that is appropriate for all groups. This is equally true for the elderly who reflect a variety of different subcultures as well as a variety of degrees of dysfunction. It is inappropriate and unwise to attempt to uncritically take a test or scale developed for use with younger populations and apply it to the elderly. Every item of the scale, regardless of whether it is designed for a self-report or rating format, should be carefully examined by a group of clinicians with extensive experience with the elderly. This should be a minimum starting point before the scales are examined for psychometric properties such as reliability and validity.

One approach to test selection for the elderly involves the construction of models that direct our attention to the kind of information we need. Toward this end, two models are proposed here.

The 3-W Model

In order to decide what kind of tests we need, we have to decide on who we want to assess and why. The *what, who,* and *why* are the 3-Ws.

From the standpoint of *why,* there are usually four reasons for assessment of the elderly: (1) selection (to meet specific criteria for entrance into a study), (2) diagnosis, (3) disposition, and (4) prognosis.

From the standpoint of *who,* there are three groups that usually need to be distinguished. One is the normal population of elderly. This includes those who live with their families or alone, those who attend senior citizen centers or "golden age" clubs, and those who either work or are retired. They may or may not have some physical impairments. However, they share the general characteristic of being able to function without special assistance from other members of society. The second group of elderly are psychiatric outpatients. They have either voluntarily sought help for psychiatric problems or been referred by social workers, medical doctors, or family members to outpatient clinics or community mental health centers. In most cases they suffer from some degree of depression and/or confusion or cognitive impairment. The third group consists of psychiatric inpatients, usually found either in state mental hospitals or special nursing care facilities. Their functional capacities are low. So too are their social and cognitive skills.

What in this model refers to the appropriateness of tests or rating scales selected. For example, it would probably be sufficient to use some kind of mental status form for selecting elderly people for research. The extensiveness of the form would depend upon whether the research was concerned with drug issues or social milieu manipulation, and also would depend on how dysfunctional the group was. For purposes of diagnosis we need tests that distinguish between a depression due to loss of a spouse and depression due to endogenous factors. The scales should identify degrees of cognitive dysfunction as well as affective disturbance.

In order to decide on an appropriate disposition we need to assess the functional capacities of a person. Two persons who are depressed to the same degree on a self-report measure of depression may be quite different in their ability to handle their lives and to function in society. This would probably reflect different levels of ego strength, different defense mechanisms, or different degrees of social supports. Therefore, any adequate assessment for purposes of disposition should include measures of strengths as well as weaknesses. In addition, the kinds of tests or scales appropriate for regressed inpatients will undoubtedly be different from those appropriate to outpatients or normal individuals.

Finally, in order to make a reasonably accurate prognosis we need the kinds of information already mentioned and scales that are somewhat like those that have been used for distinguishing between process and reactive schizophrenics. Such scales typically have been based upon a description of an individual's life history and the developmental course of presenting problems.

The Sequential Branching Model

Another way to consider the problem of test selection (and by implication, test construction) is in terms of the sequence of decisions that must be made in assessing patients. In the ordinary course of events a patient makes contact with a psychiatrist which may take place in the context of private practice, in a psychiatric emergency room or outpatient clinic, or on a medical or psychiatric ward.

At the time of initial contact the psychiatrist should make a binary decision concerning the most serious possibility, such as the presence or absence of psychosis. It is evident that such serious diagnostic possibilities tend to be relatively low probability events. The judgment as to the presence or absence of psychosis entails further decisions. For example, if the patient is diagnosed as psychotic, then the psychiatrist must decide whether to administer psychotropic drugs. When a decision has been made concerning drugs, a binary decision must be made concerning inpatient or outpatient treatment.

Alternatively, if the initial evaluation leads to the decision that the patient is not psychotic, then the next logical decision in the sequential decision tree is whether the patient has organic brain disease (OBD). If the patient is judged to have OBD, then the psychiatrist must decide whether to hospitalize the patient. If the patient is judged to be free of significant OBD, then further evaluations need to be made. Most likely the next step would be to determine if the patient is depressed.

Series of binary decisions need to be made dealing first with low-probability events and then with higher probability events. This is done in order to avoid missing an important, though infrequent, diagnosis.

It might be argued that this is what a good clinician does anyway. Perhaps that is usually true, but the possiblity of errors increases when one is trying to keep a large number of impressions in one's head. One value of the proposed Sequential Branching Model is that it makes explicit the logical operations that the clinician should pursue and thus decreases the chances of errors. Another value is that the decision-making process can be automated, in a sense, so that relatively less trained personnel can properly carry through the evaluation.

In contrast to the 3-W Model, the Sequential Branching Model does not divide patients into different levels of functional capacities. However, it is obvious that the ease of making the various decisions will vary with the type of elderly population being considered. For example, there is little difficulty in distinguishing a psychotic from a nonpsychotic person in a population of normal elderly citizens. This problem is much greater in a regressed nursing home group.

One difficulty with the Sequential Branching Model is that it requires a good deal of data on the relative frequency of occurrence of different types of psychiatric pathology in the elderly. Another problem is that the sequential branchings may become so complicated that they can only be handled by a computer. It thus appears that this model is less simple and coherent at the present time than the 3-W model, although it may be of some value in the future.

These two models are simply ways of thinking about problems of test selection, and by implication, test construction. Perhaps they will help us identify our assessment strengths and weaknesses and improve both by sharpening our conceptual boundaries and decisions.

REFERENCES

Bozzetti, L. P., & MacMurray, J. P. Contemporary concepts of aging: An overview. *Psychiatric Annals,* 1977, *7,* 117–127.

Cooper, J., Kendell, R., Gurland, B., Sharpe, L., Copeland, J., & Simon, R. *Psychiatric diagnosis in New York and London: A comparative study of mental hospital admissions.* London: Oxford University Press, 1972.

Dastoor, D. P., Norton, S., Boillat, J., Minty, J., Papadopoulou, F., & Muller, H. F. A psychogeriatric assessment program. I. Social functioning and ward behavior. *Journal of the American Geriatrics Society,* 1975, *23,* 465–469.

Evenson, R. *Geriatric Profile.* Unpublished manuscript, Missouri Institute of Psychiatry, 1971.

Gaitz, C., & Baer, P. Characteristics of elderly patients with alcoholism. *Archives of General Psychiatry,* 1971, *24,* 372–378.

1968 HEW Task Force on Prescription Drugs. *The Drug Users and the Drug Prescribers.* Washington, D.C.: U.S. Government Printing Office, 1971.

Kerlinger, F. N. Social attitudes and their criterial referents: A structural theory. *Psychological Review,* 1967, *74,* 110–122.

Kramer, M., Taube, C., & Starr, S. Patterns of use of psychiatric facilities by the aged: Current status, trends, and implications. In *The mental health of the aged* (Psychiatric Research Report 23). Washington, D.C.: American Psychiatric Association, 1968.

Kuriansky, J. B., Gurland, B. J., & Fleiss, J. L. The assessment of self-care capacity in geriatric psychiatric patients by objective and subjective methods. *Journal of Clinical Psychology,* 1976, *32,* 95–102.

Maddox, G. L., & Douglass, E. B. Self-assessment of health: A longitudinal study of elderly subjects. *Journal of Health and Social Behavior,* 1973, *14,* 87–93.

Marsella, A. J., Kinzie, D., & Gordon, P. Ethnic variations in the expression of depression. *Journal of Cross-Cultural Psychology,* 1973, *4,* 435–458.

Marsella, A. J., Sanborn, K. O., Kameoka, V., Shizuru, L., & Brennan, J. Cross-validation of self-report measures of depression among normal populations of Japanese, Chinese and Caucasian ancestry. *Journal of Clinical Psychology,* 1975, *31,* 281–287.

National Center for Health Statistics. *Characteristics of residents in nursing and personal care homes: United States, June-August, 1969.* (DHEW Publication No. HSM 73-1704-Series 12 - No. 19). Washington, D.C.: U.S. Department of Health, Education and Welfare, 1973.

Plutchik, R., & Conte, H. Change in social and physical functioning of geriatric patients over a one-year period. *Gerontologist,* 1972, *12,* 181–184.

Plutchik, R., Conte, H., Lieberman Bakur, M., Grossman, J., & Lehrman, N. Reliability and validity of a scale for assessing the functioning of geriatric patients. *Journal of the American Geriatrics Society,* 1970, *18,* 491–500.

Pollack, E. S., Locke, B. Z., & Kramer, M. Trends in hospitalization and patterns of care of the aged mentally ill. In P. H. Hoch & J. Zubin (Eds.), *Psychopathology of aging.* New York: Grune & Stratton, 1961.

Rosen, B. M., Anderson, T. E., & Bahn, A. K. Psychiatric services for the aged: A nationwide survey of patterns of utilization. *Journal of Chronic Diseases,* 1968, *21,* 167–177.

Salzman, C., Kochansky, G. E., & Shader, R. J. Rating scales for geriatric psychopharmacology: A review. *Psychopharmacology Bulletin,* 1972, *8,* 3-50.

Schwartz, C. C., Myers, J. K., & Astrachan, B. M. Comparing three measures of mental status: A note on the validity of estimates of psychological disorder in the community. *Journal of Health and Social Behavior,* 1973, *14,* 265-273.

Seiler, L. H. The 22-item scale used in field studies of mental illness: A question of method, a question of substance, and a question of theory. *Journal of Health and Social Behavior,* 1973, *14,* 252-264.

Smith, J. M., Bright, B., & McCloskey, J. Factor analytic composition of the Geriatric Rating Scale (GRS). *Journal of Gerontology,* 1977, *32,* 58-62.

Smith, J. W., Seidl, L. G., & Cluff, L. E., Studies in the epidemiology of adverse drug reactions V. Clinical factors influencing susceptibility. *Annals of Internal Medicine,* 1966, *65,* 629-640; cited in Davis, R. H. (Ed.), *Drugs and the elderly.* Los Angeles: University of California Press, 1973.

Srole, L., Langner, T. S., Michael, S. T., Opler, M. K., & Rennie, T. A. C. *Mental health in metropolis: The midtown study.* (Vol. 1). New York: McGraw-Hill, 1962.

The United Nations. *The aging: Trends and policies.* New York: ST/ESA/22, 1975.

Warheit, G. J., Holzer, C. E., & Schwab, J. J. An analysis of social class and racial differences in depressive symptomatology: A community study. *Journal of Health and Social Behavior,* 1973, *14,* 291-299.

REFERENCE NOTES

1. Peak, D. T. *Older Americans resources and services program (OARS) clinical operations.* Paper presented at the meeting of the Gerontological Society, 1973. Miami Beach, Florida, November 1973.
2. Climent, C. E., Arango, M. V., & Plutchik, R. A comparison of two symptom checklists as case finding instruments for children in developing countries. Unpublished paper prepared for World Health Organization in Coli, Colombia, 1977.
3. Marsella, A. J. *Cross-cultural studies of depression: A review of the literature.* Paper presented at the Symposium on Cross-Cultural Aspects of Depression, International Association of Cross-Cultural Psychology, Tilburg, Netherlands, 1976.
4. Evenson, R. *Geriatric Profile.* Unpublished manuscript, Missouri Institute of Psychiatry, 1971.

3

Clinical Evaluation of Depression in the Elderly

Carl Salzman and Richard I. Shader
Massachusetts Mental Health Center and Harvard Medical School

INTRODUCTION

Depression in the elderly may resemble the familiar clinical syndrome seen in younger adults. More than their younger counterparts, however, the elderly may mask their depression through a variety of ego-defensive mechanisms. They commonly are reluctant to admit depression and use denial, counterphobic defenses, or express depressive symptoms through somatic complaints and hypochondriasis. Depression may also be the first symptom of a serious medical illness or may be caused or aggravated by a variety of medical drugs that are used to treat disease common in the elderly.

The clinical evaluation of depression, therefore, is a complex and challenging task. In this chapter, we approach the evaluation of depression by dividing it into its psychological and physical components. We first consider the psychological mechanisms of depression that are particularly relevant in the elderly and the coping mechanisms that are often employed by the elderly to deal with depression or depressing circumstances of life. In turn, we examine certain diseases of the aged that include depression as part of the clinical picture, that may present as depression, or mask depression, or that are frequently followed by a reactive depression. We then look at various medical and psychiatric drugs that are used to treat illness in the elderly and the effect they have upon the production or aggravation of depressive states.

RECOGNIZING DEPRESSION IN THE ELDERLY

Psychological Mechanisms of Depression in the Elderly

In the final years of life, there is the need for accepting one's life and what has happened in it as one's own responsibility. A sense of satisfaction may be experienced as one looks back on a productive life, a sense of despair for a life of little purpose and meaning (Erikson, 1959). Commonly, the older person attempts the integration of this final stage of life in the context of declining function, limited coping strategies, loss of interpersonal supports, and stress, such as disease, over which he or she cannot exert control. It is within this complex relationship of acceptance of a past life with the acknowledgment of decline and an inability to correct past errors, a finality of no more second chances, that late life depression evolves.

Bibring (1953) has defined depression as "the emotional expression of a state of helplessness and powerlessness of the ego irrespective of what may have caused the breakdown of the mechanisms which caused his self-esteem" (p. 24). Zetzel (1965) has postulated a "depressive anxiety" that she described as a fear of loss. When loss or fear of loss causes the aging person to experience increasing difficulty or frustration in gratifying needs and reducing tension, the person is likely to experience a loss of self-esteem and feel depressed (Busse, 1975). The effect of loss is strengthened by society's willingness to devalue, ignore, or ostracize older citizens. The elderly are often the objects of prejudice and discrimination. They may accurately perceive that younger members of society wish them to die and be out of sight (Levin, 1965). This withdrawal of society's support adds further to a sense of loss, helplessness, and decreased self-esteem.

The concept of loss may be extended from interpersonal supports to anything with which there is a major narcissistic attachment. Loss of health, parts of the body or their functions, cognitive abilities, employment, mobility, and independence may each contribute to failing self-esteem. In combination with each other, multiple losses are progressive and come at a time of life when only the most resourceful and least rigid are able to develop alternate sources of need gratification. Many depressive episodes of the elderly are thus realistic responses to such loss (Busse, 1975) and may be severe enough to precipitate suicide (Payne, 1975). Past age 60, suicidal attempts are almost always genuine and involve a high degree of risk. The majority of suicide attempts are successful, which is the opposite of the case for younger adults (Payne, 1975). The suicide rate for divorced elderly white males is 150 per 100,000 people per year in the seventh decade. The rate for females is lower, peaking at 20 suicides per 100,000 people per year in the fifth decade (Schmidt, 1974).

Coping Mechanisms

Faced with inevitable loss, diminished capacity for flexible need gratification, and withdrawal of supports, a failing self-esteem and a sense of hopelessness may threaten to overwhelm the older person. In an attempt to cope with such despair, the egos of older people may employ a variety of adaptive defense mechanisms that are attempts to reduce the conscious awareness of psychic pain or increase the sources of gratification. Although depression in the elderly may have typical endogenous features of low self-esteem, vegetative signs, and mood disturbances, it may be exaggerated, denied, or transformed into other symptoms that make its recognition and evaluation more difficult. Ego defenses that were employed in earlier years may still be available and even exaggerated as a person ages, but life circumstances may change the purpose of the defense mechanism (Freud, 1946). Typical ego defenses of the elderly may be classified into three adaptive categories: (1) retreating from threat, (2) excluding threat or its significance from awareness, and (3) enhancing mastery and control (Pfeiffer & Busse, 1973; Verwoerdt, 1976).

Denial, one of the more potent of the ego's defenses, may be defined as seeing but refusing to acknowledge what is seen and hearing but negating what is actually heard (Freud, 1946; Meissner, Mack, & Semrad, 1975). This mechanism is common in elderly persons and may account for the elderly and their physicians' failure to recognize physical or psychic pathology (Busse, 1965). Mild forms of denial may be adaptive for the elderly by providing a coping mechanism to deal with sexual tensions and physical deterioration (Patterson, Freeman, & Butler, 1974; Zinberg & Kaufman, 1963). Denial may be maladaptive when it leads to worsening of physical illness or a failure to develop realistic coping mechanisms to deal with the changes that accompany the aging processes. Severe denial may lead to some restriction of the ego so that anything that produces discomfort or painful affect is avoided by an ensuing restriction of awareness. Denial in the large majority of elderly people, however, is not so severe and is usually incomplete. Thus, certain memories, cognitive abilities, and sensory functions are variably retained while others are excluded from consciousness. This makes evaluation of the elderly person's mental status and affective status a challenging, and at times, confusing task.

Certain counterphobic defenses are essentially forms of denying the process of aging with its losses, diseases, and inevitable death (Perlin & Butler, 1971). Counterphobic attitudes are overcompensations for feared situations (Fenichel, 1945) and are related to denial as a form of coping with affects about getting old. Counterphobic attitudes thus may be adaptive in maintaining adjustment and avoiding depression. The phenomenon of older people who are trying to reassure themselves against fears of aging and dying, "men who would not grow old," are a manifestation of this ego defense (Perlin & Butler, 1971).

Isolation, the intrapsychic splitting of affect from content, may also serve an adaptive function by dealing with intolerable affect (Freud, 1946; Meissner et al., 1975). It may be maladaptive by also separating the older person's feelings from friends and family in an "icy distance that interferes with relationships" (Zinberg & Kaufman, 1963). Progressive withdrawal from object relationships occurs as affective bonds with these other people are loosened and severed, a process that is termed *disengagement* (Cumming & Henry, 1961). The final stage of this process is social isolation.

Somatization is an ego process by which psychic phenomena such as depressive affects are converted into bodily symptoms. In the elderly, somatization in its severe forms may become hypochondriasis, an obsessive concern and fear of bodily ill health. In younger people, hypochondriasis is thought to be a transformation of reproach toward others into self-reproach and complaints of pain. Existent illness also may be exaggerated in an attempt to avoid unwanted affects and instinctual impulses (Meissner et al., 1975). In the elderly, true illness and bodily dysfunction may form the focus for the development of such a somatic preoccupation. Through the process of conversion of affects into bodily symptoms, depression may be disguised so that the affects are not openly felt. Rather, physical suffering is experienced. Further, such somatic hyperconcern may serve the additional function of helping the older individual avoid the responsibility for real or imagined shortcomings (Verwoerdt, 1976).

Somatization and varying degrees of hypochondriasis is common in the elderly and may provide the diagnostician with the only clues to depression. It has been found that 33% of elderly people in the community displayed an anxious preoccupation with bodily functioning (Busse, 1975).

Making a Clinical Diagnosis of Depression in the Elderly

Depression in the elderly may be complex, confusing, and difficult to diagnose. In severe cases of depression, however, the clinician should have little difficulty recognizing the disorder. The elderly patient looks and feels sad and may express a sense of helplessness, despair, and worthlessness. Guilt over real or imagined past failures, errors, or indiscretions may be a predominant part of the thought content. In general, however, guilt is not a serious problem with the elderly. Younger geriatric patients may be agitated with handwringing, pacing, and twisting of clothes or handkerchiefs and with repetition of certain phrases: "Oh my God, oh my God," or, "I have no one, no one, no one." Other elderly patients with depression may be withdrawn or mute and refuse food and drink. In the most severe cases, these patients take to bed, refuse or are unable to rise, are unable to care for body functions, and may even be incontinent. If able to speak, such patients sometimes say that any treatment efforts will be futile as they are hopeless and beyond assistance.

Bizarre and severe delusions of worthlessness, guilt, and self-depreciation are sometimes part of the clinical picture. Pessimism, hopelessness, and apathy are often prominent symptoms of early depression before severe retardation or agitation becomes evident. Delusions of somatic dysfunction, apparent in the very severe depressions, may dominate the clinical picture. In such cases, patients may claim, despite all evidence to the contrary, that parts of their body are dead, cancerous, or nonfunctional. Statements such as "My brain stopped working" or "My insides are rotted with cancer" are examples of such somatic delusions.

Paranoia, with delusions of persecution, grandiosity, and ideas of reference, may be a part of severe late life depression. Not infrequently such thought content is connected to obsessions of guilt and is clearly a projection of inner feelings toward others for whom there are ambivalent feelings. Such paranoia can be distinguished from late paraphrenia in which the paranoid thought content is not accompanied by a mood disorder.

Vegetative (somatic) signs of depression are regular components of late life affective illness and, at times, may be the earliest signals of a depressive disorder. Insomnia, anorexia with weight loss, and fatigue are a familiar triad (Pfeiffer & Busse, 1973). Constipation is the most common somatic symptom of depression (Anderson, 1971), although diarrhea has also been noted.

Other less severely depressed elderly patients may appear before the clinician as apathetic and expressionless, and with poor attention or concentration and difficulty in rapport (Caird & Judge, 1974). There may be guilt and self-belittlement: "I'm being a nuisance, doctor" or "I'm sorry to be wasting your time again" (Williamson, 1974). Some may present with histrionic, imploring, and beseeching postures and conduct. At other times, there may be rather offhand comments suggesting depressive disease. "I wish I were away from it all" (Anderson, 1971).

Repeated physical complaints, often involving the digestive tract, may provide a clue to depression. Caird and Judge (1974) have commented that in such cases the clinician has the impression that "nothing is right." Symptoms that may be the equivalent of depression or may serve to mask affective symptoms may be the only clues to depression. For those patients who, as younger adults, could not acknowledge dysphoria, the only comfortable route to seeking help may be in making somatic complaints to a "medical" doctor rather than a "mental" doctor.

Suicidal thought has already been noted as a frequent component of severe depression and must be taken seriously in the elderly. Although some thoughts of death may be associated with relief of suffering, depressive suicidal thought is often associated with decreased self-esteem, guilt, and feelings of worthlessness.

At a time of life when physical decline and disease are increasing, the elderly have somatic symptoms that may be confusing and difficult to interpret. Blinder (1966) has offered several clinical criteria for distinguishing depression preceding physical illness from other types of depression. The affective disturbance shows labile mood and is often of gradual onset with no apparent precipitant. Changes in personality, cognitive abilities, and memory may accompany the depression. Characteristically, the patient denies the symptoms and may be the last to know that anything is wrong.

Sleep and energy difficulties, which often mask or mimic depression, may be particularly difficult to evaluate (Goldfarb, 1968; Karno & Hoffman, 1974). In general, depression is accompanied by decreased sleep in the elderly. Lassitude, sleepiness, and apathy, which can be part of retarded depressions in younger adults, are more likely to be signs of physical disease, abnormal physical function, or drug toxicity in the elderly. Table 1 presents some of the other signs and symptoms of depression and summarizes some of the nonpsychological states that should be considered in evaluating the depression.

In evaluating a depressed patient, the clinician has to decide how much of a physical status evaluation to perform. Obviously, patients who seem physically ill or have specific physical complaints should be medically evaluated. Symptoms such as apathy, weight loss, and even sleepiness that persist as depression is

TABLE 1 Nonpsychological Causes of Depression in the Elderly

Common signs or symptoms of depression	Differential diagnosis
Insomnia (early morning awakening)	Normal in the elderly; particularly if daytime napping. Dyspnea secondary to congestive heart failure; pain; many medical illnesses
Constipation	Normal in elderly secondary to decreased autonomic innervation of gastrointestinal tract; dehydration; secondary to anticholinergic effects of drugs
Anorexia	Many medical diseases such as failure to thrive; chronic infection; malignancy; diabetes
Hopelessness, despair, gloom, sadness, apathy, withdrawal, of interest	Many physical diseases such as cancer of pancreas, pernicious anemia, hypo- and hyperendocrine function; reaction to severe or chronic physical disease; secondary to sedating drugs; secondary to antihypertensive drugs such as L-dopa
Memory loss	Mild forgetfulness is normal; pseudodementia; true early dementia; secondary to medical drugs, e.g., cardiac glycosides
Multiple somatic complaints and pains	Many medical diseases such as hyperparathyroidism; Addison's disease; rheumatoid arthritis
Withdrawal, mutism, retardation of affect and movement	Idiopathic parkinsonism; drugs, e.g., akinetic mutism secondary to phenothiazines; apathetic thyrotoxicosis; antihypertensives; early congestive heart failure
Irritability	Secondary to benzodiazepine drugs, alcohol, and other disinhibitors; secondary to amphetamines; hyperadrenal function or cortisol drugs; drug withdrawal states (barbiturates, benzodiazepines, antipsychotics, antidepressants); many medical diseases; reaction to chronic illness
Decreased libido	Some decrease is normal; secondary to physical illness; secondary to drugs, e.g., phenothiazines, antihypertensives
Weight loss, pallor, increasing frailty	Failure to thrive; chronic infection; diabetes; advanced metastatic cancer

lifting should be investigated for a hidden physical illness. Because of the interweaving of depression, physical illness, and drug effects, however, we suggest that all psychiatric evaluations of depressed elderly patients include: (a) a careful physical examination and noninvasive laboratory tests, (b) a careful appraisal of the prescribed and over-the-counter medications that the patients are consuming, and (c) a careful psychiatric interview with indirect and nonthreatening questions that may elicit depressive symptoms. A physical evaluation of the depressed elderly patient should include these procedures:

Physical examination including neurological status
Complete blood count
Urinalysis
BUN, serum electrolytes
Thyroid status
EKG
Fasting blood sugar
Liver function studies (LDH, SGOT, SGPT)
Pancreatic function (amylase, glucose tolerance)

An appraisal of medications used may necessitate showing patients pictures of various tablets, capsules, liquids, etc., in order to display a complete inventory of their pharmaceutical ingestion. Patients who are depressed and taking one or more of the medications potentially related to depression should be carefully evaluated for drug toxicity. An excellent guideline for psychiatric interviewing has been provided by Busse (1973). It lists the following modifications of diagnostic procedures that take account of the special needs and limitations of elderly persons:

1. Attention to nonverbal communication
2. Need for active inquiry
3. Evaluation of social relationships and activities of daily living
4. Need to speak with family members
5. Slow pacing of the psychiatric history taking and interviewing

THE RELATIONSHIP BETWEEN DEPRESSIVE SYMPTOMS AND MEDICAL DISEASE

Symptoms of depression are occasionally among the initial presenting symptoms of serious medical illness (Schwab, 1968; Walker, 1967). In elderly patients, however, the differential diagnosis of medically related depression versus the symptoms of depression of a psychogenic origin may be difficult. Apathy, anorexia, insomnia, decreased energy, decreased libido, pain, protean somatic symptoms, and hypochondriasis may be manifestations of depression in the elderly, as well as parts of a medical disease (Rice, 1959; Schwab, 1969).

Depression as a Response to Physical Illness

Between 60 and 85% of elderly subjects are able to identify the specific event or stimulus that precipitated feelings of depression (Post, 1965; Busse, 1975). There is a particularly close association between physical illness and depressive reactions in old age (Pfeiffer & Busse, 1973); older persons seem to tolerate the loss of love objects and prestige better than a decline in physical health (Busse, 1965). It is likely, therefore, that physical illness may be a frequent and recognizable precipitant of depression in the elderly. The depression that accompanies severe or life-threatening illness may dominate the clinical picture (Hackett & Adams, 1977). The severity, duration, and rate of progression of the illness are factors in determining the magnitude of the depressive response of the elderly to sickness (Verwoerdt, 1976). Additional factors that may determine the severity of a depression following physical illness are: (a) the organ system involved and its role in the maintenance of life, (b) the degree of narcissistic attachment to the lost functioning, and (c) the ability to maintain a positive body image while acknowledging the loss of parts or of function (Verwoerdt, 1973).

Cardiovascular disease is common in old age. Of all patients who died in their 80's, 85% were found to have cardiovascular and renal pathology (White, 1971). Cardiac illness regularly produces severe depressive illness; the more severe the disease is, the more profound the depression (Dovenmuehle & Verwoerdt, 1963). The depression following myocardial infarction includes a gloomy preoccupation with the future, which patients tend not to discuss with their physicians (Hackett & Adams, 1977). In cardiac disease, depression appears early in the illness. As the disease progresses and the depression increases, fatigue and exhaustion set in (sometimes falsely attributed to a failing heart by the sick patient), followed by irritability, anxiety, dependency, aimlessness, and boredom. Such increased dependency fosters further regression, greater helplessness, and social isolation, which all contribute to the maintenance of depression (Payne, 1975). Payne (1964) has presented a clinical vignette of a 62-year-old woman. Following a myocardial infarction, the woman developed an agitated depression with suicidal preoccupation, as she grew increasingly dependent on her husband for whom she had ambivalent feelings.

The inevitable result of a diagnosis of cancer is depression (Hackett & Adams, 1977). Following initial shock and depression, denial and counterphobic defenses may be employed by the patient, and depression may vanish. These rapidly emerging defenses are, in part, stimulated by the patient's fear of abandonment by physician, family, and friends should depressive affects be openly acknowledged.

However, the depression may persist for the remainder of life if basic adaptive mechanisms are disrupted (Sutherland, 1957). Such mechanisms include not only character defenses but also strategies that have been developed to achieve gratification and self-esteem. The disruption of such mechanisms can cause a plummeting of self-esteem and overwhelming feelings of helplessness that not only threaten psychic narcissism but also lead to a fear of loss of interpersonal supports.

Some of the reaction to cancer results from the loss of certain affected body parts through surgery. Loss of function of organs of sexual identity or of those involved with excretion, for example, may revive earlier psychological conflicts regarding these bodily functions with a resulting self-hatred and condemnation and a sense of worthlessness (Sutherland, 1957). A sense of weakness, mutilation, and body disfigurement leading to severe depression are often seen following bowel surgery with the establishment of a colostomy (Sutherland, Orbach, Dyk, & Bard, 1952). For a woman, the removal of a cancerous breast may produce a sense of lost sexual identification and diminished womanhood that may lead to a chronic depression. Weight loss following mastectomy has been attributed to depression rather than malignancy and is an example of a somatic expression of a profound affective disorder (Hollender, 1954).

The psychological reaction to the loss of a body part or the loss of body function in the elderly may occur as a result of natural aging processes or as a consequence of a chronic disease other than cancer. The occurrence of guilt and shame along with depression is common in elderly people with such losses (Verwoerdt, 1973). As in cancer patients, the intensity of the reaction to the loss of a body part (or function) partly depends on the representation it has in the body image (Hollender, 1958; Lipowski, 1968).

Maintenance of contact with reality requires stimulation from the environment. Loss of vision and hearing are common in the elderly and impairment or loss of these faculties may lead to depression, social isolation, and loss of independence (Goldstein, Hersperger, Wilson, & Senturka, 1971; Nicholson, 1974; Sanders & Smith, 1971). When eyes and vision have an especially important meaning to the elderly person, the depression may become severe. The case of a 70-year-old woman is illustrative (Hollender, 1955). Following a successful cataract operation, the woman became seriously depressed and required hospitalization. She felt that the surgery had ruined her body image, which was dependent on her "beautiful eyes." Decreased hearing likewise may contribute to a secondary depression, although it more commonly contributes to paranoia in the elderly (Pfeiffer & Busse, 1973).

Patients of all ages with chronic disease may suffer from reactive depressions. An overall incidence of depression that accompanies medical disease, regardless of age, suggests that depression is a relatively frequent companion to such illness. Depressive illnesses are associated with 38% of gastrointestinal illness, 21% of neurologic disease, 20% of respiratory illness, 14% of genitourinary disorder, 12% of cardiovascular disease, 12% of musculoskeletal disorder, and 7% of endocrine disorder (Schwab, Bialow, Holzer, Brown, & Stevenson, 1967). In the elderly, the already existing circumstances of reduced somatic functioning, loss, and inevitable death may raise the incidence of depression to higher levels.

The Concept of Depressive Equivalents

Although medical illness or physical decline may present as depression or with depressive-like symptoms, the opposite is true as well. Depression may present with a variety of physical symptoms. In some cases, the use of somatic complaints to communicate affective states represents an adaptive ego-coping mechanism. In other cases, somatic complaints as an expression of depression may be a manifestation of hypochondriasis that functions to acquit the elderly from responsibility for the etiology of the depression (Verwoerdt, 1973). Many elderly patients with depression present with an aggravation of a preexisting physical illness such as a stroke or a respiratory or cardiovascular malfunction (Williamson, 1974). Such patients may appear depressed but vigorously deny it (Pfeiffer & Busse, 1973).

The term *depressive equivalent* is used to describe the expression of depression through complaints of bodily malfunctions (Ewalt, 1960, 1964). The term was first used to describe patients who had various somatic complaints but did not show any apparent depressive mood (Beck, 1967; Kennedy & Wiesel, 1946). Synonyms for depressive equivalents include masked or atypical depressions. Psychoanalytic explanations of this phenomenon are derived from the theory of hypochondriasis. Anger and guilt are turned against the self and can be understood as self-punishment or even partial suicide when surgery is conducted to relieve symptoms (Ewalt, 1964; Menninger, 1938).

Fenichel (1945) has described fatigue and anorexia as symptoms of inhibited aggressiveness and thus equivalents of depression. Lopez-Ibor (1972) describes four inclusive categories of masked depressions, or depressive equivalents: (1) pains and paresthesias, (2) agoraphobia, (3) psychosomatic disturbances and hypochondria, and (4) anorexia. Gero (1953) has described at length the psychoanalytic treatment of a case of anorexia that he considered to be a depressive equivalent.

A variety of other symptoms may be unconsciously used by a patient to mask depression as well as to communicate and ask for help (Ancherson, 1961; Lundquist, 1961). Gastrointestinal symptoms are the most common. The patient is preoccupied with constipation, flatulence, and abdominal pains. The mouth may be a site of depressive equivalents with symptoms of bad taste, burning tongue, toothaches, and vague oral discomfort, often referable to ill-fitting dentures. Each attempt to make the plates fit better (or taste better) may aggravate the symptoms (Ewalt, 1964). Symptoms referable to the genitourinary tract, such as burning urination and pains in the lower abdomen, are also frequent depressive equivalents. Pain, lassitude, fatigability, and loss of strength are more vague symptoms that may be somatic expressions of depression.

In addition to psychoanalytic formulations, theoretical explanations must be sought for the development of depressive equivalents in the elderly. Busse (1975) has noted that somatic hyperconcern of older people may be a consequence of real loss of objects or means of external support. Failing physical functioning is a reality in the elderly as are the devastating effect of physical disease and the inevitable specter of death. The role of cultural differences in the identification and response to physical illness must also be considered. Zborowski (1952) has noted that Jewish and Italian patients respond to pain in an emotional fashion; Americans are more stoical; and Irish patients frequently deny pain. Such differences may extend to other symptoms and to attitudes about seeking medical help for symptom distress (Mechanic, 1972). It is likely that for many older people of differing ethnic, economic, and intellectual backgrounds, as well as with different premorbid character defense styles, the communication of affective distress may be more threatening than talk of physical illness.

Depression, Dementia, and Pseudodementia

The clinician is sometimes confronted with a perplexing differential diagnostic puzzle: the mildly or moderately demented elderly patient. Such seeming organic confusional state may be an atypical presentation of late life depression. Depression may also be superimposed on a mild or moderate senile dementia making differentiation nearly impossible (Hamilton & Cowdry, 1971).

Failing memory, like other failing bodily functions, may provoke a reactive depression depending upon the degree of narcissistic involvement the person has with cognitive abilities. For one who has taken pride in memory and has depended on mental faculties for support and gratification, failing memory may be the equivalent of a limb amputation to an athlete. At times, failing memory may present as depression (Post, 1965). If the memory loss is modest, the depression may be an exaggerated response to the forgetfulness that is common in older age. For more severe cognitive impairment, the depression may be an expression of helplessness in the face of true progressive physical loss and impairment.

At times, depression may actually present as dementia. The term *pseudodementia* has been applied to this condition (Busse, 1973; Post, 1965; Slaby & Wyatt, 1974). Such patients may appear perplexed, apathetic, listless, and disinterested. Forgetfulness and disorientation mimic an organic syndrome. The clinical differentiation between pseudodementia and true dementia is important since the underlying depression of the former may be treatable. Clinical experience suggests that the improvement of memory following treatment for pseudodementia is indicative of an affective rather than a cognitive disorder. At times the differentiation between the two etiologies may be nearly impossible and may require a therapeutic trial of antidepressant drug or electroconvulsive therapy treatment (Wang & Busse, 1971).

Differential symptoms and signs between dementia and pseudodementia/depression are summarized in Table 2. In general, pseudodemented patients seem to experience an abrupt onset of symptoms, and the mood depression often precedes the impairment of consciousness or loss of memory. Patients with an affective illness tend to be negativistic, sad, and sometimes agitated or restless. These patients show more interest in confabulating than in answering questions (Busse, 1973). Premorbid intelligence is often low, and there are often sleep disturbances and self-deprecating attitudes (Langley, 1975). The patient seems to say, "I don't want to remember" (cf. chapters 1 and 9 for additional discussions of depressive pseudodementia).

Diseases That May Present with Depression or That May Be Accompanied by Depressive Symptoms

Neurologic Illness

Idiopathic Parkinson's disease (as contrasted with postencephalitic or drug-induced Parkinson-like symptoms) is a disease of middle and late life. The decreased motility produced by this neurologic disorder may resemble the physical signs of retarded depression: lassitude, weakness, and slowness. Mask-like facies may occasionally be mistaken for depression, and decreased speech for poverty of thought or negativism. Since other signs of Parkinson's disease such as cogwheel rigidity are usually present in the elderly, it is unlikely that the movement disorder per se would be confused with an affective illness.

The occurrence of true depressive affect with Parkinson's disease, however, has been accepted as a common part of the clinical syndrome. Incidences of depression ranging from 40 to 90% have been cited (Brown & Wilson, 1972;

TABLE 2 Characteristics of Senile Dementia and Severe Depression

Characteristics	Depressed	Senile	Characteristics	Depressed	Senile
Depression	++++	++	Confusion	++	++++
Sleep and appetite disturbance	+++	++	Disorientation	+	++++
Suicidal thoughts	++	±	Impaired recent memory	+	++++
Emotional lability	+	+++	Decreased mental alertness	++	++++
Anxiety	+++	++	Unsociability	++	++++
Hostility-irritability	++	+++	Uncooperativeness	++	++++

Mindham, 1970; Mjones, 1949). In one series of 170 patients with a mean age of 65.8, 37% were considered to be depressed, with a higher prevalence among women. There was no relationship between the severity of the motor disturbance and the prevalence and severity of the depression. Furthermore, there was no correlation between the duration of the parkinsonian symptoms and the presence or absence of depression (Celesia & Wanamaker, 1972). It is a matter of debate whether the depressive symptoms are part of the neurologic etiology of the disease or are a secondary reaction to the illness and its chronic, progressive disability (Warbarton, 1967; Wilson, 1940). The depressive symtpoms of Parkinson's disease have been successfully treated with electroconvulsive therapy in a 61-year-old man with Parkinson's disease who experienced early morning awakening, ideas of guilt, worthlessness, hopelessness, suicidal ideation, and depressed mood (Asnis, 1977).

Amyotrophic lateral sclerosis is another neurologic disease that may include depression as part of the clinical picture. Although it is more common in middle-aged than in elderly persons, it does occur above the age of 60. The symptoms of depression may be masked with this disease through the rather common use of denial and the displacement to bodily symptoms (Brown & Mueller, 1970). For example, a 64-year-old man with amyotrophic lateral sclerosis denied depression and seemed cheerful and calm yet suffered from severe anorexia and insomnia that could not be attributed to the primary disease. A 71-year-old man denied being sad but would experience episodes of weeping as well as fitful sleep and increasing constipation. A 62-year-old woman denied depression or anger but suffered from anorexia and severe constipation. A 60-year-old man denied depression and was cheerful although he was planning for an "accidental" suicide. A 66-year-old man, however, admitted frank despair and suicidal thoughts in addition to anorexia and insomnia. The authors commented that mood adjective testing on paper-and-pencil tests reveals a failure to check pleasant affect adjectives rather than a checking of dysphoric items.

Brain tumors are among the most likely neurologic diseases that may present as depression (Altschule, 1965; Rossman, 1969). Primary intracranial tumors are infrequent past the age of 60 (Wilson & Bruce, 1955). Brain tumors, as a cause of depression in the elderly, are more likely to result from metastases from other primary sites of tumors that are common as people age. Carcinoma of the breast, lung, bones, stomach, and liver often metastasize to the brain. Symptoms of depression that might not necessarily be typical of the primary neoplasm can be attributed to the brain metastasis (Rossman, 1969). Gliomas are the most frequent type of primary cerebral tumor that has been implicated in depression. The rise of intracranial pressure with growth of a tumor may produce general changes in psychological functioning: inattention, indifference, decreased initiative, withdrawal, depressed or labile mood, drowsiness, and lethargy. The location of the tumor may play a role in the production of affective symptoms (Wilson & Bruce, 1955). Tumors near or within the ventricular system (e.g., frontal lobe, temporal lobe, or of the corpus callosum) are likely to produce some emotional impairment. Depression, although possible, is generally less common than dementia, the primary symptom of such growths. Other cortical tumors are also not likely to produce depression as a major symptom, although tumors in other locations have been associated with depression (Rossman, 1969).

Multiple sclerosis is also a disease more common under the age of 40 that occasionally appears in older people. Even though mania and elation are more frequently seen, depression characterized by irritability and labile mood changes are common. Occasionally, depression may be the presenting symptom (Brown & Davis, 1922; Gallineck & Kalinowsky, 1958; Goodstein & Fenrell, 1977; Surridge, 1969). Retardation and apathy are conspicuously absent from the depression of multiple sclerosis (Altschule, 1965).

There is also an increased incidence of vascular disturbances in the elderly such as small silent strokes that may produce depression. Intracranial aneurisms, another cause of depression, can occur at any age but are more likely to occur as the walls of arteries become thinner in old age (Rossman, 1969). Older people are also more susceptible to bacterial infections, such as meningitis, that may produce depressive symptoms (Strassman, 1957).

Endocrine Disturbances

Endocrine abnormalities are often associated with alterations in affective states. Although disease of endocrine organs are not among the more frequent hazards of old age, they may occur beyond age 60 and can produce depressions of alarming severity. In general, both hypo- and hyperfunctioning of the various endocrine systems have been implicated in depression.

Hypothyroidism is a disease commonly associated with early adulthood, although it occasionally appears in old age and should be considered in the care of every geriatric patient (Starr, 1971). Hypothyroid functioning is associated with an 80% incidence of depressive symptoms as well as with cognitive impairment (Brown, 1975) and a 93% incidence of psychomotor retardation and irritability (Smith, Barish, Correa, & Williams, 1972). Thyroid gland hypofunction can mirror depressions as well as mental retardation and schizophrenia. Prominent symptoms include slowness of thinking, depressive mood, facetiousness and silliness (Witzelsucht), and the physical concomitants of hypothyroidism.

Hyperthyroidism is more common than hypothyroidism in the elderly, and it is more common in females than males (Green, 1974). In a survey of 1,000 patients, 124 (12%) were over the age of 60. Of these 124 patients, weight loss was the presenting symptom in over 70%, and 32% of all patients complained of nervousness and emotionalism (Bartels & Kingsley, 1949; Iverson, 1965), although emotionalism was not specifically defined.

One form of hyperthyroid disease that may occur in the elderly and is a particularly confusing diagnostic problem is *apathetic thyrotoxicosis.* This form of the disease is nonactivating in contrast to the hyperkinetic form. It is characterized by a senile appearance in the patient, the presence of a small thyroid gland, and an absence of exophthalmos, tachycardia, and smooth skin, the usual symptoms of thyrotoxicosis (Thomas, Mazzaferri, & Skillman, 1970). These authors noted that apathetic thyrotoxicosis may be frequent in the elderly (7 of 9 patients studied), and that apathy and detached depression were prominent features. A 73-year-old woman was discussed as an example. She was described as disinterested, quiet, and almost resigned to death. Prior to a diagnosis of thyrotoxicosis, she had been diagnosed as depressed by her psychiatrist and as having old age depression by her family. The authors offered the following diagnostic criteria for apathetic thyrotoxicosis: (a) an elderly patient with apathetic appearance; (b) small goiter; (c) depression, lethargy, or apathy; (d) absence of ocular manifestation; (e) substantial muscular wasting; (f) excessive weight loss; and (g) cardiovascular dysfunction with atrial fibrillation.

Diseases of the parathyroid glands are also associated with depression. In a study by Brown (1975), 30% of patients with hypoparathyroid functioning presented with depression, irritability, and emotional lability, although tetany was a more common presenting symptom. Primary hypoparathyroidism is unusual in the elderly, although secondary hypoparathyroidism following thyroid surgery may occur in all age groups and therefore should be considered in the differential diagnosis of the elderly patient (Starr, 1971). In a series of hypoparathyroid patients, none who were over age 60 with a diagnosis of primary (idiopathic) hypoparathyroidism was described as depressed. Two elderly women, however, were described as developing depression as a concomitant to decreased parathyroid functioning following thyroid surgery (Denko & Kaelbing, 1962). In general, psychiatric symptoms of secondary hypoparathyroidism do not differ from idiopathic primary hypoparathyroidism. The symptoms include mental impairment, organic dementia, depression, and schizophrenic-like symptoms.

In 1926, test animals given parathyroid hormone seemed depressed, and in 1929 an association was made between hyperparathyroidism and depression (Gatewood, Organ, & Mead, 1975). Hyperparathyroidism in the elderly patient may present with depression or include depression as part of the clinical syndrome. Although considered to be a disease more common to middle life (ages 45-50), in one study 23% of the patients with this diagnosis were past 60 (Hellstrom & Ivemark, 1962). The depression of hyperparathyroidism has been characterized by a lack of initiative, spontaneous activity, suicidal preoccupation, fatigue, memory impairment, and irascibility (Hellstrom & Ivemark, 1962; Peterson, 1968; Smith, Barish, Correa, & Williams, 1972). One case report presented a 64-year-old woman with hyperparathyroid disease who had an agitated depression with tremulousness and anxiety (Karpati & Frame, 1964). In another series of five patients with hyperparathyroidism, four were over the age of 60 (Gatewood, Organ, & Mead, 1975). Two of the four elderly patients initially presented with a depressive syndrome that included affective symptoms as well as constipation, fatigue, and lethargy. These authors believed that the depression was due to hypercalcemia, which may dampen neurological functioning much like lithium ions. They further speculated that the depressive symptoms may have been secondary to a depletion of magnesium ions, which accompanies the hypercalcemia. Decreased serum magnesium can produce depressive symptoms as well as mental confusion.

Diminished functioning of the adrenal glands (Addison's disease) is a disorder of middle life that, like other pathological endocrine functioning, should be suspected in elderly patients who tire easily and exhibit anorexia, weight loss, and many somatic symptoms, particularly of the gastrointestinal tract (Brown, 1975; Thorn, 1955). The depression that may accompany Addison's disease has been reported in 60-80% of patients and is described as including apathy, decreased initiative, poverty of thought, and negativism (Brown, 1975; Fawcett & Bunney, 1967). The disease often starts insidiously, and depression may be the first symptom. Pigmented skin changes characteristic of Addison's disease are rarely seen at this early stage (Altschule, 1965).

Primary hyperadrenal function (Cushing's disease) may produce depression in 20% of those afflicted (Smith et al., 1972; Spillane, 1951; Starr, 1952). It may lead to suicide attempts in 10%; the suicide rate of patients with Cushing's disease has bee considered to be 1,000 times that of the normal population of the same age (Brown, 1975; Starr, 1952). Cushing's disease is a disorder principally of the third and fourth decade; although it has been diagnosed in the elderly. One series of 25 patients with Cushing's disease included a 62-year-old woman with marked lethargy, drowsiness, irritability, depressive affect, crying spells, and hypomotoric behavior (Trethoven & Cobb, 1952). Because of the frequency and severity of the depression that accompanies Cushing's disease, it should be considered in elderly patients with depression, particularly those with suicidal ideation.

Pernicious Anemia

Pernicious anemia is a disease that has its highest incidence in persons between ages 60 and 70. It is thought to be due to malabsorption of vitamin B_{12} secondary to the achlorhydria and hypochlorhydria that is common in the elderly (Tauber, Goodhart, Hsu, Blumberg, Kassab, & Chow, 1957). Depression is a common occurrence in elderly patients with pernicious anemia and it may even be the presenting symptom (Anderson, Cooper, & Naylor, 1968). Pernicious anemia is invariably associated with dementia or a fluctuating confusional state, and it is more likely to be misdiagnosed as presenile or senile dementia than as depression (Buxton, Davison, Hyams, & Irvine, 1969; Strachan & Henderson, 1965).

Diseases of the Pancreas

Diseases of the pancreas are sometimes associated with depression, a relationship noted as far back as the 17th century (Fras, Litin, & Pearson,

1967). Depression, crying spells, insomnia, and anxiety have been noted with pancreatic disease, which must therefore be considered in any elderly person with severe depression. Islet cell tumors that produce a state of hyperinsulinism may present with depression and associated fatigue (Altschule, 1965; Martin, 1975). Other symptoms including nervousness, dizzy spells, disorientation, and anxiety are also prominent, and seizures may occur as the disease progresses.

Pancreatitis is a disease that may be associated with depression (Rickles, 1945) and must be distinguished from pancreatic carcinoma, which is also associated with depression.

Carcinoma of the pancreas is a tumor that appears most frequently between the ages of 50 and 70 (Martin, 1975). This form of cancer, in contrast to all other types of abdominal neoplasia, is most regularly associated with depressive symptoms. Patients have described themselves as depressed, low down, and in the dumps, without a loss of initiative, ambition, and perseverance. Other symptoms are anorexia, insomnia, weight loss, and back pain (Perlas & Faillace, 1964). Inexplicable feelings of doom, hopelessness, and despair are sometimes the first symptoms of the disease, appearing weeks or months before the onset of physical symptoms (Hackett & Adams, 1977). Irritability occurs in a high number of patients who develop cancer of the pancreas. In this regard it resembles cancer of the stomach. The two may be differentiated, however, by a lack of insomnia and anxiety in the latter. Jacobson and Ottoson (1971) believe that depression is not the primary mental symptom with pancreatic cancer, rather they see a mild "organic-psycho-syndrome with the triad of irritability, weakness and mild depression."

Urinary Tract Disease

Urinary tract disease with decreased renal function and elevation of blood urea nitrogen are common in the elderly (Walker, 1967; Moore-Smith, 1973). Depressive mood changes, apathy, and suicidal ruminations may be emotional manifestations of uremia (Schwab, 1968; Wise, 1974). The depression of uremia, or the reactive depression that accompanies chronic renal disease, is frequently associated with a delirium of varying proportions. In the early stages, mood alteration may precede the delirium (Greenblatt & Shader, 1975). Altered electrolyte balance secondary to impaired renal function may also produce depression. Severe depressions have been noted with sodium, potassium, and magnesium depletion (Davison, 1971). With the increasing use of maintenance hemodialysis and renal transplantation for the management of chronic renal disease of the elderly, mood alterations with depression are likely to become more frequent.

Miscellaneous Disorders

Chronic lymphoid leukemia, which is rare under the age of 40, is known to be associated with depressive symptoms (Fras et al., 1967).

Systemic lupus erythematosus is a disease that frequently produces affective symptoms and may appear in later years (Guze, 1967). In a review of the literature on systemic lupus erythematosus, Heine (1969) has noted that up to 9% of all patients mentioned in clinical reports had depressive symptoms. In his own series of 38 patients ranging in age from 13 to 78, 18% (7 patients) were depressed, and 3 patients presented with depression as the initial symptom. He presented case histories of two elderly females who were depressed and demented.

Early congestive heart failure may present as depression with mood changes and fatigue. Insomnia is frequent and may be due to dyspnea. Mood elevation is often observed following digitalis treatment of the cardiac decompensation.

Failure to Thrive

Symptoms due to mental and physical deterioration or those that deplete energy may mimic some of the vegetative signs that are associated with depression or may be confused with depression. Listlessness, apathy, fatigue, anorexia, insomnia, as well as symptoms of sadness and hopelessness may accompany a decline in physical health. The pediatric term *failure to thrive* may be appropriate for insidious and progressive physical deterioration (Hodkinson, 1973). Such symptoms are commonly seen in chronic anemias (in addition to the more specific depression of pernicious anemia) and chronic infections. Chronic pulmonary tuberculosis, brucellosis, and subacute bacterial endocarditis, although uncommon, are treatable serious illnesses that may appear as depression. Lingering influenza and chronic hepatitis can also produce a physical decline that may resemble depression or depressive symptoms.

Failure to thrive with depressive-like signs and symptoms may be due to malnutrition and vitamin deficiency. The elderly who live alone sometimes eat inadequate, poorly balanced diets (Corless, 1973; Schroeder, 1971). Depression may accompany protein deficiency and vitamin B deficiencies. Pellagra, commonly associated with dementia, may also present as depression. Malnutrition secondary to malignancy similarly may produce this progressive physical decline that resembles depression. Depression with advanced carcinomatosis has been described in the elderly (Goldfarb, 1967; Greenblatt & Shader, 1975). The depressive symptoms include depressed mood, anorexia, and insomnia. These same authors described a short-lived but excellent response to ECT in a 76-year-old woman with advanced carcinomatosis and concomitant depression.

Diabetes, which often appears late in life, may produce the failure-to-thrive syndrome. The depressive-like symptoms include deteriorating social competence, weight loss, anorexia, increased frailty, decreased initiative, decreased concentration, and decreased motivation (Hodkinson, 1973).

Intermittent porphyria, although not a disease commonly associated with the elderly, occasionally presents with depression among other abnormal mental states.

DRUGS THAT MAY CONTRIBUTE TO DEPRESSION IN THE ELDERLY

Drugs, either prescribed by a physician or taken independently, are often responsible for the development of depression, the aggravation of a preexisting depression, or the production of depressive-like symptoms such as sedation, apathy, and lethargy. The elderly are particularly likely to be taking drugs for treatment of a medical or emotional disturbance and thus are likely to be predisposed to depressive side effects.

The elderly are more susceptible to unwanted toxic effects of drugs. As the human body ages, a variety of morphologic changes occur naturally that may account for this increased susceptibility. Absorption of a drug, for example, may be reduced because of (a) a decrease in stomach acid output, (b) decreases in mesenteric blood flow, (c) diminished size of the absorbing surface, and (d) a diminution in the efficiency of the enzyme systems responsible for the transport of a drug across interstitial epithelial membranes (Bender, 1974). Decreases in protein binding, circulation time, and hepatic metabolic processes may dramatically alter the pharmacokinetics of drug metabolism thereby lengthening the drug's stay in the body and the period of potential toxicity (Salzman & Shader, 1974; Salzman, Shader, & Pearlman, 1970). Impairment of renal clearance of drugs, often present in old people, may further delay the removal of drugs or their metabolites thus allowing toxic substances to accumulate in the body (Davison, 1973).

Structural changes within the central nervous system (CNS) may predispose the elderly to increased sensitivity of a drug's neuroactive clinical effect as well as unwanted side effects (Ayd, 1960; Domino, 1969; Hamilton, 1966; Jacobsen, 1964; Mann, 1965; Sieda & Muller, 1967). Drugs that depress the CNS have the potential, therefore, of producing severe depression of neurologic function. Depressed mood is often the subjective result of this increased sensitivity. Apathy, lethargy, drowsiness, and sedation are depressive-like signs that may be confused with clinical depression and are also signs of diminished CNS functioning.

Drugs used to treat a wide variety of medical conditions are capable of producing CNS or mood depression. Since many of these drugs (such as antihypertensives) are widely used in old age, the diagnosis of depression must include a careful evaluation of drug ingestion by the aged patient. Elderly people are also likely to be taking several drugs at once. The interaction between pharmaceuticals is common and sometimes productive of depressive states.

Drugs Used to Treat Medical Disease

Certain drugs may indirectly produce depression or depressive-like symptoms by inducing a secondary illness that has depression as part of the syndrome. Sulfonylurea, for example, may produce a secondary hypothyroidism, which often has depressive mood, apathy, lethargy, and fatigue as part of the syndrome (Davison, 1971). Lithium carbonate, used to treat and prevent affective illness, may similarly induce a secondary hypothyroid condition. Other examples of secondary depressions include the potassium depletion secondary to thiazide diuretics. Diuretics, widely used among the elderly to treat hypertension and other cardiovascular problems, deplete potassium, and this depletion in turn may produce lethargy and weakness that may be misperceived as depression. Diuretics may also induce or unmask a diabetic condition that may then present as failure to thrive.

Digitalis

Digitalis is widely prescribed to the elderly who are increasingly prone not only to cardiac pathology and disease but also to digitalis toxicity (Hurwitz & Wade, 1969). Reduced renal clearance of digitalis by the aging kidneys is thought to be the cause of this increased incidence of toxicity (Ely, Kapadia, Yao, & Marcus, 1969). Digitalis intoxication commonly produces a triad of nausea, vomiting, and mental confusion. Depression is sometimes reported secondary to digitalis intoxication although this is less frequent than delirium (Capella, Copeland, & Stern, 1961; Dall, 1965, 1970; Herrmann, 1966; Soffer, 1959). Weiss (1929) has described the mental changes attributable to digitalis as headache, dizziness, sleeplessness, and depression. Scattered reports have since appeared in the literature suggesting that in the elderly digitalis may induce dysphoric mood, apathy, weakness, and weight loss (Davison, 1971; Ellis & Dimond, 1966; Kleiger, 1976). Greenblatt and Shader (1972a) suggested that depression may be an early state of delirium.

Antihypertensives

Of all drugs taken by the elderly antihypertensives are the most likely to induce a true depression of mood. In patients treated with antihypertensives 50-70% have been noted to have depression characterized by sadness, weakness, apathy, agitation, and insomnia (Lewis, 1971). Older patients are particularly likely to experience such depression (Faucett, Litin, & Achor, 1957). Older patients with prior episodes of depression are the most susceptible of all to such depression (Lemieux, Davignon, & Genest, 1956).

Reserpine is the antihypertensive agent that is most responsible for producing depression. Symptoms reported with reserpine include decreased energy, depressed mood, loss of interest, crying spells, indecisiveness, hopelessness, impaired concentration, fear of physical ailments, suicidal tendencies, lethargy, agitation, insomnia, anhedonia, drowsiness, fatigue, lassitude, and loss of energy (Ayd, 1958; Faucett et al., 1957; Jensen, 1959; Kline, Barsa, & Gosline, 1956; Muller, Pryor, Gibbons, & Orgain, 1955). Characteristic features of this depressive syndrome that help distinguish it from true endogenous depression are presence of anxiety, lack of guilt, and lack of self-depreciation (Bernstein & Kaufman, 1960; Goodwin, Ebert, & Bunney, 1972). Tester-Dalderup, nevertheless, has noted that reserpine-induced depression often goes unrecognized (1977).

Methyldopa, like reserpine, is a widely prescribed antihypertensive that produces depressive side effects (McKinney & Kane, 1967). The elderly are also particularly susceptible to the depressive side effects of this drug (Davison, 1971). Symptoms of depression associated with methyldopa include drowsiness, sleepiness, fatigue, and weakness (Kennedy, 1975; Simpson, 1973; Tester-Dalderup, 1975). In patients with preexisting depression, methyldopa like reserpine may produce a severe aggravation of symptoms (Simpson, 1973).

A number of other drugs used to treat hypertension may also cause depression. Propranolol has produced depression in patients who had previously become depressed when taking reserpine (Waal, 1967). Lassitude and fatigue, and decreased exercise and tolerance have all been reported following the use of beta-adrenergic blockers like propranolol, and these symptoms may be difficult to distinguish from those of true depression (Greenblatt & Shader, 1972*b*). Guanethidine, hydralazine, clonidine are all drugs that may produce depressionlike symptoms including sedation, fatigue, anorexia, and constipation (Hollister, 1972; Tester-Dalderup, 1975). Diuretics have already been noted to produce these symptoms as a consequence of potassium depletion.

Anti-Parkinson Drugs

The elderly, particularly those over 70, are predisposed to psychiatric reactions that may accompany L-dopa therapy of Parkinson's disease (Winkelman & DiPalma, 1971). Although delirium and psychosis are more common side effects than depression, a number of reports have described severe depression with suicidal preoccupation in elderly patients (Barbeau, 1969; Celesia & Barr, 1970; Cherington, 1970; Jenkins & Groh, 1970; Mawdsley, 1970). In one series of 208 patients with a mean age of 63.8 years, 20% complained of some form of sleep disturbance and 9.5% developed overt depression (Presthus & Holmsen, 1974). Other symptoms of depression have included tearfulness, anorexia, hopelessness, apathy, petulance, negativism, and constipation (Wagshul & Daroff, 1969; McDowell, Lee, Swift, Sweet, Ogshury, & Kessler, 1970). The depression has been attributed to the elderly patient's realization that L-dopa therapy does not produce a miracle cure (Barbeau, 1969).

Other drugs used to treat Parkinson's disease have been implicated in producing depression. Bromcriptine (Calne, Teycherne, Clavera, Eastman, Greenacre, & Petrie, 1974) and Carbidopa (Lieberman, Derby, Feigenson, Goodgold, Nesbette, Resurreccion, & Valdiva, 1973), have also produced depressions. Amantadine has produced toxic psychosis with agitation and confusion, but episodes of depression are not specifically mentioned (Barbeau, Mars, Botez, and Joubert, 1971). Anticholinergic compounds likewise produce agitation, delirium, apprehension, and fear but not depression (Shader & Greenblatt, 1972).

Female Hormones

Estrogens are sometimes given to postmenopausal women to relieve depressive symptoms that sometimes accompany this stage of life (Glick, 1967; Klaiber, Broverman, Vogel, Kobayshi, & Moriarity, 1972). It is not clear whether administration of these hormones can be regarded as successful treatment for involutional disorders (Glick & Bennett, 1972). Hormonal preparations may themselves cause depression at all ages, and the elderly do not seem particularly predisposed (Hollister, 1972). Nevertheless, elderly women taking estrogen or progesterone who are depressed should have their drug and hormonal status reevaluated.

Corticosteroids

Cortisone and related compounds are used in the elderly not so much to replace missing adrenal secretions, but to treat other medical conditions, such as arthritis, common in older people (Davison, 1971). Exogenous cortisol is well known to produce euphoria (Carpenter, Strauss, & Bunney, 1972). Depressive symptoms, although less frequent, do result from adrenal hormone preparations (Bunney, 1969; Clark, Bauer, & Cobb, 1952; Clark, Quarton, Cobb, & Bauer, 1953). Fawcett and Bunney (1967) have commented that many investigators have noted that corticosteroids may be associated with depression as well as euphoria.

Antituberculosis Agents

Drugs used to treat tuberculosis have been mentioned as causing depression (Mulder-De Jong & Mulder, 1975). The literature is rather sparse in this regard, however. Iproniazid can produce a secondary vitamin B deficiency with pellagra-like condition. Depression from such an indirect cause can occur, although there is concomitant confusion and memory impairment (Olsen & Torning, 1959). Cycloserine, a newer antituberculosis agent, produces a variety of mental side effects including depression that have been characterized by drowsiness or insomnia, inability to concentrate, and symptoms of a toxic psychosis (Epstein, Nair, & Boyd, 1955; Murray, 1956; Pyle, Pfuetze, Barclary, & Kasik, 1959; Wallach & Gershon, 1972).

Anticancer Drugs

Cytostatic and immunosuppressive drugs are used as part of the treatment of cancer. All of these drugs produce toxic side effects, largely nausea and vomiting. Behavioral toxicity including depression is sometimes seen.

Depressive-like symptoms of chemotherapeutic toxicity include somnolence, apathy, lethargy, irritability, and weakness (Malpas & Whitehouse, 1977). Depressed mood has been noted (Medical Letter, 1976; Weiss, Walker, &

Wiernik, 1975) and may be part of a more generalized neurotoxicity seen particularly with vincristine vinblastine 5-flurouracil and 1-asparaginase (Kroese, 1975).

Psychotropic Drugs

Psychotropic drugs are frequently prescribed to elderly patients. In a survey of 1,276 patients over the age of 65, 61% were receiving psychoactive drugs and 25% were receiving two or more such compounds (Prien, Haber, & Caffey, 1975). Of 131 elderly patients in a long-term care facility, 29.8% were receiving neuroleptics, 22.9% hypnotics, 19.1% anxiolytics, and 9.9% antidepressants (Ingmar, Lawson, Pierpath, & Blake, 1975). Raskind and Eisdorfer (1976) has quoted one recent survey that indicated that 75% of all nursing home patients are receiving at least one (and often several) standard psychotropic medications.

Neuroleptics

Neuroleptic drugs that are used to treat psychosis in younger populations may also be used to treat agitation in the elderly (Salzman, Shader, & van der Kolk, 1975, 1976). Many neuroleptics may produce a drowsiness and sedation that may appear as depression or may be experienced as depression by the elderly (Salzman, Shader, & Pearlman, 1970). Phenothiazines have been associated with depressive symptoms since their introduction (Ayd, 1958; DiMascio, Shader, & Giller, 1970; Hollister, 1972). Old age lowers the tolerance for phenothiazines (Hamilton, 1966; Sieda & Muller, 1967) and, therefore, makes the elderly more susceptible to their depressive side effects (Hader, 1965; Salzman, 1970).

Aliphatic derivatives (e.g., chlorpromazine) and piperidine derivatives (e.g., thioridazine) of the phenothiazine nucleus are the primary offenders. These compounds have a relatively low milligram potency. As milligram potency increases (the number of milligrams needed to achieve clinical effect decreases), the sedative side effects decrease (Salzman et al., 1975). Other low milligram potency neuroleptics that may produce such depression-like sedation include chlorprothixene and loxapine. Flupenthixol, a drug not yet available in the United States, has been observed to produce severe depression in 15% of patients (Mindham, 1977). Depression also has been reported following long-acting phenothiazines (DeAlarcon & Craney, 1969).

The syndrome of akinetic mutism is sometimes confused with depression because its characteristic appearance resembles withdrawal, retardation, or apathy (Rifkin, Quitkin, & Klein, 1975). It is an extrapyramidal side effect of neuroleptics, and the elderly are increasingly sensitive to such side effects. Drugs with high milligram potency (drugs with low sedative side effects) such as the piperazine phenothiazines—thiothixene and haloperidol—are chiefly responsible, although kinetic mutism may result from large doses of any neuroleptic.

Antidepressant Drugs

Tricyclic antidepressants and monoamine oxidase inhibitors do not often produce depression per se as a side effect of their biochemical activity. The most common mental side effect of these drugs is a toxic confusional state (Kane & Keeler, 1964; Klein, 1965; Kramer, 1963). Some of the drugs, notably amitriptyline and doxepin, have considerable sedative properties. The sleepiness, drowsiness, and occasional lethargy may be misinterpreted as depression by clinician and patient alike. Depressive affect has been reported with antidepressant treatment in individuals who were not considered deeply depressed prior to treatment (Cole, Griffith, & Kaye, 1965; DiMascio, Meyer, & Stifler, 1968; DiMascio, Shader, & Giller, 1970). It is thus possible that antidepressant drugs that are given to relieve depression may cause depression or increase the depressive symptoms they were to alleviate. These effects may also be heightened because of the increased sensitivity of the elderly CNS to neuroactive drugs.

Antianxiety Agents

A great number of drugs have been given over the years to treat anxiety in all age groups. Barbiturates and later propranediols (meprobamate) were commonly used until recently replaced by benzodiazepines. The two earlier drug classes produced considerable CNS depression leading to symptoms of sedation and in some cases depressed mood and suicidal thoughts (Salzman et al., 1975; Shader & Greenblatt, 1975). The benzodiazepines are less toxic than these older substances. Drowsiness and sedation are, nevertheless, common side effects in the elderly (Boston Collaborative Study, 1973; Salzman & Shader, 1973, 1974, 1975; Salzman, Shader, & Harmatz, 1975; Salzman, Shader, Harmatz et al., 1975). Depression and sedation may also occur at lower doses than those necessary to produce this side effect in younger people.

A recent group of drugs used to treat anxiety are the beta-adrenergic blockers, exemplified by propranolol. The depressant effect of propranolol has already been noted.

Drugs to Assist Sleep Induction

Hypnotics and sedatives are sometimes given to the elderly to aid sleep. It has been previously noted that some difficulty in sleep is common as people age, and daytime napping is a frequent cause of nocturnal insomnia. Nevertheless, these drugs, which can lead to serious addictive consequences and also have strong CNS depressive effects, are used in the elderly. The aging CNS is particularly sensitive to these substances, and toxic confusional states are not uncommon side effects. The sedative symptoms may mimic depression, and the evaluation of the depressed elderly person should include an inquiry as to the ingestion of such substances.

Drug Interactions

Polypharmacy leading to drug interactions is frequent in the elderly (Prien et al., 1976; Salzman et al., 1975; Tracy & Shader, 1974). Drug interactions per se are not notable as causes of depression except for the effects of oversedation. As noted previously, the elderly CNS is increasingly sensitive to the sedative effects of many neuroactive substances. Interactions between drugs with CNS sedative properties, therefore, may markedly increase sedation. Behavioral correlates of such sedation that may be confused by the clinician with depression include drowsiness, apathy, withdrawal, and motor and speech retardation.

Any CNS depressant, such as a sleeping medication, sedative, antianxiety agent, narcotic agent, or anesthetic agent as well as alcohol will interact with a variety of other drugs with sedative action to produce increased sedation. For example, the interaction between a bedtime hypnotic and sedating phenothiazine or antidepressant drug may increase sedative symptoms. Sedative drugs added to reserpine or alpha-methyldopa antihypertensives may similarly produce increased sedation. Certain geriatric tonics or cough medication may interact with sedating medical drugs to increase sedative symptoms. Alcohol taken with antianxiety agents, sedatives, neuroleptics, or antidepressants may markedly increase sedation.

Symptoms of severe extrapyramidal nervous system involvement due to drugs (e.g., akinetic mutism) may be augmented by other drugs that also have extrapyramidal stimulating properties. This is most likely when two neuroleptic drugs are used together. Rigidity, withdrawal, sad appearance, and diminished speech are symptoms that have been confused with severe retarded depression, but are actually due to drugs or drug interactions.

Although depression is not a common result of drug interactions, other mental effects such as confusion, delirium, and psychosis can result from drug interactions. Early states of the toxic delirium sometimes appear as depression, with listlessness or agitation, self-deprecatory thought content, insomnia, and anorexia. The rapid development of an acute confusional state may serve to differentiate this syndrome from true affective symptoms. Nevertheless, the clinician must be aware of the potential for such drug interactions and their effect on cognitive as well as affective functioning of the older person.

REFERENCES

Altschule, M. D. Nonpsychologic causes of depression. *Medical Science,* 1965, *16,* 36–40.

Ancherson, P. Atypical endogenous depression. *Acta Psychiatrica Scandinavica,* 1961–62, *160–163,* 267–271. (Suppl.)

Anderson, D. C., Cooper, A. F., & Naylor, G. T. Vitamin D intoxication with hypernatremia, potassium and water depletion, and mental depression. *British Medical Journal,* 1968, *4,* 774–776.

Anderson, W. F. *Practical management of the elderly.* Oxford: Blackwell, 1971.

Asnis, G. Parkinson's disease, depression, and ECT: A review and case study. *American Journal of Psychiatry,* 1977, *134,* 191-195.

Ayd, F. J., Jr. Drug-induced depression–Fact or fallacy. *New York Journal of Medicine,* 1958, *58,* 354-356.

Ayd, F. J., Jr. Tranquilizers and the ambulatory geriatric patient. *Journal of the American Geriatric Society,* 1960, *8,* 909-914.

Barbeau, A. L-DOPA therapy in Parkinson's disease: A critical review of nine years experience. *Canadian Medical Association Journal,* 1969, *101,* 791-800.

Barbeau, A., Mars, H., Botez, M., & Joubert, M. Amantadine-HC1 (Symmetrel) in the management of Parkinson's disease: A double-blind cross-over study. *Canadian Medical Association Journal,* 1971, *105,* 42-46.

Bartels, E. C., & Kingsley, J. W. I. Hyperthyroidism in patients over sixty. *Geriatrics,* 1949, *4,* 333-340.

Beck, A. T. *The diagnosis and management of depression.* Philadelphia: University of Pennsylvania, 1967.

Bender, A. D. Pharmacodynamic principles of drug therapy in the aged. *Journal of the American Geriatric Society,* 1974, *32,* 296-303.

Bernstein, S., & Kaufman, M. R. A psychological analysis of apparent depression following Rauwolfia therapy. *Journal of Mount Sinai Hospital,* 1960, *27,* 525.

Bibring, E. The mechanism of depression. In P. Greenacre (Ed.), *Affective disorders.* New York: International Universities Press, 1953.

Blinder, M. G. The pragmatic classification of depression. *American Journal of Psychiatry,* 1966, *123,* 259-269.

Boston Collaborative Drug Surveillance Program. Clinical depression of the central nervous system due to diazepam or chlordiazepoxide in relation to cigarette smoking and age. *New England Journal of Medicine,* 1973, *288,* 277.

Brown, G. L., & Wilson, W. P. Parkinsonism and depression. *Southern Medical Journal,* 1972, *65,* 540-545.

Brown, G. M. Psychiatric and neurologic aspects of endocrine disease. *Hospital Practice,* August 1975, pp. 71-79.

Brown, S., & Davis, T. K. The mental symptoms of multiple sclerosis. *Archives of Neurology and Psychology,* 1922, *7,* 629-634.

Brown, W. A., & Mueller, P. S. Psychological function in individuals with amyotrophic lateral sclerosis. *Psychosomatic Medicine,* 1970, *32,* 141-152.

Bunney, W. E., Jr. Psychoendocrine parameters and psychopathology. In A. J. Mandell & M. P. Mandell (Eds.), *Methods and theory in psychochemical research in man.* New York: Academic Press, 1969.

Busse, E. W. Research on aging: Some methods and findings. In M. A. Berezin & S. H. Cath (Eds.), *Geriatric psychiatry: Grief, loss, and emotional disorders in the aging process.* New York: Ontario University Press, 1965.

Busse, E. W. Mental disorders in later life–organic brain syndromes. In E. W. Busse & E. Pfeiffer (Eds.), *Mental illness in later life.* Washington, D.C.: American Psychiatric Association, 1973.

Busse, E. W. Aging and psychiatric diseases of late life. In M. F. Reiser (Ed.), *American handbook of psychiatry* (Vol. 4). New York: Basic Books, 1975.

Buxton, P. K., Davison, W., Hyams, D. E., & Irvine, W. J. Vitamin B12 states in mentally disturbed elderly patients. *Gerontologia Clinica,* 1969, *11,* 22-35.

Caird, F. I., & Judge, T. C. *Assessment of the elderly patient.* London: Pitman Medical, 1974.

Calne, D. B., Teycherne, P. F., Leigh, P. N., Bamji, A. N., & Greenacre, J. K. Treatment of parkinsonism with Bromocriptine. *Lancet,* 1974, *2,* 1355.

Capella, D. V., Copeland, G. D., & Stern, T. N. Digitalis intoxication: A clinical report of 148 cases. *Annals of Internal Medicine,* 1961, *50,* 869-878.

Carpenter, W. T., Jr., Strauss, J. S., & Bunney, W. E., Jr. The psychobiology of cortisol metabolism: Clinical and theoretical implications. In R. I. Shader (Ed.), *Psychiatric complications of medical drugs.* New York: Raven Press, 1972.

Celesia, G. G., & Barr, A. N. Psychosis and other psychiatric manifestations of levodopa therapy. *Archives of Neurology,* 1970, *23,* 193–200.

Celesia, G. G., & Wanamaker, W. M. Psychiatric disturbances in Parkinson's disease. *Diseases of the Nervous System,* 1972, *33,* 577–583.

Cherington, M. Parkinsonism, L-DOPA and mental depression. *Journal of the American Geriatrics Society,* 1970, *7,* 513–516.

Clark, L. D., Bauer, W., & Cobb, S. Preliminary observations on mental disturbance occurring in patients under therapy with cortisone and ACTH. *New England Journal of Medicine,* 1952, *246,* 205–216.

Clark, L. D., Quarton, G. C., Cobb, S., & Bauer, W. Further observations on mental disturbances associated with cortisone and ACTH therapy. *New England Journal of Medicine,* 1953, *249,* 178–183.

Cole, L., Griffith, C., & Kaye, H. Anginal pain and depression: A preliminary investigation. *Diseases of the Chest,* 1965, *48,* 584–586.

Corless, D. Diet in the elderly. *British Medical Journal,* 1973, *4,* 158–160.

Cumming, E., & Henry, W. E. *Growing old: The process of disengagement.* New York: Basic Books, 1961.

Dall, J. L. C. Digitalis intoxication in elderly patients. *Lancet,* 1965, *1,* 194–195.

Dall, J. L. C. Maintenance digoxin in elderly patients. *British Medical Journal,* 1970, *2,* 705–706.

Davison, W. Drug hazards in the elderly. *British Journal of Hospital Medicine,* 1971, *6,* 83–95.

Davison, W. The hazards of drug treatment in old age. In J. C. Brockelhurst (Ed.), *Textbook of geriatric medicine.* Edinburgh: Churchill Livingston, 1973.

DeAlarcon, R., & Craney, M. W. P. Severe mood changes following slow-release intramuscular fluphenazine injection. *British Medical Journal,* 1969, *3,* 564.

Denko, J. D., & Kaelbing, R. Psychiatric aspects of hypoparathyroidism. *Acta Psychiatrica Scandinavica,* 1962, *38,* 7–70. (Suppl.)

DiMascio, A., Meyer, R. E., & Stifler, L. Effects of imipramine on individuals varying in level of depression. *American Journal of Psychiatry,* 1968, *124,* 55–58.

DiMascio, A., Shader, R. I., & Giller, D. G. Behavioral toxicity Part III: Perceptual cognitive functions and Part IV: Emotional (mood) states. In R. I. Shader & A. DiMascio (Eds.), *Psychotropic drug side effects.* Baltimore: Williams & Wilkins, 1970.

Domino, E. F. Pharmacological analysis of the pathology of schizophrenia. In D. F. Siva Sankar (Ed.), *Schizophrenia, current concepts and research.* Hicksville, New York: PJD Publications, 1969.

Dovenmuehle, R. H., & Verwoerdt, A. Physical illness and depressive symptomatology II. Factors of length and stay and severity of illness and frequency of hospitalization. *Journal of Gerontology,* 1963, *18,* 260–266.

Ellis, J. G., & Dimond, E. G. Newer concepts of digitalis. *American Journal of Cardiology,* 1966, *17,* 759–767.

Ely, G. A., Kapadia, G. G., Yao, L., & Marcus, F. S. Digoxin in the elderly. *Circulation,* 1969, *39,* 449–453.

Epstein, I. G., Nair, K. G. S., & Boyd, L. J. Cycloserine, a new antibiotic in the treatment of human pulmonary tuberculosis. A preliminary report. *Antibiotic Medicine,* 1955, *1,* 80–93.

Erikson, E. H. Identity and the life cycle. *Psychological Issues,* 1959, *1,* 50–100.

Ewalt, J. R. Somatic equivalents of depressions. *Journal of the Michigan Medical Society,* 1960, *59,* 1361–1363.

Ewalt, J. R. Somatic equivalents of depression. *Texas Journal of Medicine,* 1964, *60,* 654–658.

Faucett, R. L., Litin, E. M., & Achor, R. W. P. Neuropharmacologic action of rauwolfia compounds and its psychodynamic implications. *American Medical Association Archives of Neurology and Psychiatry,* 1957, *77,* 513-518.

Fawcett, J. A., & Bunney, W. E., Jr. Pituitary adrenal function and depression. *Archives of General Psychiatry,* 1967, *16,* 517-535.

Fenichel, O. *The psychoanalytic theory of neurosis.* New York: Norton, 1945.

Fras, I., Litin, E. M., & Pearson, S. S. Comparison of psychiatric symptoms in carcinoma of the pancreas with those in some other intra-abdominal neoplasms. *American Journal of Psychiatry,* 1967, *123,* 1553-1562.

Freud, A. *The ego and the mechanisms of defense.* New York: International Universities Press, 1946.

Gallineck, A., & Kalinowsky, L. B. Psychiatric aspects of multiple sclerosis. *Diseases of the Nervous System,* 1958, *19,* 77-80.

Gatewood, J. W., Organ, C. H., & Mead, B. T. Mental changes associated with hyperparathyroidism. *American Journal of Psychiatry,* 1975, *132,* 129-132.

Gero, G. An equivalent of depression: Anorexia. In P. Greenacre (Ed.), *Affective Disorders.* New York: International Universities Press, 1953.

Glick, I. D. Mood and behavioral changes associated with the use of the oral contraceptive agents–A review of the literature. *Psychopharmacologia,* 1967, *10,* 363-374.

Glick, I. D., & Bennett, S. E. Psychiatric effects of progesterone and oral contraceptives. In R. I. Shader (Ed.), *Psychiatric complications of medical drugs.* New York: Raven Press, 1972.

Goldfarb, A. Masked depressions in the old. *American Journal of Psychotherapy,* 1968, *21,* 791-796.

Goldfarb, C., Droesan, J., & Cole, D. Psychophysiologic aspects of malignancy. *American Journal of Psychiatry,* 1967, *123,* 1545-1552.

Goldstein, R., Hersperger, W. S., Wilson, F. B., & Senturia, B. H. Otorhinolaryngologic aspects. In E. V. Cowdry & F. U. Steinberg (Eds.), *The care of the geriatric patient.* St. Louis: Mosby, 1971.

Goodstein, R. K., & Fenrell, R. B. Multiple sclerosis–Presenting as depressive illness. *Diseases of the Nervous System,* 1977, *38,* 127-131.

Goodwin, F. K., Ebert, M. H., & Bunney, W. E., Jr. Mental effects of reserpine in man: A review. In R. I. Shader (Ed.), *Psychiatric complications of medical drugs.* New York: Raven Press, 1972.

Green, M. F. Endocrine disorders in the elderly. *British Medical Journal,* 1974, *1,* 232-236.

Greenblatt, D. J., & Shader, R. I. Digitalis toxicity. In R. I. Shader (Ed.), *Psychiatric complications of medical drugs.* New York: Raven Press, 1972. (a)

Greenblatt, D. J., & Shader, R. I. On the psychopharmacology of beta adrenergic blockade. *Current Therapeutic Research,* 1972, *14,* 615-625. (b)

Greenblatt, D. J., & Shader, R. I. Psychotropic drugs in the general hospital. In R. I. Shader (Ed.), *Manual of psychiatric therapeutics.* Boston: Little Brown, 1975.

Gurland, B. J., Ganz, V. H., Fleiss, J. L., & Zubin, J. The study of the psychiatric symptoms of systemic lupus erythematosus. *Psychosomatic Medicine,* 1972, *34,* 199-206.

Guze, S. B. The occurrence of psychiatric illness in systemic lupus erythematosus. *American Journal of Psychiatry,* 1967, *123,* 1562.

Hackett, T. P., & Adams, R. D. Grief, reactive depression, manic-depressive psychosis, involutional melancholia, and hypochondriasis. In G. W. Thorn, R. D. Adams, E. Braunwald, K. J. Isselbacher, & R. G. Petersdorf (Eds.), *Harrison's principles of internal medicine.* New York: McGraw-Hill, 1977.

Hader, M. The use of selected phenothiazines in elderly patients: A review. *Journal of Mount Sinai Hospital,* 1965, *32,* 622-633.

Hamilton, L. D. Aged brain and the phenothiazines. *Geriatrics,* 1966, *21,* 131–138.

Hamilton, S. A., & Cowdry, E. V. Psychiatric aspects. In E. V. Cowdry & F. U. Steinberg (Eds.), *The care of the geriatric patient.* St. Louis: Mosby, 1971.

Heine, B. E. Psychiatric aspects of systemic lupus erythematosus. *Acta Psychiatrica Scandinavica,* 1969, *45,* 307.

Hellstrom, J., & Ivemark, B. I. Primary hyperparathyroidism. *Acta Chirurgica Scandinavica,* 1962, *294,* 5–113. (Suppl.)

Herrmann, G. R. Digitoxicity in the aged. *Geriatrics,* 1966, *21,* 109–127.

Hodkinson, H. M. Non-specific presentation of illness. *British Medical Journal,* 1973, *4,* 94–96.

Hollender, M. H. The patient with carcinoma of the breast. *General Practice,* 1954, *10,* 74–84.

Hollender, M. H. The physician, the patient, and cancer. *Illinois Medical Journal,* 1955, *107*(1), pp. 20–23.

Hollender, M. H. *The psychology of medical practice.* Philadelphia: Saunders, 1958.

Hollister, L. E. Disorders of the nervous system due to drugs. In L. Meyler & H. M. Peck (Eds.), *Drug induced diseases* (Vol. 4). Amsterdam: Excerpta Medica, 1972.

Hurwitz, N. & Wade, O. L. Intensive hospital monitoring of adverse reactions to drugs. *British Medical Journal,* 1969, *1,* 531–536.

Ingmar, S. R., Lawson, I. R., Pierpath, P. G., & Blake, P. A survey of the prescribing and administration of drugs in a long term care institution for the elderly. *Journal of the American Geriatric Society,* 1975, *33,* 309–316.

Iverson, K. Thyrotoxicosis in aged individuals. *Journal of Gerontology,* 1965, *8,* 65–69.

Jacobsen, E. Psychopharmacology and aging. In P. F. Hansen (Ed.), *Age with a future, Proceedings of the Sixth International Congress of Gerontology, Copenhagen, 1963.* Copenhagen: Munksgaad, 1964.

Jacobson, L., & Ottoson, J. O. Mental disorders in carcinoma of the pancreas and stomach. *Acta Psychiatrica Scandinavica,* 1971, *221,* 120–127. (Suppl.)

Jenkins, R. B., & Groh, R. H. Mental symptoms in parkinsonian patients treated with L-DOPA. *Lancet,* 1970, *2,* 177–180.

Jensen, K. Depressions in patients treated with reserpine for arterial hypertension. *Acta Psychiatrica Neurologica Scandinavica,* 1959, *34,* 195.

Kane, F. S., Jr., & Keeler, M. H. Visual hallucinosis while receiving imipramine. *American Journal of Psychiatry,* 1964, *121,* 611–612.

Karno, M., & Hoffman, R. The pseudoanergic syndrome. In A. Kiev (Ed.), *Somatic manifestations of depressive disorders.* Amsterdam: Excerpta Medica, 1974.

Karpati, G., & Frame, B. Neuropsychiatric disorders in primary hyperparathyroidism. *Archives of Neurology,* 1964, *10,* 387–397.

Kennedy, F., & Wiesel, B. The clinical nature of "manic-depressive equivalents" and their treatment. *Transactions of the American Neurological Association,* 1946, *71,* 96–101.

Kennedy, R. D. Drug therapy for cardiovascular disease in the aged. *Journal of the American Geriatrics Society,* 1975, *33,* 113–120.

Klaiber, E. L., Broverman, D. M., Vogel, W., Kobayshi, Y., & Moriarity, D. Effect of estrogen therapy on plasma MAO activity and EEG driving responses of depressed women. *American Journal of Psychiatry,* 1972, *128,* 1492–1498.

Kleiger, R. E. Cardiovascular disorders. In E. V. Cowdry & F. U. Steinberg (Eds.), *The care of the geriatric patient.* St. Louis: Mosby, 1976.

Klein, D. F. Visual hallucinations with imipramine. *American Journal of Psychiatry,* 1965, *121,* 911–914.

Kline, N. S., Barsa, J., & Gosline, E. Management of the side effects of reserpine and combined reserpine-chlorpromazine treatment. *Diseases of the Nervous System,* 1956, *17,* 352.

Kramer, M. Delirium as a complication of imipramine therapy in the aged. *American Journal of Psychiatry,* 1963, *120,* 502–503.

Kroese, W. F. S. Cytostatic drugs. In M. N. G. Dukes (Ed.), *Meyler's side effects of drugs.* Amsterdam: Excerpta Medica, 1975.

Langley, G. E. Functional Psychoses. In J. G. Howells (Ed.), *Modern perspectives in the psychiatry of old age.* New York: Brunner/Mazel, 1975.

Lemieux, G., Davignon, A., & Genest, J. Depressive states during rauwolfia therapy for arterial hypertension. *Canadian Medical Association Journal,* 1956, *74,* 522–526.

Levin, S. Depression in the aged. In M. A. Berezin & S. H. Cath (Eds.), *Geriatric psychiatry: Grief, loss, and emotional disorders in the aging process.* New York: International Universities Press, 1965.

Lewis, W. H. Iatrogenic psychotic depressive reaction in hypertensive patients. *American Journal of Psychiatry,* 1971, *127,* 1416–1417.

Lieberman, A. N., Derby, B. M., Feigenson, J., Goodgold, A., Nesbette, J., Resurreccion, E. C., & Valdiva, F. MK-486 and levodopa in treatment of parkinsonism. *Diseases of the Nervous System,* 1973, *34,* 167.

Lipowski, Z. T. Review of consultation psychiatry and psychosomatic medicine. *Psychosomatic Medicine,* 1968, *30,* 395–422.

Lopez-Ibor, J. I. Masked depressions. *British Journal of Psychiatry,* 1972, *120,* 245–258.

Lundquist, G. Somatic and mental stress as causative factors in depression. *Acta Psychiatrica Scandinavica,* 1961–1962, *160–163,* 267–271. (Suppl.)

Malpas, J. S., & Whitehouse, J. M. N. Cytostatic and immunosuppressive drugs. In M. N. G. Dukes (Ed.), *Side effects of drugs* (Annual 1). Amsterdam: Excerpta Medica, 1977.

Mann, D. E., Jr. Biological aging and its modification of drug activity. *Journal of Pharmaceutical Sciences,* 1965, *54,* 499–510.

Martin, M. J. Psychiatry and medicine. In A. M. Freedman, H. I. Kaplan, & B. J. Sadock (Eds.), *Comprehensive textbook of psychiatry–II.* Baltimore: Williams & Wilkins, 1975.

Mawdsley, C. Treatment of parkinsonism with laevo-dopa. *British Medical Journal,* 1970, *1,* 331–337.

McDowell, F., Lee, J. E., Swift, T., Sweet, R. D., Ogshury, J. S., & Kessler, J. T. Treatment of Parkinson's syndrome with L-Dihydroxyphenylalanine (levodopa). *Annals of Internal Medicine,* 1970, *72,* 29–35.

McKinney, W. R., Jr., & Kane, F. J., Jr. Depression with the use of alpha-methyldopa. *American Journal of Psychiatry,* 1967, *124,* 80.

Mechanic, D. Social psychologic factors affecting the presentation of bodily complaints. *New England Journal of Medicine,* 1972, *286,* 1132–1139.

Medical Letter. *Cancer Chemotherapy,* 1976, *18,* 109–116.

Meissner, W. W., Mack, J. E., & Semrad, E. V. Classical psychoanalysis. In A. M. Freedman, H. I. Kaplan, & B. J. Sadock (Eds.), *Comprehensive textbook of psychiatry–II.* Baltimore: Williams & Wilkins, 1975.

Menninger, K. A. *Man against himself.* New York: Harcourt, Brace and Company, 1938.

Mindham, R. H. S. Psychiatric symptoms of parkinsonism. *Journal of Neurology, Neurosurgery and Psychiatry,* 1977, *33,* 188–191.

Mjones, S. H. Paralysis agitans: Clinical and genetic study. *Acta Psychiatrica Neurologica,* 1949, *54,* 1–195. (Suppl.)

Moore-Smith, B. Urinary tract diseases. *British Medical Journal,* 1973, *3,* 686–689.

Mulder-De Jong, M. T., & Mulder, R. J. Drugs used in the treatment of tuberculosis and leprosy. In M. N. G. Dukes (Ed.), *Meyler's side effects of drugs.* Amsterdam: Excerpta Medica, 1975.

Muller, J. C., Pryor, W. W., Gibbons, J. E., & Orgain, E. S. Depression and anxiety occurring during Rauwolfia therapy. *Journal of the American Medical Association,* 1955, *159,* 836.

Murray, F. J. A pilot study of cycloserine toxicity. *American Review of Tuberculosis,* 1956, *74,* 196–209.

Nicholson, W. J. Disturbances of the special senses and other functions. *British Medical Journal,* 1974, *1,* 33–35.

Olsen, P. S., & Torning, K. Psychological side-effects during long term ambulatory chemotherapy with isoniazid and PAS. *Acta Tuberculosea Scandinavica,* 1959, *37,* 89–103.

Patterson, R. D., Freeman, L. C., & Butler, R. N. Psychiatric aspects of adaptation, survival and death. In S. Granick & R. D. Patterson (Eds.), *Human aging II.* Rockville: NIMH, 1974.

Payne, E. C. Teaching medical psychotherapy in special clinical settings. In N. E. Zinberg (Ed.), *Psychiatry and medical practice in a general hospital.* New York: International Universities Press, 1964.

Payne, E. C. Depression and suicide. In J. G. Howells (Ed.), *Modern perspectives in the psychiatry of old age.* New York: Brunner/Mazel, 1975.

Perlas, A. P., & Faillace, L. A. Psychiatric manifestations of carcinoma of the pancreas. *American Journal of Psychiatry,* 1964, *121,* 182.

Perlin, S., & Butler, R. N. Psychiatric aspects of adaptation to the aging experience. In J. E. Buren, R. N. Butler, S. W. Greenhouse, L. Sokolff, & M. R. Yarrow (Eds.), *Human aging I: A biological and behavioral study.* Rockville, NIMH, 1971.

Petersen, P. Psychiatric disorders in primary hyperparathyroidism. *Journal of Clinical Endocrinology,* 1968, *28,* 1491–1495.

Pfeiffer, E., & Busse, E. W. Affective Disorders. In E. W. Busse & E. Pfeiffer (Eds.), *Mental illness in later life.* Washington: American Psychiatric Association, 1973.

Post, F. *The significance of affective symptoms in old age.* London: Oxford University Press, 1962.

Post, F. *The clinical psychiatry of late life.* London: Pergamon Press, 1965.

Presthus, J., & Holmsen, R. Appraisal of long term levodopa treatment of parkinsonism with special reference to therapy limiting factors. *Acta Neurologica Scandinavica,* 1974, *50,* 774–790.

Prien, R. F., Haber, P. A., & Caffey, E. M. The use of psychoactive drugs in elderly patients with psychiatric disorders: Survey conducted in twelve Veterans Administration hospitals. *Journal of the American Geriatrics Society,* 1976, *23,* 104–112.

Pyle, M. M., Pfuetze, K. H., Barclary, W. R., & Kasik, S. E. Cycloserine in high dosage in "salvage cases" of pulmonary tuberculosis with control of toxicity by concomitant medication: Efficacy as medical and presurgical treatment. *Trans 18th conference on the chemotherapy of tuberculosis,* Washington, D.C.: U.S. Government Printing Office, 1959.

Raskind, M., & Eisdorfer, C. Psychopharmacology in the aged. In L. L. Simpson (Ed.), *Drug treatment of mental disorders.* New York: Raven Press, 1976.

Rice, D. Somatic syndromes causing depressive state. *Practitioner,* 1959, *183,* 49.

Rickles, N. K. Functional symptoms as first evidence of pancreatic disease. *Journal of Nervous and Mental Disorders,* 1945, *101,* 566–571.

Rifkin, A., Quitkin, F., & Klein, D. F. Akinesia: A poorly recognized drug-induced extrapyramidal behavioral disorder. *Archives of General Psychiatry,* 1975, *32,* 672–674.

Rossman, P. L. Organic diseases resembling functional disorders. *Hospital Medicine,* 1969, *5,* 72–76.

Salzman, C., Shader, R. I., & Pearlman, M. Psychopharmacology and the elderly. In R. I. Shader (Ed.), *Psychotropic drug side effects.* Baltimore: Williams & Wilkins, 1970.

Salzman, C., & Shader, R. I. Response to psychotropic drugs in the normal elderly. In C. Eisdorfer & W. E. Fann (Eds.), *Psychopharmacology and aging.* New York: Plenum Press, 1973.

Salzman, C., & Shader, R. I. Research considerations in geriatric psychopharmacology. *Journal of Geriatric Psychiatry,* 1974, *7,* 165–184.

Salzman, C., Shader, R. I., & Harmatz, J. S. Response of the elderly to psychotropic drugs: Predictable or idiosyncratic. In S. Gershon & A. Raskin (Eds.), *Genesis and treatment of psychologic disorders in the elderly.* New York: Raven Press, 1975.

Salzman, C., Shader, R. I., Harmatz, J., & Robertson, L. Psychopharmacologic investigations in elderly volunteers: Effect of diazepam in males. *Journal of the American Geriatrics Society,* 1975, *23,* 451–457.

Salzman, C., Shader, R. I., & van der Kolk, B. A. Psychopharmacology and the geriatric patient. In R. I. Shader (Ed.), *Manual of psychiatric therapeutics.* Boston: Little Brown, 1975.

Salzman, C., Shader, R. I., & van der Kolk, B. A. Clinical psychopharmacology and the elderly patient. *New York State Journal of Medicine,* 1976, *76,* 71–77.

Sanders, T. E., & Smith, M. E. Opthalmic aspects. In E. V. Cowdry & F. U. Steinberg (Eds.), *The care of the geriatric patient.* St. Louis: Mosby, 1971.

Schmidt, C. W. Psychiatric problems of the aged. *Journal of the American Geriatrics Society,* 1974, *22,* 355–359.

Schroeder, H. A. Nutrition. In E. V. Cowdry & F. U. Steinberg (Eds.), *The care of the geriatric patient.* St. Louis: Mosby, 1971.

Schwab, J. J. *Handbook of psychiatric consultation.* New York: Appleton-Century-Crofts, 1968.

Schwab, J. J. Psychiatric illness produced by infections. *Hospital Medicine,* October 1969.

Schwab, J. J., Bialow, M., Holzer, C. E., Brown, J. M., & Stevenson, B. E. Sociocultural aspects of depression in medical inpatients. *Archives of General Psychiatry,* 1967, *17,* 533.

Shader, R. I., & Greenblatt, D. J. Belladonna alkaloids and synthetic anticholinergics: Uses and toxicity. In R. I. Shader (Ed.), *Psychiatric complications of medical drugs.* New York: Raven Press, 1972.

Shader, R. I., & Greenblatt, D. J. The psychopharmacological treatment of anxiety states. In R. I. Shader (Ed.), *Manual of psychiatric therapeutics.* Boston: Little Brown, 1975.

Sieda, H., & Muller, H. F. Choreiform movements as side effects of phenothiazine medication in geriatric patients. *Journal of the American Geriatrics Society,* 1967, *15,* 517–522.

Simpson, F. O. Antihypertensive drug therapy. *Drugs,* 1973, *6,* 333.

Slaby, A. E., & Wyatt, R. J. *Dementia in the presenium.* Springfield, Ill.: Charles C Thomas, 1974.

Smith, C. K., Barish, J., Correa, J., & Williams, R. H. Psychiatric disturbance in endocrinologic disease. *Psychosomatic Medicine,* 1972, *34,* 69–86.

Soffer, A. The changing clinical picture of digitalis intoxication. *Archives of Internal Medicine,* 1959, *107,* 681–688.

Spillane, J. D. Nervous and mental disorders in Cushing's syndrome. *Brain,* 1951, *74,* 72–94.

Starr, A. M. Personality changes in Cushing's syndrome. *Journal of Clinical Endocrinology,* 1952, *12,* 502–505.

Starr, P. Endocrinologic disorders. In E. V. Cowdry & F. U. Steinberg (Eds.), *The care of the geriatric patient.* St. Louis: Mosby, 1971.

Strachan, R. W., & Henderson, J. G. Psychiatric syndromes due to avitaminosis B 12 with normal blood and marrow. *Quarterly Journal of Medicine,* 1965, *34,* 303–317.

Strassman, G. Unrecognized intracranial lesions in mentally sick patients over the age of 60. *Geriatrics,* 1957, *12,* 350–354.

Surridge, D. An investigation into some psychiatric aspects of multiple sclerosis. *British Journal of Psychiatry,* 1969, *115,* 749–764.

Sutherland, A. M. The psychological impact of postoperative cancer. *Bulletin of New York Academic Medicine,* 1957, *33,* 428–455.

Sutherland, A. M., Orbach, C. E., Dyk, R. B., & Bard, M. The psychological impact of cancer and cancer surgery I. Adaptation to the dry colostomy; preliminary report and summary of findings. *Cancer,* 1952, *5,* 857–872.

Tauber, S. A., Goodhart, R. S., Hsu, J. M., Blumberg, N., Kassab, J., & Chow, B. F. Vitamin B12 deficiency in the aged. *Geriatrics,* 1957, *12,* 368–374.

Tester-Dalderup, C. B. M. Hypotensive drugs. In M. N. G. Duke (Ed.), *Meyler's side effects of drugs* (Vol. 8). Amsterdam: Excerpta Medica, 1975.

Tester-Dalderup, C. B. M. Hypotensive drugs. In M. N. G. Duke (Ed.), *Side effects of drugs* (Annual 1). Amsterdam: Excerpta Medica, 1977.

Thomas, F. B., Mazzaferri, E. L., & Skillman, T. G. Apathetic thyrotoxicosis: A distinctive clinical and laboratory entity. *Annals of Internal Medicine,* 1970, *72,* 679–685.

Thorn, G. W. Addison's disease. In R. L. Cecil & R. F. Loeb (Eds.), *Textbook of medicine.* Philadelphia: Saunders, 1955.

Tracy, M., & Shader, R. I. Drug use patterns among the elderly. *Psychopharmacology Bulletin,* 1974, *10,* 14–17.

Trethoven, W. H., & Cobb, S. Neuropsychiatric aspects of Cushing's syndrome. *American Medical Association Archives of Neurology and Psychiatry,* 1952, *67,* 283–309.

Verwoerdt, A. Emotional responses to physical illness. In C. Eisdorfer & W. E. Fann (Eds.), *Psychopharmacology and aging.* New York: Plenum Press, 1973.

Verwoerdt, A. *Clinical geropsychiatry.* Baltimore: Williams & Wilkins, 1976.

Waal, H. J. Propranolol-induced depression. *British Medical Journal,* 1967, *2,* 50.

Wagshul, A. M., & Daroff, R. B. Depression during L-DOPA treatment. *Lancet,* 1969, *2,* 592.

Walker, S., III. *Psychiatric signs and symptoms due to medical problems.* Springfield, Ill.: Charles C Thomas, 1967.

Wallach, M. G., & Gershon, S. Psychiatric sequelae to tuberculosis chemotherapy. In R. I. Shader (Ed.), *Psychiatric complications of medical drugs.* New York: Raven Press, 1972.

Wang, H. S., & Busse, E. W. Dementia in old age. In C. E. Wells (Ed.), *Dementia.* Philadelphia: Davis, 1971.

Warburton, J. W. Depressive symptoms in patients referred for thalamotomy. *Journal of Neurology, Neurosurgery and Psychiatry,* 1967, *30,* 368–370.

Weiss, H. D., Walker, M. D., & Wiernik, P. H. Neurotoxicity of commonly used antineoplastic agents. *New England Journal of Medicine,* 1975, *291,* 75–81.

Weiss, S. The effects of the digitalis bodies on the nervous system: An analysis of the mechanism of cardiac slowing, nausea, vomiting, psychosis, and visual disturbances following digitalis therapy. *Medical Clinics of North America,* 1929, *15,* 963–982.

White, P. D. Cardiovascular disorders. In E. V. Cowdry & F. U. Steinberg (Eds.), *The care of the geriatric patient.* St. Louis: Mosby, 1971.

Williamson, J. Depression. In W. F. Anderson & T. G. Judge (Eds.), *Geriatric medicine.* London: Academic Press, 1974.

Wilson, S. A. K. *Neurology.* Baltimore: Williams & Wilkins, 1940.

Wilson, S. A. K., & Bruce, A. N. *Neurology* (2nd ed.). Baltimore: Williams & Wilkins, 1955.

Winkelman, A. C., & DiPalma, J. R. Drug treatment of parkinsonism. *Seminars in Drug Treatment,* 1971, *1,* 10.

Wise, T. N. Pitfalls of diagnosing depression in chronic renal disease. *Psychosomatics,* 1974, *15,* 83–84.

Zborowski, M. Cultural components in responses to pain. *Journal of Social Issues,* 1952, *8,* 16–30.

Zetzel, E. R. Dynamics of the metapsychology of the aging process. In M. A. Berezin & S. H. Cath (Eds.), *Geriatric psychiatry: Grief, loss, and emotional disorders in the aging process.* New York: International Universities Press, 1965.

Zinberg, N. E., & Kaufman, I. Cultural and personality factors associated with aging: An introduction. In N. E. Zinberg & I. Kaufman (Eds.), *Normal psychology of the aging process.* New York: International Universities Press, 1963.

4

The Role of Electroencephalographic Techniques in the Assessment of Life-span Changes and Response to Drugs

Henry J. Michalewski
Larry W. Thompson
Julie V. Patterson
University of Southern California

Electrophysiological recordings of the kind represented by the electroencephalogram (EEG) can provide unique information about brain and behavior relationships, especially as they might be applied to assessment situations and the evaluation and treatment of senile and geriatric patients. Although EEGs are routinely performed in clinical and research settings, there has been some lag in developing neurological and psychological tests based on the electroencephalogram, or derivatives of the EEG such as evoked responses or slow potentials. Tests are expected to develop rapidly, however, as the general availability of special purpose computers increases and refined analysis procedures are developed. It is neither expected nor desirable to have EEG measures supplant other proven assessment techniques, but EEG techniques may well supplement and expand the usefulness of existing methods. It is not always practical or reasonable to subject persons to a battery of EEG tests when other assessment means are entirely adequate or more appropriate. Yet the EEG should prove useful in the development of new assessment procedures, especially those involved in sensory processes, attention, and perception, or in the evaluation of pharmacological agents on nervous system functions.

The development of any test based on measures of the EEG, with the precision and sensitivity required in applied situations, demands a thorough understanding of the phenomenon in question, its effects over the life span, and its relation to disease conditions. For the most part, our consideration here is limited to EEG activity and related events, but other electrophysiological measures may serve a similar role in assessment procedures (Reitan, 1976; Thompson & Marsh, 1973).

Even a cursory look through the recent EEG literature reveals a bewildering array of studies ranging in design and aims from very simple to very complicated. With this diversity in mind, selected studies that are representative and suggestive of many topic areas have been chosen for this chapter and should be of interest to those who wish to know more about EEG measures or wish to incorporate EEG measurements into their assessment procedures. Topic areas include ongoing EEG, localized disturbances, EEG blocking, reactive EEG, evoked potentials, slow waves, clinical application of event-related potentials, and the pharmacological effects of antidepressants on the EEG. References detailing specific information on topic areas are cited for those who wish to pursue particular interest points.

BRAIN WAVE ACTIVITY IN THE ELDERLY

The most common brain wave recorded from a resting but attentive adult is the well-known alpha rhythm. This highly synchronous rhythm has a frequency range between 8 and 13 cycles per second (cps) and is most prominently found over occipital and parietal regions of the scalp. Other forms of brain wave activity include theta waves (4–7 cps), delta waves (approximately .5–3.5 cps), and beta waves (13 cps and above). Other electrical activity may be distinguished on the basis of both amplitude and frequency and includes synchronous or asynchronous discharges, lateralized or asymmetrical differences between the cerebral hemispheres, focal discharges, abnormal slow wave complexes, phase shifts, periods of electrical silence, and direct current electrical potentials. The origins of these potentials are attributed to graded dendritic responses that are slow and sensitive to different intensities of input (Glaser, 1963; Metcalf, 1975). The generators of these rhythms are part of a complicated cortical network that is dependent upon a critical metabolic milieu for proper functioning and that is particularly sensitive to the actions of psychoactive and pharmacological agents (Fink, 1963). Several excellent texts are available that describe common electroencephalographic techniques and procedures and discuss in detail the application of these techniques in clinical settings (Cooper, Osselton, & Shaw, 1969; Kiloh, McComas, & Osselton, 1972; Kooi, 1971).

Alpha Slowing

A consistent feature in the brain wave patterns of the elderly is the slowing of the resting alpha frequency (Obrist, 1976). A normal young adult may display a mean alpha frequency in the range between 10.2 and 10.5 cps (Lindsley, 1938), whereas older subjects (over 60) show a frequency decline to levels around 9.0–9.7 cps (Obrist & Busse, 1965). This pattern of slowing in the alpha rate with age has been observed in a hospital population by Friedlander (1958). The pattern appears to occur quite slowly over the adult life span. Older males tend to have lower mean alpha frequencies than age-matched females (Mundy-Castle, 1962). The exact cause of alpha slowing in the elderly is not known, although vascular disorders (Obrist, 1963, 1964) and brain metabolism (Thompson, 1976) have been implicated. There are instances, however, (Liberson and Seguin, 1945, for example) where a substantial proportion of arteriosclerotic and senile patients tested did not show any appreciable disturbance in the EEG even though abnormalities might be expected.

Focal Disturbances

Another common disturbance in the electroencephalogram of the aged is the appearance of focal abnormalities over the temporal regions (Harvald, 1958). In a study of elderly community volunteers, Busse, Barnes, Silverman, Shy, Thaler, and Frost (1954) have found that a high percentage of the volunteers displayed focal disturbances (slowing, 3-5 cps) in temporal areas, especially left anterior temporal areas, in the resting EEG. Specific intellectual deficits have not been linked to these temporal lobe disturbances, and their origin is most likely the result of impaired cerebral circulation (Busse & Obrist, 1963). In healthy aged subjects there is generally no relation between measures of intellectual functioning and the EEG (Busse, Barnes, Friedman, & Kelty, 1956).

Patients suffering from severe dementia often display bursts of EEG activity that are different in either frequency or amplitude from the dominant rhythm in the electroencephalogram (Frey & Sjögren, 1959). Electroencephalographic abnormalities, defined in terms of rhythms slower than 8 cps or frequencies above 13 cps, have been related by Greenblatt (1944) to a U-shaped function in which irregularities in the EEG are greater at extreme ages (under 15 years and over 55 years) than in early- and mid-adult ranges (15 to 55 years).

EEG Blocking and Timing Functions

A troublesome aspect in analyzing resting EEG records is the fact that patients with obvious behavioral, physiological, or anatomical impairments often display normal brain rhythm patterns. In 1944 W. T. Liberson introduced the concept of functional electroencephalography into the examination of resting EEG recordings. The technique involved applying sensory stimulation so that changes in the activity or responsiveness of the ongoing EEG would become visible. Since that time a number of experimental procedures have been employed to activate the ongoing EEG so that latent abnormalities might be observed. Clinical techniques commonly include hyperventilation, sleep, photic stimulation, tapping noises, and the administration of drugs (Wells, 1963).

An early discovery was that the desynchronization or blocking of rhythmic alpha activity occurs in response to light. This pattern of desynchronization is interpreted as a sign of cortical arousal or mobilization and has been shown to be most likely dependent upon the brainstem reticular activating system (Lindsley, 1956; Lindsley, Schreiner, Knowles, & Magoun, 1950; Moruzzi & Magoun, 1949). Decreased cortical reactivity in older individuals may signal the onset of senescent changes in the brain. Obrist (1965) has presented evidence that habituation to repeated stimulus flashes is significantly less for older persons, meaning less cortical reactivity in terms of alpha blocking, than for a younger comparison group. On the basis of alpha reactivity (blocking) measures, Liberson (1944) has found more alpha attenuation in patients suffering functional psychosis (depression, anxiety) than in schizophrenic patients or in patients with arteriosclerosis. Elderly female psychiatric patients (mean age = 68.3 years) display less alpha desynchronization than an age-matched sample of male psychiatric patients (Andermann & Stoller, 1961).

In a series of experiments, Surwillo (1963a; 1963b) hypothesized that the ongoing fluctuations of the EEG represent a basic timing mechanism of the central nervous system. The EEG cycle was thought of as the fundamental unit of time by which events were programmed by the nervous system. Behavioral measures, such as the speed of reaction time, were functions of the time or number of brain wave cycles needed to execute a particular response. Using subjects between the ages of 29 and 99, Surwillo found a significant relation ($r = .72$) between reaction time and the average period (frequency = 1/period) of the EEG. Age did not significantly enter into this relation; however, a significant relation between age and period of brain wave was found. It was further demonstrated that reaction time variability could be accounted for by differences in the brain wave period. More complicated response situations demonstrated that longer decision times were related to slower brain waves and, conversely, that shorter decision times were associated with faster brain wave patterns (Surwillo, 1964a). Experimental manipulation of an individual's brain rhythm to speed of response was also suggested by the data presented by Surwillo (1964b). Overall, the results were interpeted as a demonstration that response slowing with age could be accounted for by brain wave frequency.

Thompson and Wilson (1966) conducted a study to investigate changes in the EEG frequency spectrum in elderly persons during photic stimulation and performance on a learning task. The 15 male subjects tested ranged in age from 63 to 85. The subjects were divided into subgroups of good and poor learners depending upon their performance on a paired-associates list. Except for learning ability, the subjects formed a homogeneous group with respect to health, socioeconomic status, intellectual level, and occupational classification. During a rest control condition, the data indicated a general, though not statistically significant, shift to the slower EEG frequencies for the poor learners compared to good learners. The peak frequencies were 9 cps and 10 cps respectively for the poor and good learners. Good learners also tended to have more frequencies above 14 cps than poor learners. Generally, the number of beta waves (> 12 cps) increased as the result of stimulation, while the number of alpha waves (8–12 cps) decreased for both groups. Good learners, however, had significantly more beta activity during "eyes open" and photic stimulation conditions than did poor learners. In terms of alpha activity, there were no signficant differences between good and poor learners during any of the experimental conditions. Although not statistically significant, more slow waves (< 8 cps) were recorded for the poor learner group than for the good learner group for all conditions. On the average, good learners appeared more cortically alert and were more reactive to sensory input than were poor learners. Thompson and Botwinick (1968) explored the manner in which an EEG activation pattern might relate both to reaction time and to conditions of mental set or expectancy by testing the experimental manipulation of a warning signal and various preparatory interval durations. The subjects tested included a group of elderly persons (62–87 years of age) and a group of young adults (19–35 years of age). Subject criteria also included the presence of measurable amounts of alpha activity in parieto-occipital locations as observed in EEG records. Each reaction time trial was initiated by the subject. Approximately 2 seconds after a key switch was pressed, a warning tone of .5-second duration (400 cps) was presented. The end of the preparatory interval was marked by the onset of another tone (1000 cps), which was terminated by a finger lift response. In both a regular and an irregular series presentation, the interval durations used were .5, 3.0, 6.0, and 15.0 seconds. Electroencephalographic recordings were simultaneously collected during behavioral testing. The findings indicated that while the two age groups did not differ with respect to an overall activation pattern (desynchronization, EEG amplitude change), they did differ in relation to preparatory interval. For both age groups, the greatest change in the EEG occurred during the .5-second preparatory duration in the regular series. In the irregular presentation, however, older subjects displayed the maximum EEG alteration with the shortest preparatory interval (.5 second), whereas for the younger subjects the minimum EEG change occurred with this interval. In terms of reaction times, older subjects were significantly slower than younger subjects, yet preparatory duration did not produce a differential effect for the two age groups. To the extent that desynchronization can be considered a nervous system sign of arousal, the evidence suggested that activation patterns based on preparatory set were different for the young and the old.

Reactive Measures in the EEG

Wells (1962) investigated alpha rhythm blocking in normal subjects and in patients with documented central nervous system disorders. The cerebral response that interested Wells was based on the fact that a tone can block alpha activity when conditionally paired with a bright flash of light. In order to investigate which anatomical structures might be implicated in conditioned alpha blockade, Wells designed his study so that he could observe the conditioning process in neurologically normal subjects and patients with a variety of disease entities, e.g., intracranial neoplasms, cerebral vascular diseases, and seizure disorders. (Many of the patients tested showed no evidence of structural disorders such as lesions.) Conditioning trials consisted of a tone followed approximately 1 second later by a long flash. Individual conditioned cerebral responses were defined as a substantial reduction in the alpha rhythm scored from EEG tracings after the tone presentation but before the occurrence of the flash.

Results from scalp records showed that the mean number of alpha blockades for 50 presentations of the tone-flash pair was 10.2 for normals and 6.1 for patients. Overall, patients with brainstem and hemispheric disorders produced significantly fewer conditioned alpha block responses than the normal subjects. In the patient group, alpha responsiveness (blockade) did not appear to be related to either the locus or size of the lesion. When the effects of single flashes (without stimulus pairing) were analyzed, normal controls demonstrated much more attenuation effects than the patient group. Further analysis showed a close relation between alpha reduction to single photic stimulation presented intermittently and contingent alpha blockade. A final subexperiment by Wells considered habituation effects of alpha blockade in normals and patients. (Habituation in this context refers to the diminishing response of alpha blocking over repetitive presentations of photic stimulation.) Responses to 100 flash presentations showed greater habituation effects in the impaired patient group than in the normal group. Although the overall results of these experiments were striking, Wells believed that as tests they had limited value in a clinical setting. Problems in scoring records and in determining blockade and the fact that only subjects with well-defined alpha patterns could be tested were some of the restrictions noted by Wells. Temporary cerebral connections of the kind illustrated by conditioned or contingent alpha blocking were studied earlier by Wells and Wolff (1960). In an experimental situation similar to later studies, groups of normals and brain-damaged patients were tested for alpha suppression to tone-flash presentations. Compared to normal subjects, patients with varying degrees of organic damage showed fewer numbers of suppressed alpha responses. Further, when blocks of paired stimulus presentations were analyzed, the brain-damaged subjects displayed less capacity for alpha attenuation, as trial pairings were repeated, than did normal subjects. Follow-up testings on patients who had undergone successful surgery for removal of neoplasms and arterial abnormalities showed no relation of the size and locus of the lesion to the number of contingent alpha blockings.

Using evocative techniques similar to Wells, Blum (1957) compared the responsiveness of the electroencephalogram of schizophrenics to the abnormal responsiveness of brain-damaged patients. One group of normal subjects, two schizophrenic groups, and one brain-damaged group were tested. (Brain-damaged patients were older than either normals or schizophrenics.) A complicated stimulation schedule was followed, which yielded measures of alpha responsiveness to visual and auditory stimulation and to synchronous photic driving. Brain wave responsiveness was scored visually from EEG tracings. Records of resting alpha activity showed no differences among the groups tested. In the test situations, normals demonstrated more alpha responsiveness (blocking or driving) than either the schizophrenic or brain-damaged groups. No significant differences were observed between the schizophrenic and brain-damaged groups. Blum concluded that the lack of cortical responsiveness found in schizophrenics was similar to the lack of responsiveness in patients with organic brain impairment.

Visser (1961) investigated the relation of contingent alpha responses (suppression) to certain characteristics of the background electroencephalogram. The subjects examined included psychiatric and epileptic patients, as well as a group of normal subjects, ranging in age from 15 to 64 years. The subjects were placed in a dark, quiet room and were exposed to a 4-second tone (contingent stimulus) and rapid flashes of light (uncontingent stimulus) presented during the final 2 seconds of the tone. Alpha scalp rhythms were recorded from parieto-occipital locations (P_3-0_1, P_4-0_2). Three separate phases of the contingent reaction were studied: (1) habituation, presentation of the tone alone (10 trials); (2) formation of the contingent response, pairing of tone and flash (20 trials); and (3) extinction, tone alone (10 trials). Most subjects demonstrated an initial alpha reaction to the tone in the first few trials that diminished greatly by the fifth trial and was almost nonexistent on the tenth trial. Development of the contingent cerebral response (tone-flash pairings) took place rapidly and reached a peak by the third trial. Responses declined and fluctuated slightly for the remaining trials. In the extinction phase, the contingent response was reduced by the fifth trial and disappeared by the tenth trial. No relationship was found between background electrical activity and estimated strength of the contingent response. However, a high alpha frequency was positively related to the strength or intensity of the contingent alpha response, whereas the actual quantity of alpha activity present in the ongoing electroencephalogram was negatively related to the responsiveness in associating tone-flash pairings.

For the most part, these early studies were based on data derived from manual scoring of the raw EEG tracings. Since these studies were conducted, significant advances in computer technology have made it possible to quantify large amounts of data and to apply special procedures for the analysis and detection of small signals. The previous experiments should, therefore, be repeated. In most of the studies on conditioned alpha blocking, a fixed interval between the contingent and uncontingent stimuli was used as an optimal time for all the subjects tested. Looked at another way, this procedure alone may have contributed to a loss of information in the EEG in that the different diagnostic groups tested, especially the senile and brain-damaged populations, may be expected to have had differential rates of conditioning dependent upon the integrity of the functioning cortical system. The assumed temporary connections formed by the process of this simple conditioning may well serve as an index to an individual's interaction with the environment and serve as a nonverbal exploration of the relation among different regions of the brain and sensory modalities.

SCALP RECORDED EVOKED POTENTIALS

Evoked responses are extracted from the background EEG in the time domain by special purpose signal averagers or by using digital computer techniques. Averaging procedures assume that the neural signal of interest is time locked in repetitive stimulus presentations while ongoing background activity is not. Scalp recordings used to gather responses to brief stimulus presentations result in an average waveform composed of several components of both positive and negative deflections. A 10-microsecond flash can produce a brain response that lasts from 250 to 300 milliseconds or longer. The initial components between 30 and 70 milliseconds are usually attributed to basic perceptual mechanisms while later components extending to 300 milliseconds and beyond are most likely related to higher integrative processes (Kooi, Guvener, & Bagchi, 1965). Characteristic waveform and latency of components are associated with average responses of different sensory modalities.

When averaging procedures are applied to the electroencephalogram in response to distinct sensory stimulation, a complex waveform emerges that seems to reflect both input conduction from receptors and integrative activity attributed to higher cortical centers. A great deal of attention has been devoted to the careful examination of brain responses to simple flashes of light (Cigànek, 1975), auditory stimulation (Storm van Leeuween, 1975), and somatosensory systems (Halliday, 1975). Several texts exist in the field of evoked responses that cover techniques, measurement methods, significance, and application (for example, Callaway, 1975; Desmedt, 1977; Donchin & Lindsley, 1969; Perry & Childers, 1969; Regan, 1972; Shagass, 1972; Thompson & Patterson, 1973–1974).

While the initial components of the evoked response are sensitive to stimulus parameters such as brightness or frequency, later components are affected by factors such as the experimental situation, subject states that include alertness and attention, and pathology. The evoked response technique is especially attractive as a diagnostic tool since averages are typically based on relatively short time intervals and, hence, are more manageable in terms of quantification; additionally, evoked potentials are reactive measures in the sense that stimulation sequences can be carefully controlled in order to evaluate nervous system reactions. The general use of digital computers and averager-computer configurations should ease earlier technical difficulties in gathering evoked responses and should allow the full development of these procedures in clinical settings.

Before proceeding to a consideration of the aging and clinical usefulness of the evoked response, some general factors known to influence cortical responses should be discussed. For this purpose, several representative experiments dealing with visual, auditory, and somatosensory responses are briefly covered.

Factors Affecting the Evoked Response

Garcia-Austt, Bogacz, and Vanzulli (1964) monitored visual evoked responses (VERs) from the scalp during experimental sessions of forced attention and during sessions with interfering stimulation. Distraction stimuli consisted either of tones or clicks at 70 dB. Results indicated that the VER waveform during sessions of focused attention had an increased number of components visible, i.e., P_1N_1, P_2N_2, P_3N_3, etc. When the subject simply counted the single flashes during stimulation, an increase in the size of the VER was observed, particularly for the later components. Distracting stimuli produced an overall decrease in the amplitude of the VER.

Satterfield (1965) conducted a study to determine the effects of attention on evoked cortical responses. Subjects were instructed to attend to either click or shock stimuli during the alternate presentation of clicks and shocks. Results indicated that averaged cortical activity was increased for the stimulus attended, whereas cortical activity for unattended stimuli was suppressed. Using three different vigilance tasks, Spong, Haider, and Lindsley (1965) recorded visual and auditory evoked responses from occipital and temporal regions of the scalp. The experimental conditions included (a) attending to a brightness change, (b) a key-pressing task, and (c) a counting task. The stimuli were simple flashes and clicks alternately presented. In the brightness and key-pressing tasks, VERs in the occipital area were larger for flashes than for clicks. However, subjects who attended clicks showed larger auditory evoked responses (AERs) in the temporal region than subjects who attended flashes. In the counting task no similar trends in evoked responses were observed. It was suggested that counting may be distracting and damaging to the attentive state. Generally, the results indicated that perceptual discriminations that demanded close subject attention were paralleled by a corresponding change in cortical activity.

In considering the information content that can be delivered by simple stimuli, Sutton, Tueting, and Zubin (1967) reported on the significance of a large positive process in evoked potentials that occurred approximately 300 milliseconds after stimulus presentation. When a subject was required to make a response to a stimulus that resolved some uncertainty, this late component, or P_{300} wave, was generally of larger amplitude than when the response did not resolve any uncertainty, e.g., when the subject had prior knowledge of the forthcoming stimulus. In the latter situation of subject certainty, the stimulus only served to mark the time of its occurrence; in the former situation, however, the uncertain stimulus provided information, albeit simple, in addition to the time of its occurrence. Further, it was found that the P_{300} component was larger when the information carrying stimulus was delivered externally than when the information was conveyed by the absence of an external event.

John, Herrington, and Sutton (1967) demonstrated that VER waveforms are not only determined by simple receptor stimulation but are also affected by the perceptual context of the stimulus. Their data were based on monopolar scalp recordings from a location on the midline 3 cm above the inion, the most prominent point of the external occipital protuberance. Four pairs of stimuli were compared: (1) a blank field versus a field containing some geometric shape, (2) one geometric shape versus a different shape of equal area, (3) two figures of the same shape but different areas, and (4) the words *circle* and *square* (equated for letter areas). The VERs to blank fields and geometric shapes were different, as were the VERs for dissimilar shapes of equal area. Figures of identical shape but unequal areas, however, produced VERs that were very similar to each other. The VER results for different words indicated dissimilar waveforms.

In a continuous vigilance task, subjects normally attend to all the stimuli that are presented (Ritter & Vaughan, 1969). Evoked responses that are recorded during a continuous vigilance situation, therefore, may not always register changes in subject attention. However, small stimulus changes randomly embedded in a series of repetitive stimuli evoked a prominent positive component (P_{300}) in the average response. The appearance of this late component is considered the result of attentional shifts or orienting responses. Ritter and Vaughan (1969) used both visual and auditory stimulation in their investigation of attention and evoked response activity. In the visual portion, repetitive flashes, 1 every 3 seconds, were presented. Randomly interspersed among the regular flashes were signal flashes of slightly dimmer intensity. The subject pressed a key whenever a signal flash was detected. In the auditory portion, tone bursts of a standard level, 40 dB, were presented; embedded among the regular tones was a signal tone at 35 dB. Again, a pressed key indicated detection of the signal. Averaged responses from scalp recordings disclosed that the vertex and occipital sites exhibited a late positive component (latencies ranged from 300 to 500 milliseconds) to the detected signals. Averages for nonsignals or detected signals did not display this late component. As soon as the discrimination was made more difficult, a late component was found for both the signal and the standard stimuli. Making the discrimination easy resulted in the disappearance of the late components for both signal and standard stimuli. This demonstrated that the late component in the different vigilance tasks was most likely dependent on central processing mechanisms for assessing the cognitive significance of the stimulus.

Given that adequate control can be gained over attentive subject states, other factors can influence the average cortical response. For example, the visual evoked response is sensitive to the sites of retinal stimulation (Eason, Groves, White, & Oden, 1967; Eason & White, 1967), intensity, and wavelength (Eason, Oden, & White, 1967). Target structure also affects the VER as shown by Lehmann and Fender (1967) who presented a flashing blank field stimulus to the right eye while the left eye observed fields of differing complexity (e.g., a dot, a cross, and a grid). Averaged records indicated that the amplitude of the VER was reduced as field structure in the contralateral eye was increased. Asymmetries in the evoked response related to language functions have also been demonstrated (Buchsbaum & Fedio, 1970; Matsumiya, Tagliasco, Lombroso, & Goodglass, 1972; McAdam & Whitaker, 1971; Wood, Goff, & Day, 1971). However, clear asymmetries in the evoked response related to verbal processing have not been demonstrated consistently (Friedman, Simson, Ritter, & Rapin, 1975; Galambos, Benson, Smith, Schulman-Galambos, & Osier, 1975).

Velasco and Velasco (1972) investigated the psychological significance of stimuli and the amplitude of the average somatic evoked response (SER). The stimuli consisted of threshold levels of shock delivered to the left median nerve. Scalp recordings were collected from right somatosensory areas and the vertex. The significance of the stimulus was manipulated by instructing subjects (a) to ignore the stimulus, (b) to press a key after each stimulus, or (c) to attend to another extraneous stimulus and ignore the shock stimulus. Results for the SER amplitudes indicated that the early components of the SER remained the same during the three experimental conditions. The late components of the SER, however, were at a maximum during attention and were at a minimum during distraction.

Evoked Response Correlates of Aging and Disease Processes

In contrast to auditory and somatosensory responses, the most notable changes related to maturation and aging are found in the VER (Beck, Dustman, & Schenkenberg, 1975). The amplitude of the VER increases from infancy to 5-8 years of age, declines slightly at approximately 13-14 years of age, stabilizes at 15 or 16 years, and apparently declines in amplitude until age 40 (Beck & Dustman, 1975). There are further decreases in the VER in later life to senescence, but at a much reduced rate. The primary changes in the VER occur in the later components (after 250 milliseconds) as can be seen from the overlaid averages in Figure 1, and the representative VERs from different ages in Figure 2. Several extracerebral events that might influence VER amplitudes in later years have been eliminated as possible sources of the attenuated response (e.g., refractive properties of the lens, slower pupillary responses, and differences in skull thickness) (Dustman & Beck, 1969). In

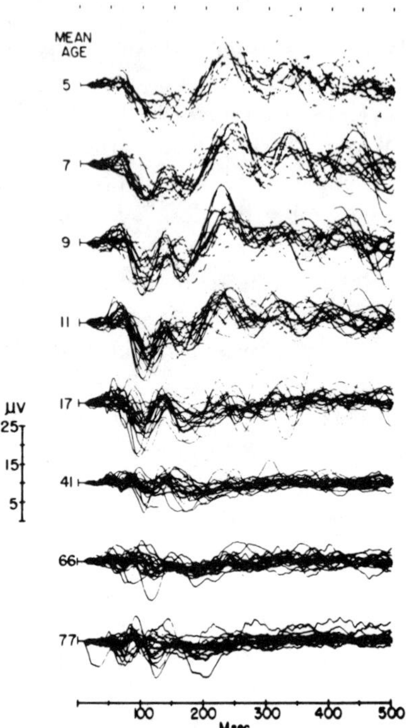

FIGURE 1 Age-related changes in the normal visual evoked response from groups of individuals ranging in age from 4 to 86 years (from Beck et al., 1975).

geriatric patients marked differences appear in the amplitude, number of components, and latency of deflections in the evoked response (Beck et al., 1975). There is also some recent evidence to suggest that the defective cognitive processes associated with the senile individuals may also be reflected in coordination differences between the cerebral hemispheres as detected by measures of evoked response characteristics (Gerson, John, Bartlett, & Koenig, 1976).

Another feature that many times accompanies photic stimulation is the appearance of an afterdischarge in the alpha frequency range (8–13 cps) over occipital sites. The discharge begins after the later components of the evoked response and may persist for several hundred milliseconds. Beck et al. (1975) have reported that the afterdischarge declines after 9 years of age and steadily decreases to senescence. Examples from our own laboratory are shown in Figures 3 and 4. The existence of the afterdischarge is quite apparent for the younger individual while it is absent in the older subject. Trials with two or three repetitive flashes separated by 200-millisecond intervals do not appear to

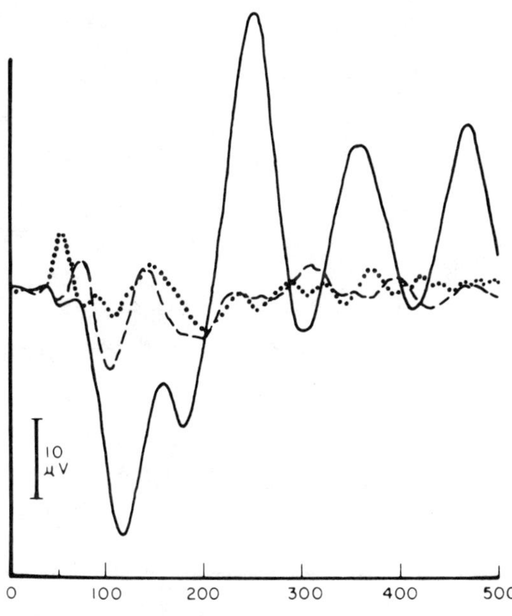

FIGURE 2 The visual evoked response of three separate subjects of different ages: —— = 6; - - - = 16; • • • = 60. (From Dustman and Beck, 1966. Copyright 1966 by the American Association for the Advancement of Science.)

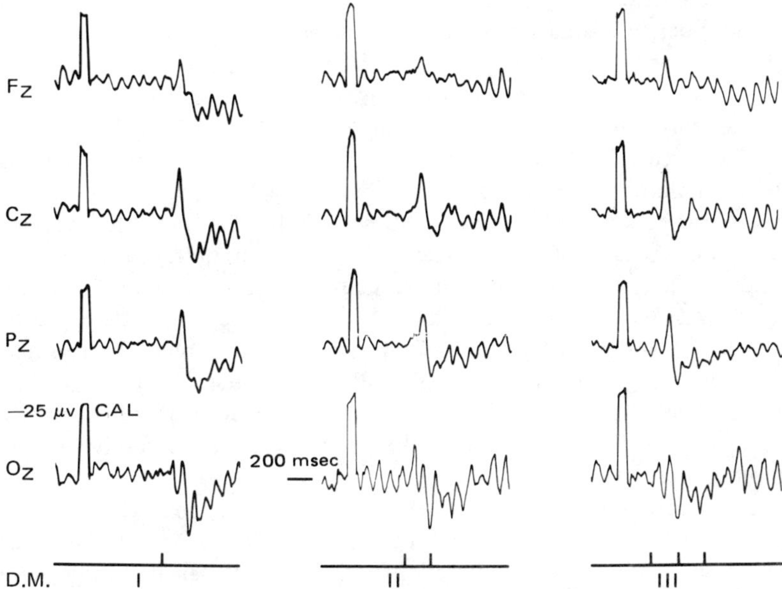

FIGURE 3 Visual evoked responses of subject D.M. (18 years of age).

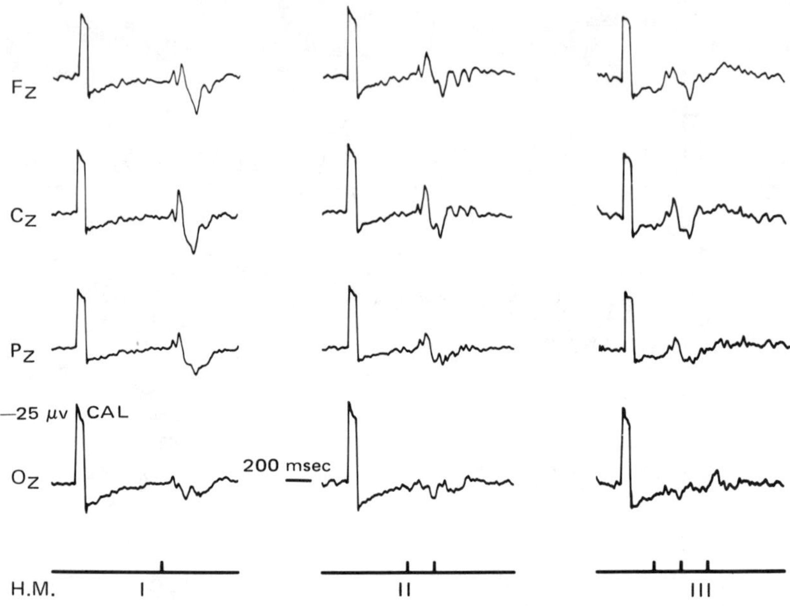

FIGURE 4 Visual evoked responses of subject H.M. (65 years of age).

change or enhance the afterdischarge effect in either the younger or older subjects. (Repetitive presentations were not synchronized with ongoing EEG.) The change in the appearance of the afterdischarge may reflect subtle alterations in the underlying neural substrate and should be explored more thoroughly in older individuals and selected clinical patients.

A technique used in testing younger subjects but that has not received much attention in aging research deals with the cortical integration of compound sensory stimulation. For example, Shipley (1970) has sought evoked response correlates of mental deficiency in retarded children using bimodal stimulation procedures. It was hypothesized that some of the differences observed in intellectual abilities may be the result of varying efficiency in the recognition and perceptual integration of sensory information. By presenting two stimuli simultaneously in two different sensory modalities, it was hypothesized that changes in the evoked response could be related to nervous system interactions. Scalp averages were recorded to single flashes of light, single auditory clicks, and simultaneous flash and click presentations. The results indicated that compared to normals, intellectually retarded subjects had bimodal responses that were less than the combined sum of the unimodal responses.

In an investigation of the somatosensory evoked response (SER) using subjects between the ages of 19 and 69, Lüders (1970) found that SER amplitudes described a U-shaped function with age. Smaller responses were recorded for the 30–45 year age group than for earlier or later age levels.

Similar findings in the SER were reported earlier by Shagass and Schwartz (1965).

Liberson (1966) examined cortical potentials in patients who suffered thrombosis of the left middle cerebral artery. For the patients studied the resulting right hemiplegia was also accompanied by aphasia. The results of somatic responses to median nerve stimulation were related to the degree of speech impairment. Patients with slight verbal impairment showed smaller responses over the ipsilateral hemisphere whether stimulated from the left or right sides. In a patient with severe aphasia, right median stimulation indicated that essentially no response was recorded from either hemisphere, whereas left side stimulation showed little or no ipsilateral response but a contralateral wave was evident.

Visser, Stam, Van Tilburg, OpDen Velde, Blom, and DeRijke (1976) studied the visual evoked response in groups of senile and presenile (Alzheimer type) dementia patients. The age range of the patients tested was 52-88 years. Common clinical features included disorientation, memory disturbances, intellectual deterioration, and language deficits. Scalp potentials were collected from left and right parieto-occipital derivations, and left and right occipital leads referred to an average potential reference. Photic stimulation was delivered to the patients at irregular intervals in an eyes closed condition. Generally six waves (I-VI) in the average evoked response were identified. Latency and amplitude measures were collected from the different peaks. When compared to normal subjects, the results indicated that senile and presenile patients had longer latencies for all peaks except for an early component (I) around 70 milliseconds. Amplitude measures revealed some increases in later peaks (III and VI). These results are comparable with the few studies conducted in this area of research. Early components of the visual evoked response may be altered by disease processes such as multiple sclerosis and affect the overall recognizability of the VER, especially in the later components (Feinsod & Hoyt, 1975).

Several investigators have pointed out the potential usefulness of recording cortical evoked responses in patients with unilateral lesions due to cerebrovascular disorders and brainstem lesions (Halliday, 1967; Nöel & Desmedt, 1975; Tsumoto, Hirose, Nonaka, & Takahashi, 1973; Williamson, Goff, & Allison, 1970). Diagnostically interesting changes in the visual evoked response have also been observed in the later stages of Jakob-Creutzfeldt disease (Lee & Blair, 1973). Processes that alter the normal conduction of electrical responses have drastic effects on the size and waveform of the averaged response. With more data regarding the effects of different disease processes, from onset to recovery, many tests based on averaged responses should be possible. Additionally, evoked potentials have encompassed studies of twins, handedness, effects of Down's syndrome, effects of alcohol, and epileptic disturbances (Beck, Dustman, & Lewis, 1976). Consideration should also be given to the fact that many older patients are under different regimens of medication that can have a variety of effects on the evoked response and can affect the overall interpretation of changes in response patterns (Borbèly, 1973; Robinson & Sabat, 1975; Skinner & Shimota, 1975).

Brainstem Evoked Potentials

Another category of electrical response that is receiving wide attention by investigators in audition are the Jewett waves or brainstem potentials (Jewett, 1970; Jewett, Romano, & Williston, 1970; Jewett & Williston, 1971). These are a series of submicrovolt deflections occurring within the first 2–12 milliseconds of an auditory response to brief acoustic stimulation (Davis, 1976). Usually the responses to 1000 or 2000 stimuli are collected in order to form an average. However, excessive experimental time is not involved since stimulus rates vary from 1 to 10 presentations per second. When recorded from remote sites such as the vertex, these very early potentials are thought to reflect far-field responses from the auditory pathways and brainstem (Starr & Achor, 1976). Considerable effort is being made in the clinical application of these techniques in diagnostic audiometry for assessing hearing loss (Ruben, Elberling, & Salomon, 1976). Starr and Hamilton (1976) have been able to associate abnormalities, i.e., specific components, in the average brainstem potential with various pathologies of the brainstem network. These potentials appear useful for diagnostic purposes in patients with neurological diseases affecting the auditory system and the related pathways to the cortex.

Habituation Effects in the Elderly

In our own studies of the normal auditory evoked potential, we have been interested in comparing young and old subjects on features of orientation, specifically habituation and dishabituation (Brent, Smith, Thompson, & Michalewski, 1977). The experimental sessions we have used consist of 15 blocks of trials with 30 tones in each block. All tones in each block are identical except for three novel tones (different pitch) that are randomly interspersed. Further, both younger and older experimental subjects are subdivided into two groups; one group actively attends the tone presentation by counting each of the tones (attend condition), while the second group concentrates on reading a short essay during the presentation of the tones (ignore condition). The results so far have shown consistent differences in the evoked potential between young and old subjects. During the first 100 milliseconds of the auditory response, amplitude but not latency differences are observed. When components beyond 100 milliseconds were considered, significantly longer latencies occurred for the older subjects. Both young and old subjects have shown dishabituation to novel tones but the form of the response was quite different. In younger subjects the response consisted of a large positive component at around 300 milliseconds (P_{300}). For older subjects no clear P_{300} was apparent, rather the dishabituation response was characterized by a large

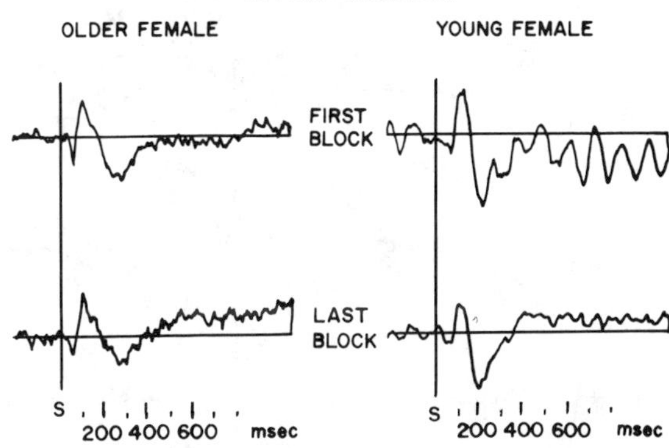

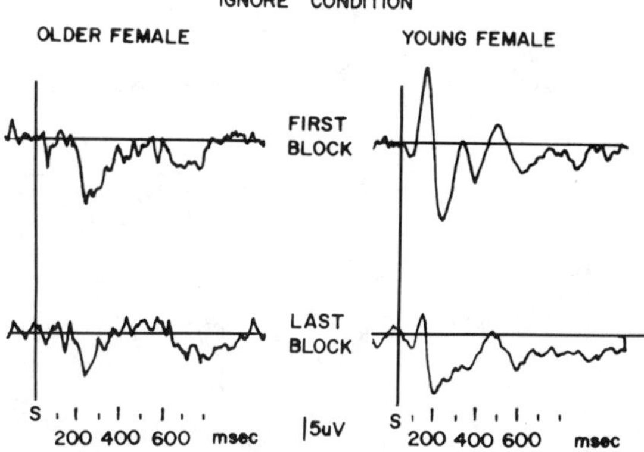

FIGURE 5 Auditory evoked responses (AERs) of younger and older subjects.

slow wave return to baseline levels. The evoked responses shown in Figure 5 illustrate the differences between younger and older subjects in the attend and ignore conditions in the first block of tones compared to the last block. The responses shown in Figure 6 demonstrate the typical changes in the waveform we have observed between younger and older subjects to the tone presented just prior to the novel tone (N − 1), to the novel tone (N), and to the tone presented just after the novel tone (N + 1). Possible explanations for the difference in waveform might include differential rates of habituation for the young and old or that the flattened and prolonged appearance of the positive going component is the result of faulty time-locking mechanisms in older subjects.

THE CONTINGENT NEGATIVE VARIATION AND RELATED SLOW SCALP POTENTIALS

The initial impetus for the experimental study of slow scalp potentials in humans was provided by Walter and his colleagues at the Burdern Neurological

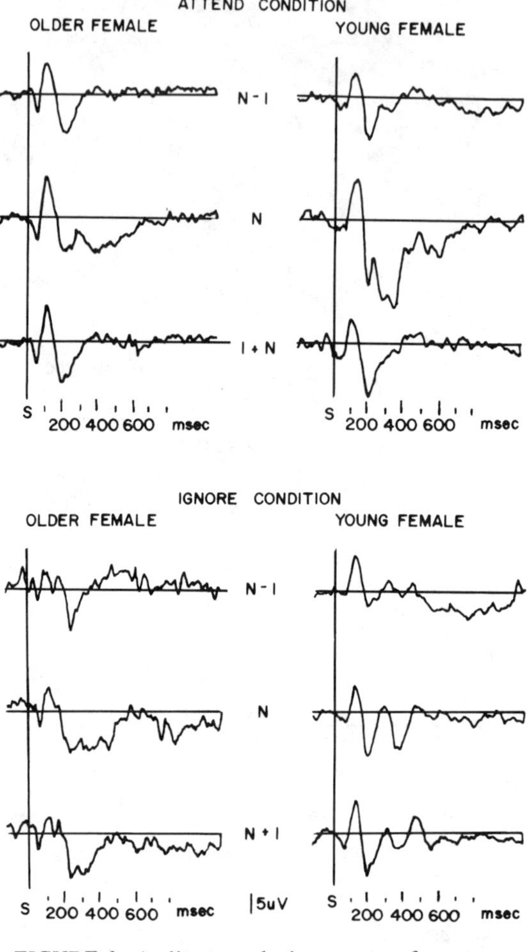

FIGURE 6 Auditory evoked responses of younger and older subjects to tones before the novel tone (N — 1), to the novel tone (N), and after the novel tone (N + 1).

Institute (Walter, Cooper, Aldridge, McCallum, & Winter, 1964). In their original report, the expectancy wave (E-wave) or contingent negative variation (CNV) was recorded using d.c. (direct-coupled) or long-time constant recordings in the interval (or empty period) of what appeared as a foreperiod reaction time (RT) task. The procedure used for eliciting slow potentials was simply a warning stimulus (S_1) followed a few seconds later by an imperative stimulus (S_2). The imperative stimulus usually signals that some particular response (e.g., a button press) is to be made by the subject. Many investigations have been conducted on the CNV phenomenon since its discovery (Tecce, 1972), and its potential for clinical application is still being weighed (Weinberg, 1975).

CNV Genesis

Normally the CNV is symmetrically distributed between the hemispheres with maximum amplitudes recorded from frontal and central regions. The slow wave builds up quickly after S_1 (about .5 seconds) and can be sustained for several seconds (Walter, 1967) although more commonly for 1.5 to 2.0 seconds. CNV potentials appear more dependent on information delivered to the subject by the S_1-S_2 situation than particular stimulus parameters, sensory modality, or critical S_1-S_2 time interval. The overall shape of the CNV can sometimes be distinguished for different individuals by the rising portion of the slow potential following the S_1 stimulus. A quick rise in the negative wave, called a Type A CNV, has been contrasted to a slow or ramp-like growth of negativity, called a Type B CNV (Tecce, 1972). The CNV is sustained from the beginning of the S_1-S_2 interval until a response is made to S_2. However, the return or resolution of the CNV to prestimulation levels has been reported to be bilaterally symmetrical even though a motor or mental response might be required of the subject (Lombroso, 1969). Evidence suggests that frontal CNVs are different from either vertex or parietal CNVs in both amplitude and waveform (Weinberg & Papakostopoulos, 1975). This difference may be the result of different processing strategies used by the subject, since the normal anterior-posterior gradients of the CNV can be altered by experimental manipulation (Järvilehto & Frühstorfer, 1970; Poon, Thompson, Williams, & Marsh, 1974).

Because the generation of the CNV usually involves a motor response by the subject, many experimenters have felt that premotor and motor responses were essential components or actual elements of the CNV waveform. Yet, CNVs have been recorded when no overt response was required of a subject following the imperative stimulus (S_2) (Donchin, Gerbrandt, Leifer, & Tucker, 1973), and even when the imperative stimulus was absent (Weinberg, Walter, Cooper, & Aldridge, 1974). Even tones presented regularly and without instructions to subjects produce CNV-like activity (Järvilehto & Frühstorfer, 1973). Having a subject actively terminate a series of flashes or clicks at S_2 decreases reaction times to the imperative stimulus, increases the magnitude of the CNV, and provides feedback about the subject's performance (Peters, Knott, Miller, Van Veen, & Cohen, 1970).

Maturational differences in the CNV have been observed by several investigators. Recordings from frontal, central, and posterior regions in children and adolescents from 5 to 18 years of age showed the earlier age groups with lower CNV amplitudes and CNVs that were not well developed (Cohen, 1970; 1973). In addition, the spatial distribution of the CNV was more prominent in frontal and central regions with increased age levels. Low and Stoilen (1973) found well-developed CNVs, vertex dominant, in children over 10 years of age; below 8 years of age, however, CNV activity was minimal or nonexistent. Yet CNV activity has been recorded from 3-year-olds with the use of novel and more interesting S_1 and S_2 stimuli (Gullickson, 1973). Although CNV activity has been recorded from subjects of a wide age range, a thorough investigation of the scalp topography of the CNV in the elderly has yet to be reported. The early maturational differences observed in the CNV in early childhood may have a counterpart in later years as cognitive abilities change and the integration of cortical functions is altered.

Each investigator of the CNV has had a particular characterization of the critical ingredients necessary for the development of the CNV. For some, the CNV reflects a complex physiological state that includes components of activation, mobilization-to-act, and preparation set. This third construct, preparation set, has been investigated by Low, Frost, Maulsby, and McSherry (1968). In their experiment, subjects were required to respond at S_2 with a specific force on a graded, hand-operated plunger; the amount of force with which the subject was to respond was indicated by a number at S_1 corresponding to the specific force level. It was found that CNV shifting between S_1 and S_2 increased in magnitude with the force required to make the response. The CNVs generated were additive with force but not linearly.

Waszak and Obrist (1969) used a disjunctive RT task to examine the relationship between motivational states and the generation of CNV potentials. An analysis of vertex averages indicated that the fastest RTs were accompanied by the largest CNVs. Evoked potentials to S_1 under instructed high motivation were significantly greater than under instructed low motivation; CNVs between motivational states, however, did not show amplitude differences. McAdam, Knott, and Rebert (1969) performed two studies to examine the effects of RT foreperiods on CNV amplitude. The experimental paradigm involved a single click as the S_1 and a single click as the S_2 signal. Three different S_1-S_2 intervals were used and simple RTs to the onset of S_2 were measured. The CNV amplitudes for the 800- and 1600-millisecond intervals were significantly larger than for the 4800-millisecond S_1-S_2 interval; there were no significant statistical differences between 800- and 1600-millisecond CNV amplitudes. When short but equally probable foreperiods (500–900 milliseconds) were used in the CNV interval, Loveless (1973) found that CNV activity increased monotonically with foreperiod duration. Gaillard and Näätänen (1973) concluded that overall CNV activity in a choice RT task paralleled the preparedness to react to S_2; in their study, however, amplitude measures of the CNV just prior to S_2 only approximated the RTs to S_2.

Slow Potentials in Voluntary Movements

Another slow potential that can be recorded from the scalp and has been directly related to voluntary motor activity is the readiness potential (RP) (Kornhuber & Deecke, 1965). The RP is bilaterally distributed over the cortex and reaches a maximum amplitude at the vertex for simple movements (Deecke, Scheid, & Kornhuber, 1969). The RP can be distinguished from a later negative potential, the motor potential, which displays a maximum contralateral to the responding limb over precentral areas. In addition to simple motor parameters, the amplitude of the RP can be varied by different motivational states (McAdam & Seales, 1969) and by experimental situations that require perceptual accuracy (McAdam & Rubin, 1971).

Studies by Loveless and Sanford (1975) and Weerts and Lang (1973) have suggested that the normal CNV is composite in waveform and made up of an initial orienting response at S_1 and a readiness potential prior to S_2. Rohrbaugh, Syndulko, and Lindsley (1976) have supplied evidence of the composite nature of the CNV by using S_1-S_2 intervals of 4 seconds duration. CNVs obtained with a 4-second interval contain elements of orienting and readiness potentials that are similar to individually averaged responses to S_1 tone signals and separate S_2 key presses.

Autonomic Concomitants

Somatic variables have been implicated in CNV generation. Gullickson and Darrow (1973) have examined the influence of respiratory cycles on slow potential changes in a CNV experiment. CNV trials were presented randomly during respiration cycles. From a vertex recording site, larger CNV shifts were observed when S_1 coincided with the starting phases of inspiration. By comparison, a positive shifting was observed with expiration at S_1 with lowered CNV activity. In contrast with these findings, Papakostopoulos and McCallum (1973) have found that multichannel recordings of various autonomic measures fail to show any relationship with CNV activity (except heart rate) including respiration. Lacey and Lacey (1973) have found a phasic bradycardia with the intention to respond and occurring along with the CNV. From the results of RT studies, Papakostopoulos (1973) has inferred that there may be some relationship between eye pupil activity and slow wave activity. Videotaped recordings of pupil activity during a typical slow wave experiment indicated that mydriasis indeed did occur during the S_1-S_2 CNV interval (Michalewski, 1976). While there appeared to be a close relationship between the onset and duration of pupil dilitation with development of the CNV, the pupil remained dilated for a long period after the CNV had been resolved to baseline levels. The pupil recordings suggest that the balance of sympathetic (dilation) and parasympathetic (constriction) activity was, at least in part, temporarily altered during and after the CNV interval.

McAdam (1969) interpreted slow wave shifts as increased excitability in the central nervous system. McAdam tested this hypothesis by using the late components of the somatosensory evoked response as an index of cortical excitability. The results showed that evoked response latencies to shock stimuli injected as probe stimuli in the CNV interval were shorter than responses recorded outside the paradigm. The faster resolution of the evoked response components was attributed to the increased cortical excitability during the period of increased scalp negativity. Rebert, Berry, and Merlo (Note 1) observed that muscle tension can be used to alter experimentally the arousal level in subjects. These investigators reasoned that if induced muscle tension was introduced between CNV trials, the transient increase in arousal level might also enhance CNV activity. In their report, induced muscle tension consisted of lifting a hand carrier with either 0-, 15-, 30-, or 45-pound weights; lifting preceded a standard S_1-S_2 CNV interval by 5 seconds. Results of amplitude measures of the CNV indicated no changes at 0- and 15-pound levels, but a marked increase in CNV potentials was observed for 30- and 45-pound levels.

Distraction Effects and Information Processing

Subject stress and anxiety may well affect arousal levels. Tecce and Hamilton (1973) have attempted to demonstrate that slow wave activity, in terms of CNVs, are inversely related to arousal. Support for this hypothesis came from the fact that distraction, deliberately introduced in the S_1-S_2 interval, reduces CNV amplitude. It is assumed that the additional attentional load imposed by the processing of these extra stimuli also accounts for the increased reaction times to S_2 signals. In their study, distraction consisted of having the subjects add 7s aloud during CNV trials. Other studies by Tecce and his associates have considered several types of distracting events, e.g., mental calculation and short-term recall for letters (Tecce & Cole, 1976; Tecce, Savignano-Bowman, & Meinbresse, 1976; Tecce & Scheff, 1969). Earlier, McCallum and Walter (1968) demonstrated that extraneous stimuli interjected between trials also had the effect of reducing the size of the CNV. Difficult discriminations may act as a distraction factor and affect the amplitude of the CNV (Delse, Marsh, & Thompson, 1972).

Not all stimulation presented in the CNV interval results in a reduction of the slow potential. If two S_1-S_2 CNV intervals are combined into one situation, the overall CNV generated is an approximate superimposed version of the CNVs taken separately (Low & McSherry, 1968). Michalewski and Weinberg (1976) have presented a study in which CNV potentials were recorded while subjects listened to tone patterns presented for 3-second CNV periods. Subjects made a perceptual judgment at an S_2 signal about whether the two tone pairs just heard were the same or different. Tone frequencies were selected so that the task was not difficult but did require attention to stimulation during the CNV buildup and simple retention of the tones. Compared to a standard S_1-S_2 CNV paradigm (empty interval), the results indicated significant increases in the amplitude of the CNV during the tone presentations. It was also noted that CNVs at lateral placements (F_3, F_4, T_3, and T_4), in contrast to the vertex (C_z), declined during the last tone. This reduction in the CNV was most likely related to stimulus processing and corresponded to a period in time when sufficient information about the tones was present in order to make a decision.

Clinical Use of the CNV in Psychiatric and Brain-Damaged Patients

A number of studies have included clinical examination of slow potential activity in hospitalized psychiatric patients (Dubrovsky & Dongier, Note 2). Timsit-Berthier, Koninckx, Dargent, Fontaine, and Dongier (1970) have surveyed CNV amplitude and waveform in 160 patients. The patients were classified as normal (45), neurotic (70), and psychotic (45). The CNV amplitude alone could not statistically distinguish between the three patient categories; however, there was a relationship between categories and the persistence of a negative afterpotential following the S_2 signal. Only 9% of the patients classified as normal displayed the sustained negativity after S_2, whereas 34% of the neurotics and 91% of the psychotics demonstrated the existence of the prolonged CNV. In another report involving neurotic and psychotic patients, Timsit-Berthier, Delaunoy, Koninckx, and Rousseau (1973) have considered three parameters of CNV activity: amplitude, morphology, and duration. Neurotics and psychotics produced small amplitude CNVs; morphology, in terms of Type A or Type B CNV classification, was equally represented in the patient groups; however, duration, or post-S_2 negativity, again appeared more often in the psychotic grouping. A different-from-normal motor potential has also been observed among psychiatric patients (Timsit-Berthier, Delaunoy, & Rousseau, 1973).

Tecce and Cole (1974) used measures of the CNV to explore the effects of amphetamine in normal subjects. Although alerting effects of amphetamine were observed in some subjects, an opposite effect was observed in others. Some subjects displayed a drowsiness and described an inability to remain alert after administration of the drug. During the drug testing, the group that was aroused by the action of the drug showed higher CNVs than during predrug testing, whereas the paradoxical responders showed a decline in the CNV compared to predrug administration. Behavioral and physiological measures indicated to the investigators that the effects of amphetamine need to be reviewed in terms of its role as a central stimulant.

The potential diagnostic value of applying the CNV technique to brain-damaged populations has received some attention. McCallum and Cummins (1973) have presented an interesting report on the effects of various brain lesions on the CNV. The patients tested included those with documented brain lesions (e.g., tumors and head injuries), localized lesions (cerebrovascular conditions), and diffuse lesions covering extensive areas of one or both cerebral hemispheres (e.g., hydrocephalus and Parkinson's disease). Brain-impaired patients were compared to a group of normal subjects and psychiatric patients without brain damage. In general, the results showed that there were marked asymmetries in the CNV associated with the damaged brain areas. CNVs were reduced or greatly suppressed over lesion sites. Diffuse cerebral impairment resulted in a general reduction of the CNV potentials over the entire scalp. In those cases where it was possible to compare recordings before and after surgery, CNV potentials following surgery recovered in amplitude with time along with an increased symmetry between the hemispheres.

Jones, Binnie, Bown, Lloyd, & Watson (1976) investigated the possibility that the CNV might yield useful clinical information for detecting latent chronic hepatic encephalopathy (CHE). The patient groups studied were formed from overt CHE patients and patients with mild hepatic insufficiency. Testing involved recording CNVs before and after administration of a provocative agent, morphine. CNVs were recorded during the period of a flash (S_1) followed 1 second later by clicks (S_2). Scalp electrical activity was collected from the vertex (C_z). The results showed that the average amplitude of the CNV in overt CHE patients was greatly reduced after morphine administration. On the other hand, no differences in amplitude of the CNV were observed for mild CHE patients between pre- and postadministrations of morphine. Despite these findings, the investigators did not feel that the CNV was sufficiently sensitive for use as a practical clinical test of CHE. However, successive testings over several days with additional placements might increase the sensitivity of the CNV in detecting CHE in patients with less severe symptoms.

Hemispheric Asymmetries

Another direction in experimentation combining both information systems and slow wave electrophysiology is the investigation of hemispheric asymmetries. There is mounting clinical (Milner, 1971) and psychophysical evidence (Dimond & Beaumont, 1974) that the cerebral hemispheres of humans process certain stimulus materials differentially. Verbal skills and associated functions are broadly localized to the left hemisphere, and spatial and pattern recognition capacities are attributed to the right hemisphere. The production of asymmetrical CNVs corresponding to some of these hemispheric differences has been demonstrated in neurologically normal individuals and has included the manipulation of numeric information (Butler & Glass, 1974), language production (Low, Wada, & Fox, Note 3), and verbal and nonverbal psychological set (Marsh & Thompson, 1973). Differences in hemispheric CNVs have also been reported between normal speakers and stutterers (Zimmermann & Knott, 1974). On the other hand, Hillyard (1973) has not observed asymmetries in the CNV in commisurotomized patients even though stimuli were directed to either the left or right hemispheres. In normal subjects, asymmetries in the CNV were not systematically found over the areas of Broca or

Wernicke in experimental conditions that required simple verbal processing and speech production (Michalewski, 1976; Michalewski, Weinberg, & Patterson, 1977).

CNVs in the Elderly

In most instances, the CNVs recorded from younger and older subjects are comparable with respect to both amplitude and general waveform (Thompson & Nowlin, 1973). Loveless and Sanford (1974) have analyzed the effects of various S_1-S_2 foreperiod durations (.5 to 15 seconds) on the CNV in a group of younger and a group of older subjects. There was a noticeable difference in the shape of the CNV between younger and older subjects, particularly at the longer S_1-S_2 intervals. Younger subjects showed an anticipatory response during long foreperiods that was indicated by an increasing shift of negativity near S_2. Older subjects did not show this increased negativity approaching S_2, but rather displayed an even level of shifting throughout the CNV interval. A possible explanation offered by the investigators for the difference between the two groups, presumably reflected in the waveform of the CNV, was that older individuals may lack the necessary control of timing sequences in order to meet response demands. In an interesting paper, Deecke, Englitz, and Schmitt (Note 4) have indicated that readiness potentials (RPs) may be absent or greatly attenuated in older individuals. The absence of an RP in older persons may account for the altered appearance (missing anticipatory negativity near S_2) of the observed CNV in older subjects. Schaie and Syndulko (1977) have presented preliminary results that indicate, contrary to the Loveless and Sanford report, well-defined negative shifts prior to S_2 in the elderly for relatively long S_1-S_2 durations.

We have been interested in the relation between experimenter-initiated CNV trials and subject-initiated CNV trials. Our paradigm is similar to the one described by Hamilton, Peters, and Knott (1973). By a method of reverse time averaging, it is possible to examine electrical potentials prior to voluntary movements. In addition to the slow CNV shift, then, a self-initiated trial also includes readiness activity corresponding to the start of the trial. Representative records from a younger subject (26 years old) and an older subject (65 years old) are shown in Figure 7. For both subjects, vertex (C_z) CNVs in the experimenter-initiated trials were quite noticeable. In the subject-initiated trials, however, the older subject showed little CNV activity during S_1-S_2 compared to the younger subject. It should also be noted that a substantial shift occurred several seconds prior to pressing the key to start the trials in the record of the older subject. This prior shifting may have limited further shifts in negativity leading to a smaller CNV. Readiness potentials prior to task initiation were only hinted at in the younger subject and were probably obscured in the older subject by the slow shifting prior to pressing the key to start the trials. Since the averages were based on 16 trials, it may be that

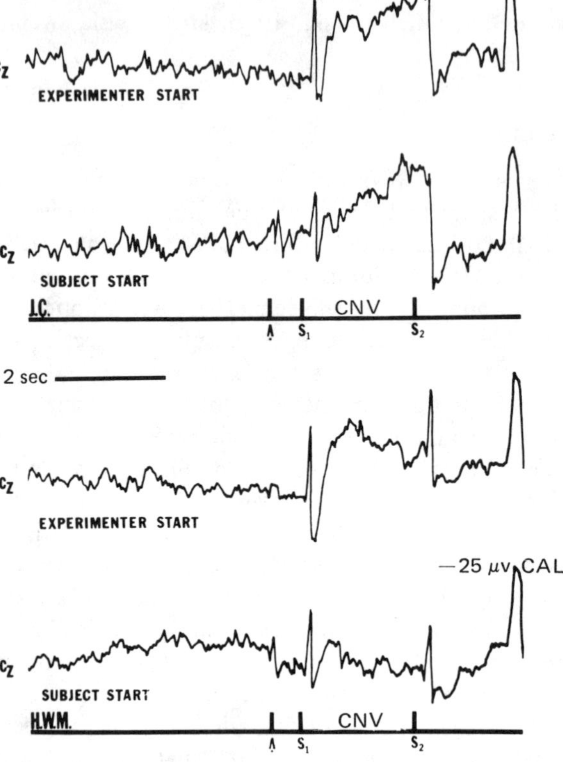

FIGURE 7 Slow potential activity of a younger subject (J.C.) and older subject (H.W.M.) under conditions of experimenter-initiated and subject-initiated CNV trials.

additional trials are necessary to distinguish readiness components in the records. The trials were started with the same button that stopped the S_2 clicks. Similar averages were observed for both younger and older subjects when a different motor movement (e.g., the right foot) was required both for initiation of the individual experimental trials and the termination of the clicks.

THE EEG AND PHARMACOLOGICAL AGENTS: ANTIDEPRESSANTS

An increasingly important area, one that promises to yield contributions in the future, is the effects of drugs on the EEG. As might be expected, a voluminous and complicated literature has developed around this topic. So many psychopharmacological agents have been studied in relation to the electroencephalogram that a complete or even partial review is not possible here. Instead, we have chosen to focus mainly on the EEG effects of the two major classes of antidepressant medication, namely the tricyclic antidepressants and MAO inhibitors. Although these drugs have been commonly used in the treatment of depressive disorders in the elderly, aging effects were generally not the major interest of the studies sampled. Older individuals were often included as either subjects or patients in studies, but little attempt was made to evaluate age differences. We believe that these selected investigations are representative of the field generally, and serve to point out the strengths and weaknesses of this type of inquiry.

Even though other classes of psychotropic drugs such as stimulants, major tranquilizers, and lithium have been used in the treatment of depression, they are usually not preferred except for short-term use, when there is an underlying psychosis, or in cases of bipolar depression (Fann, 1976). The tricyclics as well as the MAO inhibitors have been cited as the primary drugs used in treating a variety of depressive syndromes. Studies of the comparative therapeutic effectiveness of the various classes are lacking, particularly for the aged. However, due to their reputation of causing less serious side effects, tricyclics have generally been the preferred treatment in older subjects (Ban, 1975; Fann, 1976). Although 10 different classes of tricyclic antidepressants are recognized (Ban, 1975), most of the research concerned with EEG effects has concentrated on only a select few of these, principally imipramine and amitriptyline. Others such as doxepin, chlorimipramine, iprindole, trimipramine, and desipramine have also been studied in relation to the EEG, but to a lesser extent. Some of the MAO inhibitors studied include iproniazid, isocarboxazid, phenelzine, mebanazine, and tranylcypromine.

Antidepressants and Patterned Alterations of the EEG

Early attempts to describe the EEG effects accompanying administration of antidepressant drugs were primarily qualitative in nature. More recent studies have used quantitative measures of the electroencephalogram including frequency and period analysis and averaging procedures. The researchers in this area were eager to use the EEG in a number of ways (e.g., as a means to classify various groups of psychotropic drugs with known clinical effects; to predict the therapeutic value of new drugs; to identify onset, duration, and intensity of drug effects; and as an independent index of neurohumoral changes in studies of biochemical mechanisms of psychiatric disorders) (Fink, 1974). Although not all of these uses have been realized, significant advances have been made.

Qualitative Changes

Several qualitative investigations of imipramine and its effects on the EEG reported consistent patterns of EEG change. Zappoli (1959) studied the effects of acute administrations of imipramine (300–400 mg/24 hr) in depressive patients, some of whom were both hypertensive and elderly. There was evidence of EEG desynchronization with a reduction of the occipital alpha rhythm, accentuation of beta activity in central and anterior areas, and the appearance of diffuse cerebral hyperexcitability patterns including accentuated theta dysrhythmia. Delay and Deniker (1959) investigated the effects of imipramine on the EEGs of patients with various types of depression including late depression occurring after the age of 45. The subjects ranged in age from 19 to 79. Dosages varied from 50 to 300 mg/day, and treatment duration varied from 3 days to 5 months with most patients receiving treatment for several weeks. The EEG results found by Delay and Deniker indicated "a marked increase in amplitude of the basic alpha rhythm" (p. 109) in contrast to pretreatment, a tendency toward hypersynchronization, and an acute irritative pattern with higher doses. Kiloh, Davison, and Osselton (1961) observed diffuse theta activity and moderately increased fast activity after acute intramuscular administrations of imipramine to depressive patients.

Fink (1959) administered 40–125 mg imipramine intravenously to patients diagnosed as depressive, schizophrenic, or psychoneurotic. A second group of patients with similar clinical classifications was studied before and during chronic oral doses of imipramine (75–250 mg) given for 4 weeks or longer. Patients ranged in age from 17 to 58. EEG changes observed during acute imipramine administration included: decreased percent time alpha and decreased alpha voltage, increased percent time beta and increased beta voltage, and the appearance of random theta frequencies. Chronic administration of imipramine was associated with minimal changes, but reduced voltages, more prominent well-defined fast activity, and low voltage theta were observed.

Early studies using amitriptyline showed less consistent findings, although several replicated patterns were noted. After both acute intravenous and chronic administrations of amitriptyline to depressive patients, Serra, Municchi, and Logoluso (1963) observed a decrease in the mean EEG frequency and an increase in the regularity and amplitude of background activity. Davidson (1965) studied EEG changes after intravenous injections of amitriptyline in depressed subjects ranging in age from 18 to 65. In some subjects bitemporal diffuse theta activity and increased fast activity were observed, while in other subjects a reduction or disappearance of the alpha rhythm was seen. Lechner (1963), on the other hand, found no drug-specific EEG effects in patients diagnosed as endogenous depressives using chronic intramuscular injections of imipramine and amitriptyline and chronic oral doses of thioridazine. EEG measures were collected after acute administrations and at 2- and 3-day intervals during testing. Patterns of activity were discernible, but these were not consistent for any of the drugs. These alterations (Lechner, 1973) included an "increase in abundance of alpha, a slowing of mean alpha frequency and decrease in amplitude, decreased alpha abundance and increase in beta activity, occipital theta with slowing of mean alpha frequency or decreased abundance, and generalized paroxysmal rhythms" (pp. 134-135).

Quantitative Changes

Later quantitative studies also reported several consistent EEG effects due to antidepressant drug administration. Electronic frequency analysis was applied to studies of the EEG effects of psychotropic drugs by Fink (1961) and Fink, Pollack, Klein, Blumberg, Belmont, Karp, Kramer, and Willner (1962). Male and female depressive and schizophrenic patients, referred for drug therapy, were randomly administered imipramine (increased weekly to dose levels of 300 mg), a placebo, or a combination of chlorpromazine and procyclidine (increased weekly to dose levels of 1200 mg and 15 mg, respectively). EEG records of fronto-occipital activity were taken prior to treatment and during the fifth week. Results indicated that imipramine reduced percent time alpha and total activity and increased theta and fast beta activity. Statistical tests from the predrug period showed that the increase in fast activity (22-33 cps) was significant. Fink differentiated this pattern from the pattern exhibited by chlorpromazine, which showed (a) an increase in total activity, (b) an increase in percent time delta, theta, and alpha, and (c) a decrease in alpha frequency from 12 to 10.5 cps.

These results were supported in a later report by Fink (1963), who used patients from the same psychiatric facility, referred for drug treatment. Patients ranged in age from 17 to 65, and the most common diagnoses included depression, psychoneurosis, and schizophrenia. The EEG records obtained prior to drug treatment, after acute injections at fixed rates per minute, and at intervals during chronic treatment were analyzed visually and with frequency analysis techniques. Included in the wide variety of drugs used were imipramine, chlorpromazine, and iproniazid (an MAO inhibitor). The results were similar to those reported in the studies by Fink (1961) and Fink et al. (1962) described above. Imipramine induced an increase in percent time beta and an increase in slowing for some subjects. Again this pattern could be distinguished from changes resulting from other drugs such as chlorpromazine, which was associated with increased percent time alpha, slowing of central alpha frequencies, and diminution of percent time beta. Administration of iproniazid induced increased amounts of EEG activity and increased synchronization.

Results concerning the EEG effects of chlorpromazine, imipramine, chlordiazepoxide, or saline administered in random order intravenously for 10 minutes were reported by Itil, Shapiro, and Fink (1968) and Itil, Shapiro, Fink, Kiremitci, and Hickman (1969). Subjects were normal volunteers and patients with schizophrenic and neurotic reactions, all of whom had been drug free for at least a 6-month period. After an initial 20-minute resting EEG, recordings were taken at set time intervals up to 1.5 hours following drug injection, using right occipital to right ear or right occipital to right frontal leads. Subject vigilance was maintained by button-pressing responses to acoustic stimulation presented at randomly varying intervals. The results were analyzed visually, using electronic frequency analysis (24 frequencies between 3 and 33 cps), and with period analysis.

Frequency analyzer results indicated an increase in very slow activity (theta and delta frequency bands), a decrease of alpha and slow beta activity during the second, third, and fourth time periods for the volunteers, and a decrease of alpha in the second and fourth time periods for the patients after imipramine. Itil et al. (1968) and Itil et al. (1969) noted that the clearest differences were in the slower frequency bands due to noise and electromyographic effects on the higher frequency bands. As found in earlier studies, however, chlorpromazine and imipramine could be distinguished according to fast frequencies, especially in the later time periods. Results for period analysis (examined for a single subject) showed an increase of 0–3 cps activity 30 minutes after imipramine, an increase of 8–12 cps activity, and an initial increase in the 22–40 cps frequency band of the first derivative. Amplitude increased 20 minutes after injection of imipramine. Changes due to imipramine administration were distinguished from those induced by the other drugs both by characteristics and by time of occurrence, and the results were interpreted as supportive of the use of EEG measures to predict therapeutic value and determine central effectiveness of various classes of drugs.

Although the effects of drugs on behavior have not always been examined systematically in the studies reported, it appears that the differential behavioral responsivity to drugs shows some correspondence to the specific effects of various drugs on the EEG. For example, in acute administrations, Fink (1963) has observed that chlorpromazine is associated with "sedation, increased drowsiness, denial, and euphoria, decreased agitation, panic, excitement, and delusional activity, and the minimization and displacement of symptoms" (p. 188). Behavioral effects associated with acute administrations of imipramine included increased agitation and tension followed by relaxation and drowsiness. Chronic imipramine administration was followed by a decrease in depression and an increase in well-being, sleeping, and ward participation. As reviewed earlier, distinct patterns of EEG change have usually been observed for these drugs. Chlorpromazine has shown increased alpha activity, slowing of central alpha frequencies, and a reduction of beta activity. In contrast, imipramine has shown increased fast beta activity, a reduction of alpha activity, and the appearance of random theta frequencies. Observations such as these have encouraged some workers in this area to argue that the EEG holds promise as a means of classifying individuals with respect to drug responsivity, given that other factors such as age, diagnosis, years of illness, and principal symptoms are controlled. Although this approach offers guidelines for continued clinical EEG research and application, more extensive and detailed parametric investigations are required to establish the feasibility of this type of model. This suggestion is especially justified in view of the variety of individual differences that have been observed due to differences in initial pretreatment EEG records and in response to varying dosage levels (Fink, 1959). It is also important to consider other evidence concerning the dissociation of EEG and behavior that has been found in several lesion and drug studies (Bradley, 1958; Lacey, 1967; Mirsky & Cardon, 1962; Routtenberg, 1968).

EEG and the Classification of Psychotropic Drugs

Despite the problems outlined above, there has been continued interest in the development of the EEG as a tool to predict classification of antidepressant drugs and other medications used in the treatment of behavioral disorders (Fink, 1968, 1974; Itil, 1968, 1974). Itil (1968) has recognized the difficulty in classifying the psychotropic drugs due to the size of the changes and their dependency on factors such as individual sensitivity, configuration of predrug resting records, and time-dosage relationships. However, both Fink (1968, 1974) and Itil (1968, 1974) have persistently maintained that every drug that is effective therapeutically or induces characteristic alterations in psychomotor behavior also produces a predictable accompanying pattern of EEG change.

Itil (1968) placed the clinically useful psychotropic drugs in six groups based on their characteristic or signature EEG pattern: (1) drugs that induce sleep-like patterns, increase average frequency, decrease amplitude, and induce fast, rhythmical spindle activity in the anterior area (minor tranquilizer reaction type); (2) drugs that increase slow and decrease fast activity, induce sleep patterns with spindles, decrease frequency, and increase amplitude (neuroleptic, major tranquilizer reaction type); (3) drugs that increase alpha, enhance synchronization, increase amplitude, and decrease frequency (major neuroleptic reaction type); (4) drugs that increase slow and fast activity, initially increase then decrease alpha, initially increase then decrease frequency, slightly increase amplitude, and are characterized by slow waves with superimposed fast activity (thymoleptic reaction type); (5) drugs that abolish alpha, increase slow and fast activity, flatten amplitude, are characterized by low voltage slow activity with superimposed fast activity, and produce only slight EEG alterations after drug tolerance develops (anticholinergic reaction type, including some of the MAO inhibitors); and (6) drugs that accelerate frequency, induce desynchronization, decrease rhythmicity, and flatten amplitude (hallucinogenic reaction type). In a later discussion (Itil, 1974), items (4) and (5) were combined.

The EEG classification of the psychotropic drugs given by Fink (1968) is presented in Table 1. This table also illustrates Fink and Itil's (1968) differentiation of the major types of drugs used clinically as antidepressants according to the induced EEG changes. Discrepancies in drug classifications are attributed by Itil (1968) to differences in experimental methodology. According to Fink (1968), these drug-related EEG changes

TABLE 1 EEG Patterns of Psychoactive Drugs

Class	EEG pattern	Frequency (cps)						Amplitude		Bursts		Example
		Δ (0–3.5)	θ (3.5–7.5)	α (7.5–13)	β_1 (13–22)	β_2 (22–33)	Variability	Integration	Variability	ΔB[a]	Spikes	
Ia	Slowing	+[b]	++	±[e]	0	—	—	+	0	+	+	Chlorpromazine
Ib	Slowing with inc. alpha	+	++	++	0	±	—	+	—	0	0	Butaperazine
Ic	Slowing with inc. seizure	+	+	—	0	0	±	+	—	+	+	Reserpine
IIa	Fast activity, inc. ampl.	0[c]	+	0	++	+	—	+	—	0	—	Amobarbital
IIb	Fast activity, dec. ampl.	0	—[d]	—	+	++	+	—	+	—	+	Amphetamine; LSD
IIIa	Fast and slow activity	++	+	—	+	++	+	—	+	—	±	Ditran, atropine
IIIb	Fast and slow activity, inc. seizure	+	++	—	+	+	+	—	+	+	0	Imipramine
IVa	Alpha variation, increase	0	+	+	0	0	—	+	—	±	0	Morphine, alcohol
IVb	Alpha variation, decrease	0	0	—	0	0	+	—	0	0	0	Iproniazid

Note. From Table 1 of Fink (1968).
[a] ΔB = Change in burst activity.
[b] + = increase.
[c] 0 = no effect.
[d] — = decrease.
[e] ± = variable.

> appear in systematic relation to conventional usage and to the induced behavioral changes. . . . shifts in the EEG pattern in the direction of increased fast and slow activity, usually with increased variability of frequencies and amplitudes, are associated with euphoria, increased psychomotor activity, alertness and irritability; at higher dosages, with confusion, memory defect, illusions and thought disorder, confabulation and delirium. In this pattern change, increasing the slow wave component is associated with increasing stupor and decreased excitement, while increasing the fast component is associated with increased psychomotor activity and irritability. (p. 503)

Studies conducted to verify these drug classifications have typically used a methodology similar to the following example. Male volunteers between the ages of 21 and 35 were selected as subjects in an effort to control prior drug history and subject variables. Period analysis techniques provided 22 measurements including average absolute amplitude, amplitude variability, average frequency, frequency deviation, and 8 frequency bands of the primary waves (i.e., 1.3-3.5, 3.5-7.5, 7.5-13, 13-20, 20-26.6, 26.6-40, 40-90, and over 90 cps), and average frequency, frequency deviation, and 8 frequency bands of the first derivative measurements (i.e., 1.3-10, 10-16.6, 16.6-20, 20-26.6, 26.6-40, 40-50, 50-90, and over 90 cps) (Itil, 1974). EEG was recorded using right and left frontal, central, parietal, and occipital leads. Vigilance was maintained by button-pressing responses to acoustic stimulation presented at randomly varying intervals. The foregoing study incorporates several components considered essential by Itil (1974), who stated that certain aspects of the EEG commonly disregarded by electroencephalographers (i.e., frequencies over 20 cps, multiband frequency analysis, and amplitude variability), are often the most sensitive in detecting the effects of psychotropic drugs.

Later reports by Itil (1973, 1974) and Fink (1974, 1977) upheld the EEG classifications of the psychotropic drugs. Itil (1973) investigated the EEG effects of 13 psychotropic drugs with known clinical effectiveness and a placebo. Imipramine and amitriptyline were differentiated from the other classes of drugs (minor tranquilizers, barbiturates, central stimulants, and major tranquilizers) by an increase in slow and fast activity. In another study by Itil (1974) the EEG effects of amitriptyline and imipramine (.62 mg/kg and 50 mg, respectively) were compared 3 hours after single dose administration to predrug recordings. The results indicated an increase in slow waves, decreased alpha and slow beta activity, and an increase in fast beta waves. Fink (1974) reported a study in which male volunteers were given doxepin (.2 mg/kg), imipramine (.45 mg/kg), and a placebo. Imipramine increased 4-7.5 cps and 18-22.5 cps activity, the placebo showed no effects, and doxepin increased activity in the 1.1-4 cps, 4-7.5 cps, and 18-22.5 cps frequency bands. The correlation between the profiles for doxepin and imipramine was .76. Other studies cited by Itil (1974) indicated that EEG measures are useful for predicting effective therapeutic doses of amitriptyline and the duration of drug effects.

Quantitative Pharmaco-Electroencephalography

Itil (1974) and Fink (1974) have promoted "quantitative pharmaco-electroencephalography" for establishing the central effectiveness of new compounds, predicting their clinical usefulness, and estimating effective dose ranges. Itil, Polvan, and Hsu (1972) studied the EEG profiles of two new compounds, GB-94 and GC-46, in comparison to amitriptyline, imipramine, and placebo in 12 normal volunteers and 30 depressive patients. Subgroups of the volunteers received doses of GB-94 or GC-46 spread over a period of up to several weeks (totaling up to 52.5 mg), or single oral doses of GB-94 (15 mg), GC-46 (30 mg), placebo, and imipramine (25 mg). EEGs were recorded predrug and at varying postdrug intervals (ranging from 1 hour to 144 hours following drug administration). The patients, who ranged in age from 17 to 77, were randomly assigned to GB-94 (20–72.4 mg daily in increasing doses for 3 weeks), or amitriptyline (60.7–200 mg daily in increasing doses for 3 weeks) after a placebo period. EEG records were obtained predrug and at intervals of 7 days and 21 days following drug treatment. Results indicated that GC-46 and GB-94 exhibited thymoleptic profiles similar to amitriptyline and imipramine, i.e., an increase of slow waves and superimposed fast activity after both acute and chronic administration, although these changes were decreased during the third week. The changes were observed after low doses (5 mg) and increased in magnitude with increasing doses. Further, GC-46 exhibited a profile more similar to imipramine, while GB-94 resembled amitriptyline (more slow waves and less fast activity). Measures of clinical improvement (clinical global scores, and scores on the Itil Depression Rating Scale, Hamilton Anxiety Rating Scale, and Itil Self-Rating Scale for Anxiety-Depressive-Drive) showed that GB-94 in doses of 30–55 mg induced clinical improvement that increased during the third week in a manner similar to that obtained with amitriptyline.

Antidepressants and Changes in the Sleep EEG

Another experimental strategy used to investigate the effects of psychotropic drugs is the sleep EEG. Dunleavy, Brezinova, Oswald, Maclean, and Tinker (1972) studied the effects of placebo, imipramine, desipramine, chlorimipramine, doxepin, iprindole, and trimipramine on measures of sleep EEG in healthy young males. Baseline (placebo) EEG recordings (fronto- and parieto-occipital midline positions) were collected for 4–5 nights, and up to 14 nights of recording distributed over 4 weeks were conducted during the administration of 75 mg daily of the tricyclic drugs. EEG records were scored in terms of sleep stages. Results indicated an immediate decrease in duration of rapid eye movement (REM) sleep for imipramine, desipramine, chlorimipramine, and doxepin; this decrease was reduced by the fourth week, although still present, and was followed by a rebound increase following drug withdrawal. Iprindole and trimipramine had no apparent effects on REM sleep. It is interesting to note that biochemical studies have shown that iprindole does not affect reuptake mechanisms in the same manner as other tricyclics, although it is structurally related and is an effective antidepressant (Berger, 1977; Leonard, 1975). Measures of intrasleep restlessness (frequency of spontaneous shifts into Stage 1 sleep [drowsiness] or wakefulness from other stages of sleep) indicated increases for imipramine, desipramine, and chlorimipramine, slight decreases for doxepin and trimipramine, and no apparent effect for iprindole. Similarly, Hata (1975) found decreased percent REM period after 25 mg doses of imipramine.

Kupfer, Foster, Reich, Thompson, and Weiss (1976) investigated the effects of amitriptyline administration on sleep EEG in 18 unipolar depressive patients with a mean age of 51.4 years. EEG recordings were taken on 3 consecutive nights before drug administration (baseline), the first 2 nights of drug administration, and 4 consecutive nights during the third week of treatment. Dosage levels ranged from 150 to 250 mg daily. EEG records were categorized for sleep stages, and each minute of REM sleep was scored on a 9-point scale for intensity of REM patterns (amplitude and number of conjugate eye movements). Subjects were divided into good responders and poor responders to amitriptyline therapy based on clinical assessments performed during the third week of study. It was found that amitriptyline induced an immediate decrease in REM sleep percent, a marked increase in REM latency, and a decrease in REM activity. The changes were more pronounced for good responders but were present in both groups. These effects persisted during the third week of study in both groups but were still more evident for the good responders. However, "regardless of the clinical response, there were obvious drug-induced changes in the sleep of both groups" (Kupfer et al., 1976).

Hartmann (1974) studied the effects of chronic amitriptyline and placebo administration on the desynchronized sleep patterns of normal subjects. Medication was discontinued at 28 days but recordings were continued up to 55 days following start of treatment. Amitriptyline induced an immediate decrease in amount of desynchronized sleep that continued until the drug was withdrawn. After discontinuation of medication, a rebound or increase in desynchronized sleep was evident for 6 days, followed by a return to placebo levels. Hartmann (1974) cited supporting studies that found similar decreases in desynchronized sleep for imipramine, desipramine, and some of the MAO inhibitors for depressed patients as well as for normals. Hartmann also suggested that increased availability of central catecholamines may be important in the regulation of desynchronized sleep time.

Itil, Saletu, and Akpinar (1974) have studied the effects of psychotropic drugs on EEG using computer "sleep prints." EEG recordings of night sleep using a right occipital to anterior vertex lead were analyzed using period analysis of the primary wave (zero cross) and its first derivative. Each epoch was classified into 1 stage of a 3-stage, 5-stage, and 9-stage sleep classification based on the frequency distribution in 8 primary wave bands. The sleep print plotted at the end of each night showed the percentage of time spent in each sleep stage. It was found that either imipramine (35 mg) or amitriptyline (35 mg), administered to a normal volunteer, resulted in an increase of deep sleep stages as compared to placebo, while REM activity was suppressed. The changes were contrasted with those produced by other psychotropic drugs, e.g., anxiolytics, neuroleptics, hallucinogens, and stimulants. An increase of deep sleep stages was also found following the administration of 25 mg imipramine 2 hours before sleep onset, as contrasted with placebo (Itil, 1968). Other studies (Itil et al., 1974) have supported these findings by reporting increased deep sleep and attenuated REM sleep in normal and depressed subjects after 75 mg desimipramine; increased Stage 2 sleep and decreased REM in enuretic patients after 50 mg imipramine; decreased REM in normals after 75 mg amitriptyline; and decreased REM but no effects on other sleep stages of normal and depressed subjects after the administration of several MAO inhibitors.

Wyatt, Kupfer, Scott, Robinson, and Snyder (1969) investigated the effects of five MAO inhibitors on REM sleep in three young normal male volunteers and two middle-aged depressed female patients. Subjects were given isocarboxazid (maximum 60 mg), mebanazine (maximum 15 mg), phenelzine (maximum 45 mg), isoniazid (maximum 400 mg), or paragyline hydrochloride (maximum 100 mg). MAO platelet activity was decreased and urinary tryptamine levels were increased for four of the drugs, indicating that tissue MAO inhibition was induced by all drugs except isoniazid. Parietal EEG, horizontal eye movement, and submental electromyogram records were collected predrug, during drug, and postdrug administration. Results indicated decreased REM time and REM percent, and increased REM latency for all drugs except isoniazid especially after the sixth drug night. Isoniazid also decreased REM time but not significantly. Mebanazine produced a significant rise in REM time above baseline postdrug.

In a later study, Wyatt, Fram, Kupfer, and Snyder (1971) studied the effects of the MAO inhibitor phenelzine (up to 75 mg/24 hr) on sleep in anxious, depressed patients (five middle-aged and one young) by means of EEG, electro-oculograms, and submental electromyograms. Drug administration was continued until total REM suppression was observed in each patient (from 6 to 47 nights) and for the duration of total REM suppression (from 14 to 40 nights). After discontinuation of the drug, REM sleep increased as much as 250% above baseline levels. Behavioral changes associated with REM suppression included reduced anxiety and depression as indicated in ratings on behavioral checklists completed by nurses. Two of the four patients studied after MAOI discontinuation showed increased anxiety with REM rebound, a third exhibited recurrence of initial symptoms, while the fourth became hypomanic.

Antidepressants and Changes in the Evoked Potential

Several researchers have used evoked potentials in studying the EEG effects of psychopharmacological compounds. Saletu, Saletu, and Itil (1973) studied the effects of 2 tricyclic antidepressants, amitriptyline and imipramine, on somatosensory evoked potentials (SEPs) in 3 groups of male volunteers ranging in age from 21 to 36. Using a statistically randomized design, 1 single oral dose of placebo and (at least 1 week later) 1 of imipramine (.45 mg/kg) were given to the first group of subjects; the second group received placebo and amitriptyline (.42 mg/kg); and the third group received placebo, imipramine (.62 mg/kg) and amitriptyline (.62 mg/kg). SEPs to electrical stimuli applied to the median nerve were recorded before and 2 hours after oral drug administration. Vigilance was maintained by subject interviewing and EEG monitoring and by a push button device that activated a tone if vigilance declined and the button were released. Within the evoked potential waveform 11 peaks were identified following stimulus onset; latency and peak-to-peak amplitudes were analyzed from predrug and drug conditions.

Results were most marked in terms of statistical significance for the latency measures, although the amplitude measures showed some consistent changes. Amitriptyline and imipramine both induced latency decreases in the first three peaks and increases thereafter, at both dosage levels. Amplitudes were generally attenuated, especially at the higher dosage level, with the exception of the increased amplitudes for Peaks 3 and 4. Saletu et al. (1973) concluded that these SEP changes could be considered characteristic for the tricyclic antidepressants, since they were consistent with (as well as distinguishable from) changes induced by other classes of psychotropic drugs. The latency findings indicated to Saletu et al. that these drugs have both stimulatory and inhibitory properties, a finding supported by the EEG studies that have described the "thymoleptic reaction type" (Itil, 1968, 1974). In addition, Saletu et al. (1973) pointed out that since the latency decrease in the early peaks was more marked for imipramine and the latency increase in the late peaks was greater for amitriptyline, "amitriptyline is an antidepressive compound with more sedative properties, while imipramine is an antidepressant with more stimulatory properties" (p. 10). Clinical studies have supported this observation (Fann, 1976).

Saletu (1974) proposed SEP profiles for MAO inhibitors such as isocarboxazid, tranquilizers, and central stimulants. Isocarboxazid produced latency decreases in both the early and late components of the SEP. Amplitude changes were nonsignificant, but were generally in the direction of attenuation, especially in the later components. Saletu also suggested classifications for newly developed compounds and for predicting their therapeutic value. Saletu emphasized, however, that such classifications and predictions are dependent on careful controls of such variables as dosage, route and rate of administration, drug specificity, and subject factors as age, weight, height, baseline EEG, psychiatric status, and state of alertness. According to Saletu, intraindividual SEP changes were small and nonsignificant over the 5 trials performed during each recording session, as well as over a period of 4 weeks, indicating some degree of response consistency. Changes from predrug to placebo were small, nonsystematic, and not statistically significant.

Lader (1977) investigated the auditory evoked potential (AEP) response to clicks of 70 dB intensity in 12 normal subjects given .50 and .75 mg/kg of imipramine or placebo. Subjects were required to press a key in response to the clicks. The N_1 component was the only portion of the response that was altered and its amplitude increased while latencies remained unchanged. Lader also administered imipramine (50 mg every 8 hours) to 10 depressed patients for 28 days and recorded AEPs predrug and at weekly intervals during drug treatment. The latency of the P_2 component increased during the first week but then returned to baseline levels by the fourth week of therapy. The amplitude of the N_1 and P_2 components increased. Lader's findings for normal subjects are somewhat in conflict with those of Saletu et al. (1973), who found latency decreases in the early components and a tendency toward reduced amplitudes using SEP responses. The reduced amplitudes were noted particularly for the later components after imipramine administration, however, with the amplitude of peaks 3 and 4 (approximately 35–40 msec) increasing significantly at the higher dosage level. The latency decreases in the early components were significant only at the high dosage level (.62 mg/kg). A number of factors could be contributing to the conflicting findings reported here, e.g., different modalities, varying dosages, possible differences in subject samples, and variations in procedures to control for vigilance and other cognitive processes. This emphasizes Lader's (1977) conclusion regarding drug effects on the evoked potential, namely that sufficient research providing drug response data, systematic variations of potentially critical variables, and replications of findings are needed to permit sound inferences regarding the clinical applicability or theoretical interpretations of the evoked potential.

Shagass and his colleagues approached some of these problems by examining psychiatric diagnosis and psychoactive drug administration in relation to the SEP, with particular emphasis on the SEP recovery function (Shagass & Schwartz, 1962; Shagass, Schwartz, & Amadeo, 1962). In this procedure paired stimulus pulses (.13 msec duration) were delivered to the ulnar nerve at the wrist, while the interval between stimuli was varied from 2.5 to 190 msec. Secondary components of the primary response to the first stimulus were subtracted out in order to allow for analysis of the response to the second stimulus of the pair. The relative size of the second response compared to the first provided an index of the recovery function. Results were examined by computing the ratio R_2/R_1 such that a ratio of 1 indicated complete recovery. Subjects were nonpatient controls and psychotic depressives (most of whom were female) ranging in age from 23 to 68.

Results for normals indicated that a period of full recovery took place by 20 msec, followed by diminished responsiveness, with a second peak of recovery and "supernormality" by about 120 msec. Psychotic depressives showed diminished recovery that was most prominent at the 20 msec phase. Shagass et al. (1962) and Shagass and Schwartz (1962) concentrated their analyses on this recovery at 20 msec since it was the most consistent phase of the response. In a later report, Shagass (1972) noted that in comparison to controls, a diverse group of psychiatric patients also displayed slower recovery with "absence of diagnostic specificity" (p. 216) when visual evoked potentials were used.

Included in the sample of psychotic depressives used by Shagass et al. (1962) and Shagass and Schwartz (1962) was a subsample of patients who were receiving either drugs alone or drugs in combination with electroconvulsive therapy (ECT). Retests after successful treatment with either drugs or drugs plus ECT revealed a significant shift toward the recovery function that had been exhibited by normal controls. One subject (female) received imipramine alone and was retested approximately 3 weeks and 5 months after the pretreatment test. The recovery function at 20 msec was improved at both retest times ($R_2/R_1 = .87$ at 3 weeks and .98 at 5 months) when contrasted with pretreatment ($R_2/R_1 = .50$). In a later study, Shagass and Schwartz (1964) reported the nonspecificity of some aspects of the SEP. They found that the increase in the negative deflection following the positive peak of the initial SEP response frequently observed after drug administration could be produced by diverse treatment agents.

Evidence gathered during these studies indicated to Shagass et al. (1962) that imipramine probably did not act directly on mechanisms regulating recovery function. Two depressive patients who had been receiving a MAO inhibitor and two who had received imipramine for 3 weeks without therapeutic effect were compared with depressive patients who had received no drugs and with nonpatients. The recovery curves of the patients receiving drugs and not receiving drugs were very similar, while both differed markedly from those of the nonpatients. Two nonpatient volunteers who were given imipramine for several weeks showed reduced recovery at 20 msec in comparison with their predrug recovery curves. The intensity-response gradient, which related the intensity of the stimulus to the amplitude of the SEP, was found to be steeper among psychiatric patients than among normal subjects. A reduced intensity-response curve was observed in one subject with a psychotic depressive reaction who was retested after taking imipramine for 6 weeks, while two nonpatient subjects who received imipramine for several weeks displayed increased intensity-response gradients. Shagass et al. (1962) and Shagass (1968) concluded from these findings that the psychiatric condition of the patient was probably the critical factor influencing the evoked response effects observed, since the antidepressant medications studied induced differential effects depending on the presence or absence of depression and amount of depression.

A later study presented data on amitriptyline in relation to a modified version of the recovery function (Shagass, Straumanis, & Overton, 1973). This procedure used a fixed stimulus interval but varied the intensity of the conditioning stimulus while keeping the test stimulus intensity constant. Subjects were depressed patients (75% female) ranging in age from 23 to 59 who had been taking about 200 mg/day of amitriptyline for approximately 40 days between predrug and drug tests. Amplitude measurements obtained after the stimulus at four time intervals were reduced by amitriptyline, and these reductions involved both the early and late portions of the response. Differences between predrug and drug conditions were not found for amplitude variations as a function of conditioning stimulus intensity (dynamic range). These findings could be distinguished from those obtained for lithium carbonate, which induced amplitude increases, especially in the early portions of the SEP, and increased dynamic range. Shagass et al. (1973) speculated about the relationship between these amplitude decreases and the proposed tricyclic-induced increase in the functional level of norepinephrine at the postsynaptic adrenergic receptors. The reduced amplitude of the SEP with amitriptyline might be related to greater inhibitory activity resulting from increased norepinephrine "if it is assumed that the relevant effects involve predominantly inhibitory norepinephrine receptors" (Shagass et al., 1973, p. 195). This interpretation is in contrast with the earlier conclusion by Shagass et al. (1962) and Shagass and Schwartz (1962) that the changes in SEP recovery functions with imipramine probably do not involve direct effects on cortical activity but rather are related to psychiatric status. In a later report, Shagass (1974) noted that when SEP responses were separated into 4–28 Hz and 32–500 Hz bands using Fourier analysis techniques, amitriptyline was found to reduce amplitudes in the 4–28 Hz portion of the response. By contrast, lithium induced amplitude increases mainly in the 32–500 Hz portion of the response.

CONCLUSION

Several consistent changes in electrophysiological activity have been observed after the administration of antidepressant drugs, and these appear to have specific behavioral concomitants. This interrelationship has been interpreted, by some, as confirmatory evidence that the EEG can be used to classify psychotropic medications in terms of their possible mechanisms and therapeutic effectiveness (Itil, 1974; Fink, 1974). Others have been less enthusiastic about this use of the EEG. Longo (1977), for example, points out that EEG studies should be considered "only as complementary to other techniques of research; in particular it is difficult to interpret the EEG data in the light of the biochemical hypothesis of mechanisms of action since studies which provide a correlation between the neurophysiological effects and the postulated blockade of the catecholamine uptake in the CNS are lacking" (p. 7C-54). Past studies have included a diversity of experimental procedures, patient groups, and drug manipulations; future studies must use a greater systematization of research paradigms before any convincing conclusions can be drawn.

Although this might seem discouraging, given the quantity of studies reported, the measures in question are exquisitely sensitive to a variety of effects, ranging from biochemical differences at the cellular level to attitudinal differences in interpersonal processes. However, the very factors that make the investigation of these phenomena so complex also render them compelling as potential analytic tools. These factors (e.g., the apparent lawfulness of changes in evoked potentials, the various manipulations in both the behavioral and biological realm, and the ease of measurement during ongoing functions) may provide a unique and highly practical methodology for the study of brain behavior relationships at the human level and for a possible clinical assessment device.

It is worthwhile to encourage continued research in this area with the expectation that progress may appear slow in the near future. Developments in EEG research could be enhanced by standardization of procedures in laboratories and control of individual differences in group composition. Perhaps a more important problem at the moment, particularly for the relationship of EEG to psychopharmacologic effects, is the paucity of theoretical direction. Greater implementation of models can facilitate standardization in laboratories and provide direction for systematic investigation, whereas continued empirical studies that lack conceptual framework cannot. In addition, careful control should be exercised over the measurement problems associated with electrophysiological investigations of drug effects. As noted earlier, there are several factors that can affect the recordings, such as route and rate of drug administration, drug specificity, and subject variables such as predrug resting EEG, age, weight, height, and psychiatric status. The continued exploration of monoamine effects on the interrelationship of electrophysiological measures, psychiatric status, and aging seems worthwhile in view of recent studies of the relationship of brain amines to the pathogenesis of the affective disorders (Schildkraut, 1965; Schildkraut, Draskoczy, Gershon, Reich, & Grab, 1971), as well as prior investigations of changes in central catecholamines and indoleamines with aging (Finch, 1977).

It is noteworthy that many early studies did not control age factors adequately, and later studies on drug effects emphasized EEG changes only in healthy young subjects. Clinical studies have indicated that older subjects are more likely to exhibit the side effects associated with the tricyclic antidepressants (e.g., confusion, visual and auditory hallucinations, hypotension, twitching, ataxia, and atropine-like delirium) and with the MAO inhibitors (Fann, 1976; Salzman, Shader, & Harmatz, 1975). Older subjects are also more sensitive to lower doses of these antidepressant medications. Imipramine, for example, has been shown to produce more sedation among elderly research volunteers (Salzman et al., 1975). A relationship may exist between the higher incidence of depression found for the elderly (Lipton, 1976; Stotsky, 1975) and the evidence concerning lowered levels of brain amines and increased MAO activity during aging (Finch, 1977; Lipton, 1976). The important finding that some antidepressants take several weeks to produce a clinical effect yet induce immediate alterations in catecholamine and indoleamine reuptake must be explored. The EEG could be a useful measure in future studies focusing on these issues. It may become a meaningful index in studies of aging, biochemical changes, and the affective disorders.

REFERENCES

Andermann, K., & Stoller, A. EEG in hospitalized and non-hospitalized aged. *Electroencephalography and Clinical Neurophysiology,* 1961, *13,* 319. (Abstract)

Ban, T. A. Pharmacotherapy of depression–A critical review. *Psychosomatics,* 1975, *16,* 17–20.

Beck, E. C., & Dustman, R. E. Developmental electrophysiology of brain function as reflected by changes in the evoked response. In J. W. Prescott, M. S. Read, & D. B. Coursin (Eds.), *Brain function and malnutrition.* New York: Wiley, 1975.

Beck, E. C., Dustman, R. E., & Lewis, E. G. The use of the averaged evoked potential in the evaluation of central nervous system disorders. *International Journal of Neurology,* 1976, *9,* 211–232.

Beck, E. C., Dustman, R. E., & Schenkenberg, T. Life span changes in the electrical activity of the human brain as reflected in the cerebral evoked response. In J. M. Ordy & K. R. Brizzee (Eds.), *Neurobiology of aging.* New York: Plenum Press, 1975.

Berger, P. A. Antidepressant medications and the treatment of depressions. In J. P. Barchas, P. A. Berger, R. D. Ciaranello, & G. R. Elliott (Eds.), *Psychopharmacology: From theory to practice.* New York: Oxford, 1977.

Blum, R. H. Alpha-rhythm responsiveness in normal, schizophrenic, and brain damaged persons. *Science,* 1957, *126,* 749–750.

Borbèly, A. A. *Pharmacological modifications of evoked brain potentials.* Stuttgart: Hans Huber, 1973.

Bradley, D. B. The central action of certain drugs in relation to the reticular formation of the brain. In H. H. Jasper, L. D. Proctor, R. S. Knighton, W. C. Noshaw, & R. T. Costello (Eds.), *Reticular formation of the brain.* Boston: Little Brown, 1958.

Brent, G. A., Smith, D. B. D., Thompson, L. W., & Michalewski, H. J. Differences in the evoked potential in young and old subjects during habituation and dishabituation procedures. *Psychophysiology,* 1977, *14,* 96. (Abstract)

Buchsbaum, M., & Fedio, P. Hemispheric differences in evoked potentials to verbal and nonverbal stimuli in the left and right visual fields. *Physiology and Behavior,* 1970, *5,* 207–210.

Busse, E. W., Barnes, R. H., Friedman, E. L., & Kelty, E. J. Psychological functioning of aged individuals with normal and abnormal electroencephalograms. *Journal of Nervous and Mental Diseases,* 1956, *124,* 135–141.

Busse, E. W., Barnes, R. H., Silverman, A. J., Shy, G. M., Thaler, M., & Frost, L. L. Studies of the aging process: Factors that influence the psyche of elderly persons. *American Journal of Psychiatry,* 1954, *110,* 897–903.

Busse, E. W., & Obrist, W. D. Significance of focal electroencephalographic changes in the elderly. *Postgraduate Medicine,* 1963, *34,* 179–182.

Butler, S. R., & Glass, A. Asymmetries in the CNV over left and right hemispheres while subjects await numeric information. *Biological Psychology,* 1974, *2,* 1–16.

Callaway, E. *Brain electrical potentials and individual psychological differences.* New York: Grune & Stratton, 1975.

Cigànek, L. Visual evoked responses. *The handbook of electroencephalography and clinical neurophysiology.* In P. Buser (Ed.), *Electrical reactions of the brain and complementary methods of evaluation.* Amsterdam: Elsevier, 1975.

Cohen, J. Maturation of the contingent negative variation. *Electroencephalography and Clinical Neurophysiology,* 1970, *28,* 99. (Abstract)

Cohen, J. The CNV in children with special reference to learning disabilities. In W. C. McCallum & J. R. Knott (Eds.), *Event-related slow potentials of the brain: Their relations to behavior.* Amsterdam: Elsevier, 1973.

Cooper, R., Osselton, J. W., & Shaw, J. C. *EEG technology.* London: Butterworths, 1969.

Davidson, K. EEG activation after intravenous amitriptyline. *Journal of Electroencephalography and Clinical Neurophysiology,* 1965, *19,* 298–300.

Davis, H. Brain stem and other responses in electric response audiometry. *Annals of Otology, Rhinology, and Laryngology,* 1976, *85,* 1-12.

Deecke, L., Scheid, P., & Kornhuber, H. Distribution of readiness potential, pre-motion positivity, and motor potential of the human cerebral cortex preceding voluntary finger movements. *Experimental Brain Research,* 1969, *7,* 158–168.

Delay, J., & Deniker, P. Efficacy of Trofanil in the treatment of various types of depression: A comparison with other antidepressant drugs. *Canadian Psychological Association Journal,* 1959, *4,* 100–112. (Suppl.)

Delse, F. C., Marsh, G. R., & Thompson, L. W. CNV correlates of task difficulty and accuracy of pitch discrimination. *Psychophysiology,* 1972, *9,* 53–62.

Desmedt, J. E. *Visual evoked potentials: New developments.* Oxford: London, 1977.

Dimond, S. J., & Beaumont, J. G. *Hemisphere function in the human brain.* London: Paul Elek, 1974.

Donchin, E., Gerbrandt, L. K., Leifer, L., & Tucker, L. R. Contingent negative variations and motor responses. In W. C. McCallum & J. R. Knott (Eds.), *Event-related slow potentials of the brain: Their relations to behavior.* Amsterdam: Elsevier, 1973.

Donchin, E., & Lindsley, D. B. *Average evoked potentials: Methods, results, and evaluations.* Washington, D.C.: U.S. Government Printing Office, 1969.

Dunleavy, D. L. F., Brezinova, V., Oswald, I., Maclean, A. W., & Tinker, M. Changes during weeks in effects of tricyclic drugs on the human sleeping brain. *British Journal of Psychiatry,* 1972, *120,* 663–672.

Dustman, R. E., & Beck, E. C. The effects of maturation and aging on the wave form of visually evoked potentials. *Electroencephalograpy and Clinical Neurophysiology,* 1969, *26,* 2–11.

Dustman, R. E., and Beck, E. C. Visually evoked potentials: Amplitude changes with age. *Science,* 1966, *151,* 1013–1015.

Eason, R. G., Groves, P., White, C. T., & Oden, D. Evoked cortical potentials: Relation to visual field and handedness. *Science,* 1967, *156,* 1643–1646.

Eason, R. G., Oden, D., & White, C. T. Visually evoked potentials and reaction time in relation to site of stimulation. *Electroencephalography and Clinical Neurophysiology,* 1967, *22,* 313–324.

Eason, R. G., & White, C. T. Averaged occipital responses to stimulation in the nasal and temporal halves of the retina. *Psychonomic Science,* 1967, *7,* 309–310.

Fann, W. T. Pharmacotherapy in older depressed patients. *Journal of Gerontology,* 1976, *31,* 304–310.

Feinsod, M., & Hoyt, W. F. Subcortical optic neuropathy in multiple sclerosis. *Journal of Neurology, Neurosurgery, and Psychiatry,* 1975, *38,* 1109–1114.

Finch, C. E. Neuroendocrine and autonomic aspects of aging. In C. E. Finch & L. Hayflick (Eds.), *Handbook of the biology of aging.* New York: Van Nostrand, 1977.

Fink, M. Electroencephalographic and behavioral effects of Trofanil. *Canadian Psychological Association Journal,* 1959, *4,* 166–171. (Suppl.)

Fink, M. Quantitative electroencephalography and human psychopharmacology I: Frequency spectra and drug action. *Medicina Experimentales,* 1961, *5,* 364–369.

Fink, M. Quantitative EEG in psychopharmacology: II. Drug patterns. In G. H. Glaser (Ed.), *EEG and behavior.* New York: Basic Books, 1963.

Fink, M. EEG classification of psychoactive compounds in man: Review and theory of behavioral associations. In D. H. Efron (Ed.), *Psychopharmacology: A review of progress 1957–1967* (U.S. Public Health Service Publication No. 1836). Washington, D.C.: U.S. Government Printing Office, 1968.

Fink, M. EEG profiles and probability measures of psychoactive drugs. In T. M. Itil (Ed.), *Psychotropic drugs and the human EEG.* Basel: S. Karger, 1974.

Fink, M. Quantitative EEG analysis and psychopharmacology. In A. Rèmond (Ed.), *EEG informatic: A didactic review of methods and applications of EEG data processing.* Amsterdam: Elsevier, 1977.

Fink, M., & Itil, T. M. EEG and human psychopharmacology: Clinical antidepressants. In D. H. Efron (Ed.), *Psychopharmacology: A review of progress 1957–1967* (U.S. Public Health Service Publication No. 1836). Washington, D.C.: U.S. Government Printing Office, 1968.

Fink, M., Pollack, M., Klein, D. F., Blumberg, A. G., Belmont, I., Karp, E., Kramer, J. C., & Willner, A. Comparative studies of chlorpromazine and imipramine. I. Drug discriminating patterns. In P. B. Bradley, F. Flugel, & P. H. Hock (Eds.), *Neuropsychopharmacology* (Vol. 3). New York: Elsevier, 1962.

Frey, T. S., & Sjögren, H. The electroencephalogram in elderly persons suffering from neuropsychiatric disorders. *Acta Psychologica et Neurologica,* 1959, *34,* 438–450.

Friedlander, W. J. Electroencephalographic alpha rate in adults as a function of age. *Geriatrics,* 1958, *13,* 29–31.

Friedman, D., Simson, R., Ritter, W., & Rapin, I. Cortical evoked potentials elicited by real speech words and human sounds. *Electroencephalography and Clinical Neurophysiology,* 1975, *38,* 13–19.

Gaillard, A. W., & Näätänen, R. Slow potential changes and choice reaction time as a function of interstimulus interval. *Acta Psychologica,* 1973, *37,* 173–186.

Galambos, R., Benson, P., Smith, T. S., Schulman-Galambos, C., & Osier, H. On hemispheric differences in evoked potentials to speech stimuli. *Electroencephalography and Clinical Neurophysiology,* 1975, *39,* 279–283.

Garcia-Austt, E., Bogacz, J., & Vanzulli, A. Effects of attention and inattention upon visual evoked response. *Electroencephalography and Clinical Neurophysiology,* 1964, *17,* 136–143.

Gerson, I. M., John, E. R., Bartlett, F., & Koenig, V. Average evoked response (AER) in the electroencephalographic diagnosis of the normally aging brain: A practical application. *Clinical Electroencephalography,* 1976, *7,* 77–91.

Glaser, G. H. The normal electroencephalogram and its reactivity. In G. H. Glaser (Ed.), *EEG and behavior.* New York: Basic Books, 1963.

Greenblatt, M. Age and electroencephalographic abnormality in neuropsychiatric patients. *American Journal of Psychiatry,* 1944, *101,* 82–90.

Gullickson, G. R. CNV and behavioral attention to a glide-tone warning of interesting non-moving or kaleidoscopic visual or auditory patterns in 2- and 3-year-old children. In W. C. McCallum & J. R. Knott (Eds.), *Event-related slow potentials of the brain: Their relations to behavior.* Amsterdam: Elsevier, 1973.

Gullickson, G. R., & Darrow, C. W. Contingent negative variation modified by respiratory phase. In W. C. McCallum & J. R. Knott (Eds.), *Event-related slow potentials of the brain: Their reactions to behavior.* Amsterdam: Elsevier, 1973.

Halliday, A. M. Changes in the form of cerebral evoked responses in man associated with various lesions of the nervous system. In L. Widen (Ed.), *Recent advances in clinical neurophysiology.* Amsterdam: Elsevier, 1967.

Halliday, A. M. Somatosensory evoked responses. *The handbook of electroencephalography and clinical neurophysiology.* In P. Buser (Ed.), *Electrical reactions of the brain and complementary methods of evaluation.* Amsterdam: Elsevier, 1975.

Hamilton, C. E., Peters, J. F., & Knott, J. R. Task initiation and amplitude of the contingent negative variation (CNV). *Electroencephalography and Clinical Neurophysiology,* 1973, *34,* 587–592.

Hartmann, E. Effects of psychotropic drugs on desynchronized sleep. In T. M. Itil (Ed.), *Psychotropic drugs and the human EEG.* Basel: S. Karger, 1974.

Harvald, B. EEG in old age. *Acta Psychologica et Neurologica,* 1958, *33,* 193–196.

Hata, H. Dissociation between the tonic and the phasic events during REM sleep by the administration of some neuroactive drugs. *Journal of Electroencephalography and Clinical Neurophysiology,* 1975, *39,* 543.

Hillyard, S. A. The CNV and human behavior. In W. C. McCallum & J. R. Knott (Eds.), *Event-related slow potentials of the brain: Their relations to behavior.* Amsterdam: Elsevier, 1973.

Itil, M. Electroencephalography and pharmacology. In F. A. Freyhan, W. Petrilovitsch, & P. Pinchot (Eds.), *Clinical psychopharmacology.* Basel: S. Karger, 1968.

Itil, M. Quantitative pharmaco-EEG–A new approach to the discovery of a psychotropic drug. In T. A. Ban (Ed.), *Psychopharmacology, sexual disorders, and drug abuse.* New York: Elsevier, 1973.

Itil, M. Quantitative pharmaco-electroencephalography. Use of computerized cerebral potentials in psychotropic drug research. In T. M. Itil, (Ed.), *Psychotropic drugs and the human EEG.* Basel: S. Karger, 1974.

Itil, T. M., Polvan, N., & Hsu, N. Clinical and EEG effects of GB-94, a "tetracyclic" antidepressant (EEG model in discovery of a new psychotropic drug). *Current Therapeutic Research,* 1972, *14,* 395–413.

Itil, T. M., Saletu, B., & Akpinar, S. Classification of psychotropic drugs on digital computer sleep prints. In T. M. Itil (Ed.), *Psychotropic drugs and the human EEG.* Basel: S. Karger, 1974.

Itil, T. M., Shapiro, D., & Fink, M. Differentiation of psychotropic drugs by quantitative EEG analysis. *Agressologie,* 1968, *9,* 267–279.

Itil, T. M., Shapiro, D. M., Fink, M., Kiremitci, N., & Hickman, C. Quantitative EEG studies of chlordiazepoxide, chlorpromazine, and imipramine in volunteers and schizophrenic subjects. In W. O. Evans & N. S. Kline (Eds.), *The psychopharmacology of the normal human.* Springfield, Ill.: Charles C Thomas, 1969.

Järvilehto, T., & Frühstorfer, H. Differentiation between slow cortical potentials associated with motor and mental acts in man. *Experimental Brain Research,* 1970, *11,* 309–317.

Järvilehto, T., & Frühstorfer, H. Is the sound-evoked DC potential a contingent negative variation? In W. C. McCallum & J. R. Knott (Eds.), *Event-related slow potentials of the brain: Their relations to behavior.* Amsterdam: Elsevier, 1973.

Jewett, D. L. Volume conducted potentials in response to auditory stimuli as detected by averaging in the cat. *Electroencephalography and Clinical Neurophysiology,* 1970, *28,* 609–618.

Jewett, D. L., Romano, M. N., & Williston, J. S. Human auditory evoked potentials: Possible brainstem components detected on the scalp. *Science,* 1970, *167,* 1517–1518.

Jewett, D. L., & Williston, J. S. Auditory evoked far-fields averaged from the scalp of humans. *Brain,* 1971, *94,* 681–696.

John, E. R., Herrington, R. N., & Sutton, S. Effects of visual form on the evoked response. *Science,* 1967, *155,* 1439–1442.

Jones, D. P., Binnie, C. D., Bown, R. L., Lloyd, D. S. L., & Watson, B. W. The contingent negative variation and psychological findings in chronic hepatic encephalopathy. *Electroencephalography and Clinical Neurophysiology,* 1976, *40,* 661–665.

Kiloh, L. G., Davison, K., & Osselton, J. W. An electroencephalographic study of the analeptic effects of imipramine. *Journal of Electroencephalography and Clinical Neurophysiology,* 1961, *13,* 216–223.

Kiloh, L. G., McComas, A. J., & Osselton, J. W. *Clinical electroencephalography.* New York: Appleton-Century-Crofts, 1972.

Kooi, K. A. *Fundamentals of electroencephalography.* New York: Harper & Row, 1971.

Kooi, K. A., Guvener, A. M., & Bagchi, B. K. Visual evoked responses in lesions of the higher optic pathways. *Neurology,* 1965, *15,* 841–854.

Kornhuber, H. H., & Deecke, L. Hirnpotentialanderungen bei Willkurbewegungen und passiven Bewegungen des Menschen: Bereitshaftspotential und reafferente Potentiale. *Pflugers Archiv für die gesamte Physiologie des Menchen und der Tiere,* 1965, *284,* 1–17.

Kupfer, D. J., Foster, F. G., Reich, L. Thompson, K. S., & Weiss, B. EEG sleep changes in depression. *American Journal of Psychiatry,* 1976, *133,* 622–626.

Lacey, J. I. Somatic response patterning and stress: Some revisions of activation theory. In M. H. Appley & R. Turnbull (Eds.), *Psychological stress: Some issues in research.* New York: Appleton-Century-Crofts, 1967.

Lacey, J. I., & Lacey, B. C. Experimental association and dissociation of phasic bradycardia and vertex-negative waves: A psychophysiological study of attention and response-intention. In W. C. McCallum & J. R. Knott (Eds.), *Event-related slow potentials of the brain: Their relations to behavior.* Amsterdam: Elsevier, 1973.

Lader, M. Effects of psychotropic drugs on auditory evoked potentials in man. In J. E. Desmedt (Ed.), *Auditory evoked potentials in man. Psychopharmacology correlates of EPs.* Basel: S. Karger, 1977.

Lechner, H. EEG changes with thymoleptic drugs in endogenous depressive psychosis: Clinical correlations. *Journal of Electroencephalography and Clinical Neurophysiology,* 1963, *15,* 134.

Lee, R. G., & Blair, R. D. G. Evolution of EEG and visual evoked response changes in Jakob-Creutzfeldt disease. *Electroencephalography and Clinical Neurophysiology,* 1973, *35,* 133–142.

Lehmann, D., & Fender, D. H. Monocularly evoked electroencephalogram potentials: Influence of target structure presented to the other eye. *Nature,* 1967, *215,* 204–205.

Leonard, B. E. Neurochemical and neuropharmacological aspects of depression. *International Review of Neurobiology,* 1975, *18,* 357–387.

Liberson, W. T. Functional electroencephalography in mental disorders. *Diseases of the Nervous System,* 1944, *5,* 357–364.

Liberson, W. T. Study of evoked potentials in aphasics. *American Journal of Physical Medicine,* 1966, *45,* 135–142.

Liberson, W. T., & Seguin, C. A. Brain waves and clinical features in arteriosclerotic and senile mental patients. *Psychonomic Medicine,* 1945, *7,* 30–35.

Lindsley, D. B. Electrical potentials of the brain in children and adults. *Journal of General Psychology,* 1938, *19,* 285–306.

Lindsley, D. B. Physiological psychology. *Annual Review of Psychology,* 1956, *7,* 323–348.

Lindsley, D. B., Schreiner, L. H., Knowles, W. B., & Magoun, H. W. Behavioral and EEG changes following chronic brain stem lesions in the cat. *Electroencephalography and Clinical Neurophysiology,* 1950, *2,* 483–498.

Lipton, M. A. Age differentiation in depression: Biochemical aspects. *Journal of Gerontology,* 1976, *31,* 293–299.

Lombroso, C. T. The CNV during tasks requiring choice. In C. R. Evans & T. B. Mulholland (Eds.), *Attention in neurophysiology.* London: Butterworths, 1969.

Longo, V. G. Effects of drugs on the EEG. In V. G. Longo (Ed.), *Handbook of electroencephalography and clinical neurophysiology,* 1977, Whole No. 7 (Pt. C).

Loveless, N. E. The contingent negative variation related to preparatory set in a reaction time situation with variable foreperiod. *Electroencephalography and Clinical Neurophysiology,* 1973, *35,* 369-374.

Loveless, N. E., & Sanford, A. J. Effects of age on the contingent negative variation and preparatory set in a reaction-time task. *Journal of Gerontology,* 1974, *29,* 52-63.

Loveless, N. E., & Sanford, A. J. Slow potential correlates of preparatory set. *Biological Psychology,* 1975, *2,* 217-226.

Low, M. D., Frost, J. D., Maulsby, R. L., & McSherry, W. Electroencephalographic correlates of preparation set. *Electroencephalography and Clinical Neurophysiology,* 1968, *24,* 286. (Abstract)

Low, M. D., & McSherry, A. B. Further observations of psychological factors involved in CNV genesis. *Electroencephalography and Clinical Neurophysiology,* 1968, *25,* 203-207.

Low, M. D., & Stoilen, L. CNV and EEG in children: Maturational characteristics and findings in the MCD syndrome. In W. C. McCallum & J. R. Knott (Eds.), *Event-related slow potentials of the brain: Their relations to behavior.* Amsterdam: Elsevier, 1973.

Lüders, H. The effects of aging on the wave form of the somatosensory cortical evoked potential. *Electroencephalography and Clinical Neurophysiology,* 1970, *29,* 450-460.

Marsh, G. R., & Thompson, L. W. Effect of verbal and non-verbal psychological set on hemispheric asymmetries in the CNV. In W. C. McCallum & J. R. Knott (Eds.), *Event-related slow potentials of the brain: Their relations to behavior.* Amsterdam: Elsevier, 1973.

Matsumiya, Y., Tagliasco, V., Lombroso, C. T., & Goodglass, H. Auditory evoked response: Meaningfulness of stimuli and interhemispheric asymmetry. *Science,* 1972, *175,* 790-792.

McAdam, D. W. Increases in CNS excitability during negative cortical slow potentials in man. *Electroencephalography and Clinical Neurophysiology,* 1969, *26,* 216-219.

McAdam, D. W., Knott, J. R., & Rebert, C. S. Cortical slow potential changes in man related to interstimulus interval and to pre-trial prediction of interstimulus interval. *Psychophysiology,* 1969, *5,* 349-358.

McAdam, D. W., & Rubin, E. H. Readiness potential, vertex, positive wave, contingent negative variation, and accuracy of perception. *Electroencephalography and Clinical Neurophysiology,* 1971, *30,* 511-517.

McAdam, D. W., & Seales, D. M. Bereitshaftspotential enhancement with increased level of motivation. *Electroencephalography and Clinical Neurophysiology,* 1969, *27,* 73-75.

McAdam, D. W., & Whitaker, H. A. Language production: Electroencephalographic localization in the normal brain. *Science,* 1971, *172,* 499-502.

McCallum, W. C., & Cummins, B. The effects of brain lesions on the contingent negative variation in neurosurgical patients. *Electroencephalography and Clinical Neurophysiology,* 1973, *35,* 449-456.

McCallum, W. C., & Walter, W. G. The effects of attention and distraction on the contingent negative variation in normal and neurotic subjects. *Electroencephalography and Clinical Neurophysiology,* 1968, *25,* 319-329.

Metcalf, D. R. Electroencephalography. In J. W. Prescott, M. S. Read, & D. B. Coursen (Eds.), *Brain function and malnutrition.* New York: Wiley, 1975.

Michalewski, H. J. *Lateralized cerebral processing and the development of hemispheric slow potentials—The CNV.* Unpublished doctoral dissertation, Simon Fraser University, Burnaby, British Columbia, 1976.

Michalewski, H. J., & Weinberg, H. Observations of the CNV during a simple auditory task. *Physiological Psychology,* 1976, *4,* 451-456.

Michalewski, H. J., Weinberg, H., & Patterson, J. The contingent negative variation (CNV) and speech production: Slow potentials and the area of Broca. *Biological Psychology,* 1977, *5,* 83-96.

Milner, B. Interhemispheric differences in the localization of psychological processes. *British Medical Bulletin,* 1971, *27,* 272-277.

Mirsky, A. F., & Cardon, P. V. A comparison of the behavioral and physiological changes accompanying sleep deprivation and chlorpromazine administration in man. *Electroencephalography and Clinical Neurophysiology,* 1962, *14,* 1-10.

Moruzzi, G., & Magoun, H. W. Brain stem reticular formation and activation of the EEG. *Electroencephalography and Clinical Neurophysiology,* 1949, *1,* 455-473.

Mundy-Castle, A. C. Central excitability in the aged. In H. T. Blumenthal (Ed.), *Medical and clinical aspects of aging.* New York: Columbia University Press, 1962.

Nöel, P., & Desmedt, J. E. Somatosensory cerebral evoked potentials after vascular lesions of the brain-stem and diencephalon. *Brain,* 1975, *98,* 113-128.

Obrist, W. D. The electroencephalogram of healthy aged males. In *Human aging: A biological and behavioral study* (U.S. Public Health Service Publication No. 986). Washington, D.C.: U.S. Government Printing Office, 1963.

Obrist, W. D. Cerebral ischemia and the senescent electroencephalogram. In E. Simonson & T. H. McGavack (Eds.), *Cerebral ischemia.* Springfield, Ill.: Charles C Thomas, 1964.

Obrist, W. D. Electroencephalographic approach to age changes in response to speed. In A. T. Welford & J. E. Birren (Eds.), *Behavior, aging and the nervous system.* Springfield, Ill.: Charles C Thomas, 1965.

Obrist, W. D. Problems of aging. *The handbook of electroencephalography and clinical neurophysiology,* A. Remond, Editor-in-chief. In E. G. Chatrian & G. C. Lairy (Eds.), *The EEG of the waking adult.* Amsterdam: Elsevier, 1976.

Obrist, W. D., & Busse, E. W. The electroencephalogram in old age. In W. P. Wilson (Ed.), *Applications of electroencephalography in psychiatry.* Durham, N.C.: Duke University Press, 1965.

Papakostopoulos, D. CNV and autonomic function: A review. In W. C. McCallum & J. R. Knott (Eds.), *Event-related slow potentials of the brain: Their relations to behavior.* Amsterdam: Elsevier, 1973.

Papakostopoulos, D., & McCallum, W. C. The CNV and autonomic change in situations of increasing complexity. In W. C. McCallum & J. R. Knott (Eds.), *Event-related slow potentials of the brain: Their relations to behavior.* Amsterdam: Elsevier, 1973.

Perry, N. W., & Childers, D. G. *The human visual evoked response.* Springfield, Ill.: Charles C Thomas, 1969.

Peters, J. F., Knott, J. R., Miller, L. H., Van Veen, W., & Cohen, S. Response variables and magnitude of the contingent negative variation. *Electroencephalography and Clinical Neurophysiology,* 1970, *29,* 608-611.

Poon, L. W., Thompson, L. W., Williams, R. B., & Marsh, G. R. Changes of anterio-posterior distribution of CNV and late positive component as a function of information processing demands. *Psychophysiology,* 1974, *11,* 660-673.

Regan, D. *Evoked potentials in psychology, physiology and clinical medicine.* New York: Wiley, 1972.

Reitan, R. M. Neurological and physiological bases of psychopathology. *Annual Review of Psychology,* 1976, *27,* 189-216.

Ritter, W., & Vaughan, H. G. Averaged evoked responses in vigilance and discrimination: A reassessment. *Science,* 1969, *164,* 326-328.

Robinson, D. N., & Sabat, S. R. Sensory psychopharmacology. *Current developments in psychopharmacology* (Vol. 2). New York: Spectrum, 1975.

Rohrbaugh, J. W., Syndulko, K., & Lindsley, D. B. Brain wave components of the contingent negative variation in humans. *Science,* 1976, *191,* 1055-1057.

Routtenberg, A. The two-arousal hypothesis: Reticular formation and limbic system. *Psychological Review,* 1968, *75,* 51–80.

Ruben, R. J., Elberling, C., & Salomon, G. *Electrocochleography.* Baltimore: University Park Press, 1976.

Saletu, B. Classification of psychotropic drugs based on human evoked potentials. In T. M. Itil (Ed.), *Psychotropic drugs and the human EEG.* Basel: S. Karger, 1974.

Saletu, B., Saletu, M., & Itil, T. M. Effects of tricyclic antidepressants on the somatosensory evoked potential in man. *Psychopharmacologia,* 1973, *29,* 1–12.

Salzman, C., Shader, R. I., & Harmatz, J. S. Response of the elderly to psychotropic drugs: Predictable or idiosyncratic? In S. Gershon & A. Raskin (Eds.), *Aging* (Vol. 2). New York: Raven, 1975.

Satterfield, J. H. Evoked response enhancement and attention in man: A study of responses to auditory and shock stimuli. *Electroencephalography and Clinical Neurophysiology,* 1965, *19,* 470–475.

Schaie, J. P., & Syndulko, K. CNV component and cardiac correlates of time estimation and reaction time performance in the elderly. *Psychophysiology,* 1977, *14,* 92. (Abstract)

Schildkraut, J. J. The catecholamine hypothesis of affective disorders: A review of supporting evidence. *American Journal of Psychiatry,* 1965, *122,* 509–522.

Schildkraut, J. J., Draskoczy, P. R., Gershon, E. S., Reich, P., & Grab, E. L. Effects of tricyclic antidepressants on norepinephrine metabolism: Basic and clinical studies. In B. T. Ho & W. McIsaac (Eds.), *Brain chemistry and mental disease.* New York: Plenum Press, 1971.

Serra, C., Municchi, L., & Logoluso, R. Electroencephalographic and clinical changes induced by acute and chronic administration of amitriptyline to psychotic patients. *Journal of Electroencephalography and Clinical Neurophysiology,* 1963, *15,* 920.

Shagass, C. Pharmacology of evoked potentials in man. In D. H. Efron (Ed.), *Psychopharmacology: A review of progress 1957-1967* (U.S. Public Health Service Publication No. 1836). Washington, D.C.: U.S. Government Printing Office, 1968.

Shagass, C. *Evoked brain potentials in psychiatry.* New York: Plenum Press, 1972.

Shagass, C. Effects of psychotropic drugs on human evoked potentials. In T. M. Itil (Ed.), *Psychotropic drugs and the human EEG.* Basel: S. Karger, 1974.

Shagass, C., & Schwartz, M. Cerebral cortical reactivity in psychotic depressions. *Archives of General Psychiatry,* 1962, *6,* 235–242.

Shagass, C., & Schwartz, M. Evoked potential studies in psychiatric patients. *Annals of the New York Academy of Sciences,* 1964, *112,* 526–542.

Shagass, C., & Schwartz, M. Age, personality, and somatosensory cerebral evoked responses. *Science,* 1965, *148,* 1359–1361.

Shagass, C., Schwartz, M., & Amadeo, M. Some drug effects on evoked cerebral potentials in man. *Journal of Neuropsychiatry,* 1962, *3,* 549–558.

Shagass, C., Straumanis, J. J., & Overton, D. A. Effects of lithium and amitriptyline therapy on somatosensory evoked response "excitability" measurements. *Psychopharmacologia,* 1973, *29,* 185–196.

Shipley, T. Evoked brain potentials and sensory interaction in the retarded child. *American Journal of Mental Deficiency,* 1970, *74,* 517–523.

Skinner, P., & Shimota, J. A comparison of the effects of sedatives on the auditory evoked cortical response. *Journal of the American Audiology Society,* 1975, *1,* 71–78.

Spong, P., Haider, M., & Lindsley, D. B. Selective attentiveness and cortical evoked responses to visual and auditory stimuli. *Science,* 1965, *148,* 395–397.

Starr, A., & Achor, J. Auditory brain stem responses in neurological disease. *Archives of Neurology,* 1975, *32,* 761–768.

Starr, A., & Hamilton, A. E. Correlation between confirmed sites of neurological lesions and abnormalities of far-field auditory brainstem responses. *Electroencephalography and Clinical Neurophysiology,* 1976, *41,* 595–608.

Storm van Leeuween, W. Auditory evoked potentials. *The handbook of electroencephalography and Clinical Neurophysiology.* In P. Buser (Ed.), *Electrical reactions of the brain and complementary methods of evaluation.* Amsterdam: Elsevier, 1975.

Stotsky, B. A. Psychoactive drugs for geriatric patients with psychiatric disorders. In A. Gershon & A. Raskin (Eds.), *Aging* (Vol. 2). New York: Raven, 1975.

Surwillo, W. W. The relation of simple response time to brain wave frequency and the effects of age. *Electroencephalography and Clinical Neurophysiology,* 1963, *15,* 105–114. (a)

Surwillo, W. W. The relation of response-time variability to age and the influence of brain wave frequency. *Electroencephalography and Clinical Neurophysiology,* 1963, *15,* 1029–1032. (b)

Surwillo, W. W. The relation of decision time to brain wave frequency and to age. *Electroencephalography and Clinical Neurophysiology,* 1964, *16,* 510–514. (a)

Surwillo, W. W. Some observations of the relation of response speed to photic stimulation under conditions of EEG synchronization. *Electroencephalography and Clinical Neurophysiology,* 1964, *17,* 194–198. (b)

Sutton, S., Tueting, P., & Zubin, J. Information delivery and the sensory evoked potential. *Science,* 1967, *155,* 1436–1439.

Tecce, J. J. Contingent negative variation (CNV) and psychological processes in man. *Psychological Bulletin,* 1972, *77,* 73–108.

Tecce, J. J., & Cole, J. O. Amphetamine effects in man: Paradoxical drowsiness and lowered electrical brain activity (CNV). *Science,* 1974, *185,* 451–453.

Tecce, J. J., & Cole, J. O. The distraction-arousal hypothesis, CNV, and schizophrenia. In D. I. Mostofsky (Ed.), *Behavior control and modification of physiological activity.* Englewood Cliffs, N.J.: Prentice-Hall, 1976.

Tecce, J. J., & Hamilton, B. T. CNV reduction by sustained cognitive distraction. In W. C. McCallum & J. R. Knott (Eds.), *Event-related slow potentials of the brain: Their relations to behavior.* Amsterdam: Elsevier, 1973.

Tecce, J. J., Savignano-Bowman, J., & Meinbresse, D. Contingent negative variation and the distraction-arousal hypothesis. *Electroencephalography and Clinical Neurophysiology,* 1976, *41,* 277–286.

Tecce, J. J., & Scheff, N. M. Attention reduction and suppressed direct-current potentials in the human brain. *Science,* 1969, *164,* 331–333.

Thompson, L. W. Cerebral blood flow, EEG, and behavior in aging. In R. D. Terry & S. Gershon (Eds.), *Neurobiology of aging.* New York: Raven Press, 1976.

Thompson, L. W., & Botwinick, J. Age differences in the relationship between EEG arousal and reaction time. *The Journal of Psychology,* 1968, *68,* 167–172.

Thompson, L. W., & Marsh, G. R. Psychophysiological studies of aging. In C. Eisdorfer & M. P. Lawton (Eds.), *The psychology of adult development and aging.* Washington, D.C.: American Psychological Association, 1973.

Thompson, L. W., & Nowlin, J. B. Relation of increased attention to central and autonomic nervous system states. In L. F. Jarvik, C. Eisdorfer, & J. E. Blum (Eds.), *Intellectual functioning in adults.* New York: Springer, 1973.

Thompson, L. W., & Wilson, S. Electrocortical reactivity and learning in the elderly. *Journal of Gerontology,* 1966, *21,* 45–51.

Thompson, R. F., & Patterson, M. M. (Eds.). *Bioelectric recording techniques* (3 vols.). New York: Academic Press, 1973–1974.

Timsit-Berthier, M., Delaunoy, J., Koninckx, N., & Rousseau, J. C. Slow potential changes in psychiatry. I. Contingent negative variation. *Electroencephalography and Clinical Neurophysiology,* 1973, *35,* 355–361.

Timsit-Berthier, M., Delaunoy, J., & Rousseau, J. C. Slow potential changes in psychiatry. II. Motor potential. *Electroencephalography and Clinical Neurophysiology,* 1973, *35,* 363–367.

Timsit-Berthier, M., Koninckx, N., Dargent, J., Fontaine, O., & Dongier, M. Variations Contingentes Negatives en Psychiatrie. *Electroencephalography and Clinical Neurophysiology,* 1970, *28,* 41–47.

Tsumoto, T., Hirose, N., Nonaka, S., & Takahashi, M. Cerebrovascular disease: Changes in somatosensory evoked potentials associated with unilateral lesions. *Electroencephalography and Clinical Neurophysiology,* 1973, *35,* 463–473.

Velasco, M., & Velasco, F. Correlation between the psychological significance of stimuli and the amplitude of the cortical somatic evoked potential in man. *Electroencephalography and Clinical Neurophysiology,* 1972, *33,* 239. (Abstract)

Visser, S. L. Correlations between the contingent alpha blocking, EEG characteristics and clinical diagnosis. *Electroencephalography and Clinical Neurophysiology,* 1961, *13,* 438–446.

Visser, S. L., Stam, F. C., Van Tilburg, W., OpDen Velde, W., Blom, J. L., & DeRijke, W. Visual evoked response in senile and presenile dementia. *Electroencephalography and Clinical Neurophysiology,* 1976, *40,* 385–392.

Walter, W. G. Slow potential changes in the human brain associated with expectancy, decision, and intention. In W. Cobb & C. Morocutti (Eds.), *The evoked potentials.* Amsterdam: Elsevier, 1967.

Walter, W. G., Cooper, R., Aldridge, V. J., McCallum, W. C., & Winter, A. L. Contingent negative variation: An electric sign of sensorimotor association and expectancy in the human brain. *Nature,* 1964, *203,* 380–384.

Waszak, M., & Obrist, W. D. Relation of slow potential changes to response speed and motivation in man. *Electroencephalography and Clinical Neurophysiology,* 1969, *27,* 113–120.

Weerts, T. C., & Lang, P. J. The effects of eye fixation and stimulus and response locations on the contingent negative variation. *Biological Psychology,* 1973, *1,* 1–19.

Weinberg, H. The contingent negative variation: Its clinical past and future. *American Journal of EEG Technology,* 1975, *15,* 51–67.

Weinberg, H., & Papakostopoulos, D. The frontal CNV: Its dissimilarity to CNVs recorded from other sites. *Electroencephalography and Clinical Neurophysiology,* 1975, *39,* 21–28.

Weinberg, H., Walter, W. G., Cooper, R., & Aldridge, V. J. Emitted cerebral events. *Electroencephalography and Clinical Neurophysiology,* 1974, *36,* 449–456.

Wells, C. E. Response of alpha waves to light in neurologic disease. *Archives of Neurology,* 1962, *6,* 478–491.

Wells, C. E. Alpha responsiveness to light in man. In G. H. Glaser (Ed.), *EEG and behavior.* New York: Basic Books, 1963.

Wells, C. E., & Wolff, H. G. Formation of temporary cerebral connections in normal and brain-damaged subjects. *Neurology,* 1960, *10,* 335–340.

Williamson, P. D., Goff, W. R., & Allison, T. Somato-sensory evoked responses in patients with unilateral cerebral lesions. *Electroencephalography and Clinical Neurophysiology,* 1970, *28,* 566–575.

Wood, C. C., Goff, W. R., & Day, M. Auditory evoked potentials during speech perception. *Science,* 1971, *173,* 1248–1251.

Wyatt, R. J., Fram, D. H., Kupfer, D. J., & Snyder, F. Total prolonged drug-induced REM sleep suppression in anxious-depressed patients. *Archives of General Psychiatry,* 1971, *24,* 145–155.

Wyatt, R. J., Kupfer, D. J., Scott, J., Robinson, D. S., & Snyder, F. Longitudinal studies of the effect of monoamine oxidase inhibitors on sleep in man. *Psychopharmacologia* 1969, *15,* 236–244.

Zappoli, R. Electroencephalographic study of patients affected by depressive state treated with imipramine hydrochloride. *Journal of Electroencephalography and Clinical Neurophysiology,* 1959, *11,* 849.

Zimmerman, G. N., & Knott, J. R. Slow potentials of the brain related to speech processing in normal speakers and stutterers. *Electroencephalography and Clinical Neurophysiology,* 1974, *37,* 599–607.

REFERENCE NOTES

1. Rebert, C. S., Berry, R., & Merlo, J. *DC potential consequences of induced muscle tension: Effects on contingent negative variation.* Paper presented at the Third International Congress on Event-Related Slow Potentials of the Brain, Bristol, August 1973.
2. Dubrovsky, B., & Dongier, M. *Evaluation of ERSP in selected groups of psychiatric patients.* Paper presented at the Third International Congress on Event-Related Slow Potentials of the Brain, Bristol, August 1973.
3. Low, M. D., Wada, J. A., & Fox, M. *Electroencephalographic localization of conative aspects of language production in the human brain.* Paper presented at the Third International Congress on Event-Related Slow Potentials of the Brain, Bristol, August 1973.
4. Deecke, L., Englitz, H. G., & Schmitt, G. *Age-dependence of the Bereitschaftspotential.* Paper presented at the Fourth International Congresss on Event-Related Potentials of the Brain, Henderson, North Carolina, April 1976.

5

Psychiatric Rating Scales for Assessing Psychopathology in the Elderly: A Critical Review

Gerald E. Kochansky
Massachusetts Mental Health Center

"You are old, Father William," the young man said,
"And your teeth are beginning to freeze.
Your favorite daughter has wheels in her head,
And the chickens are eating your knees."

"You are right," said the old man, "I cannot deny
That my troubles are many and great.
But I'll butter my ears on the Fourth of July,
And then I'll be able to skate."

Gertrude Crampton (1950)[1]

INTRODUCTION

Through charmingly absurd images the poem about Father William touches upon some of the primary clinical and methodological issues of this chapter: the physical and psychological stresses of the elderly and the assessment of the elderly by the young. Father William's physical condition is deteriorating, he faces disappointment in his favorite offspring who is far from perfect, and he lives in an environment (the chickens) that is downright hostile toward him. The poem raises the issue of assessing impairment in the elderly, for how can we be certain that Father William's teeth are not really freezing? How can we know whether the young man's observations of the old man's teeth are valid or what the interrater reliability of his judgments is? What do Father William's butter and skating ideas indicate about his mental status? The poem also deals with the physical and psychological effects of stress upon the elderly and with

[1] From *The Little Golden Funny Book* by Gertrude Crampton. Copyright 1950 by Western Publishing Company, Inc. Used by permission of the publisher.

the ego defenses available to them for coping with impairment, loss, and disappointment. For a moment Father William seems to acknowledge cognitively and affectively the seriousness of his plight, but then he seems to slip into denial and unrealistic planning for the July Fourth holiday. Finally, the crucial issue of treatment for the elderly is seen in the butter strategy. Surely the butter will be no less efficacious than many of the treatments used over the centuries to retard or reverse the effects of aging, but what methodological problems must be overcome to accurately assess its effects?

Demographic, epidemiological, and clinical data that establish the extent and seriousness of psychiatric problems of the elderly are well documented elsewhere (e.g., Busse, 1975). Suffice it to say here that the older population of the United States has increased greatly in recent years and so have the incidence and severity of a host of physical, psychological, and social problems within this population. The stresses, vulnerabilities, and ultimate impairments of the elderly require extensive and intensive study. Such research should generate a wide range of effective, preventive, and primary therapeutic services to minimize and alleviate the ill effects of the aging processes.

The human desire to control (stop or reverse) the damaging effects of the aging processes has for centuries led man to seek out antiaging potions and drugs. The development of an armamentarium of psychotropic drugs, which empirically affect the psychological functioning of humans of varying ages, has rekindled old hopes and generated a large number of geriatric psychopharmacological investigations.

As noted by Lehmann and Ban (1975), many of these studies represent attempts to investigate "empirically, in geriatric patients, the effects of psychotropic drugs whose pharmacotherapeutic profiles have already been established in other patient groups" (p. 196). Generally speaking, the psychotropic drugs used in those studies were the established antianxiety, antidepressant, or antipsychotic agents, and the targets were symptoms of the classical psychiatric disorders (i.e., the neuroses, affective disorders, and schizophrenia). Thus, the major difference between these psychotropic drug studies with elderly patients and those focusing on younger patients was the age of the population.

The other category of psychotropic drug investigations of the elderly involves drugs that were not originally developed for treating human psychological functions and behavior. Investigators empirically explored whether such drugs might improve impaired psychological functioning of the elderly by affecting physiological processes thought to mediate such impairments. Thus, many studies of the effects of cerebral vasodilators in cognitively impaired elderly patients were generated by the hypothesis that arteriosclerotic dementia is associated with an abnormal reactivity of the cerebral blood vessels and a reduced cerebral blood flow, both of which result in a chronic state of hypoxia (Sathananthan & Gershon, 1975). The effects of hyperbaric oxygen for treatment of the hypoxic state and cognitive impairments of elderly patients suffering from dementia have also been empirically explored (Thompson, 1975). Studies of the effects of Gerovital-H3 (a buffered procaine hydrochloride) on the elderly could be included in this category of geriatric psychopharmacology investigation (Jarvik & Milne, 1975).

Despite the differences inherent in both categories of psychopharmacological studies in the elderly, both are generated by the common goal: the discovery of drugs that will produce significant therapeutic psychotropic effects in psychologically impaired elderly people. This goal requires the appropriate use of extant drugs, the discovery of new drugs that produce such effects, and a methodology to accurately assess their merits or inadequacies in the target population. This latter requirement is the central theme of this chapter.

One critical factor in the development of an adequate methodology for geriatric psychopharmacology is the availability of assessment procedures that provide an accurate (i.e., valid and reliable) measurement of relevant changes in the psychological functioning of elderly research subjects. The instruments currently available for geriatric psychopharmacological research vary considerably in focus, approach, and format. In an earlier review of rating scales for geriatric psychopharmacology, the author and his colleagues (Salzman, Kochansky, & Shader, 1972) proposed that such scales primarily focused on the behavior, mood, or cognitive functioning of elderly research subjects. At the same time, other dimensions can be used to differentiate and categorize these rating scales.

In this chapter psychiatric rating scales are defined as instruments designed to assess psychopathology that use observer ratings (usually by professional mental health workers, who are often trained in the use of the rating system) instead of self-ratings or reports (cf. chapter 6). Although rating scales for assessing nursing home and ward behavior, or what has been termed "community adjustment," usually involve observer ratings and often psychopathology assessment, these instruments are reviewed in other sections of this book. This chapter is limited to scales that assess psychopathology through (a) observer ratings of affective symptomatology, (b) observer ratings of multiple psychopathological symptomatology, and (c) mental status examinations.[2]

Before launching into a review of the rating scales, a brief description of some of the important general problems inherent in the assessment of psychopathology in research with the elderly may be helpful.

GENERAL PROBLEMS IN THE ASSESSMENT OF PSYCHOPATHOLOGY IN THE ELDERLY

Although most of the basic problems inherent in the assessment of psychopathology in the elderly are not unique to this subject population, they

[2] Mental status examinations are not necessarily observer rating scales, since parts of many mental status examinations involve questions with right or wrong answers and thus are tests.

are very much colored by important characteristics of the elderly. Some of these methodological problems are relatively minor and readily overcome, but others confront geriatric psychopharmacological researchers with formidable challenges for achieving adequate reliability and validity of their assessment instruments.

The issues that follow frequently arise in the assessment phase of geriatric psychopharmacological research. Mastery over them would greatly enhance the psychopharmacologist's ability to evaluate accurately the effects of psychotropic agents on elderly individuals.

Establishing and Maintaining Rapport with Elderly Research Subjects

Establishing and maintaining rapport with subjects of any age is important in psychopharmacological research. Self- or observer-rating systems that intimidate, fatigue, or offend research subjects jeopardize the validity and/or reliability of assessment procedures. For example, geriatric researchers have pointed out that the elderly often have limited attention spans and decreased tolerance for ambiguity (Salzman & Shader, 1975); an abhorrence of mechanical gadgetry including stopwatches (Harmatz, Note 1); and impatience or anger with items they view as irrelevant to their stage of the life cycle (many elderly subjects place items inquiring into their sexual functioning in this category) (Salzman et al., 1972).

Variable Levels of Symptomatology and Impairment in the Elderly

Although variable levels of symptomatology and impairment are not unique to the elderly population, they do make for significant problems in geriatric psychopharmacological research. Psychopharmacologists must pay careful attention to this issue when developing or selecting appropriate instruments for assessing psychopathology in the elderly.

For example, there are dramatic differences between an elderly subject who is mildly depressed or mildly demented but functioning in the community and an elderly inpatient who is severely depressed or severely demented. Self-rating scales may provide valid and reliable assessments of depression and prove to be an economical approach to mildly or moderately depressed elderly outpatients but utterly worthless for severely depressed inpatients who are psychomotorically retarded, withdrawn, negativistic, and uncooperative (Salzman et al., 1972). In a similar manner, rating scales that are highly sensitive to one part of a spectrum of psychopathology in the elderly may be virtually blind to another part. Rating scales capable of fine discriminations within the range of mild to moderate depressive symptomatology may be minimally sensitive to differences within the range of severe depressive symptoms. All-purpose rating scales would be a boon to geriatric psychopharmacology; the instruments currently available must be selected (in most instances) according to the elderly subpopulation being studied.

Age-Specific Patterns of Psychopathological Symptomatology

Clinical and research data indicate that the symptom patterns associated with the various psychiatric disorders of elderly people may differ from those characterizing other age groups. Busse (1975), for example, compared the modal depressive reaction of elderly people (the awareness of precipitants, the processes leading to depressive episodes, and symptom patterns) with that of younger individuals and concluded that their modal profiles differ in important ways. This conclusion raises doubt about the assumption that rating scales designed for and standardized on younger patient populations can be effectively used for assessing psychopathology in elderly patients. The development in recent years of rating systems designed specifically for the elderly population is helping to solve this problem, but there are relatively few scales available, and they have not been in use long enough to be fully evaluated, modified, and refined. Although the review of rating scales that follows focuses upon those designed for the elderly, scales that were designed for younger patients (especially those found to be sensitive to drug effects in psychopharmacological studies of elderly patients) are also included.

Suppression and Denial of Psychopathological Symptoms and Psychological Impairment

The suppression and/or denial of psychopathological symptoms compromises the validity of assessment instruments with all age groups. How can psychotropic drug effects be adequately evaluated when research subjects refuse to acknowledge symptoms that are the targets of the psychotropic agents? My colleagues in the Psychopharmacology Research Laboratory of the Massachusetts Mental Health Center and Harvard Medical School have observed and reported this difficulty in recent laboratory psychotropic drug studies with elderly volunteers. They (Harmatz, Note 1; Harmatz & Shader, 1975) have discussed the problem of self-presentation of many elderly research subjects, noting that this problem can compound the effects of denial, thus restricting the subject's (and the researcher's) awareness of dysphoric inner experiences. These elderly subjects had difficulty acknowledging to others certain symptomatology, especially feelings of depression, anxiety, and hostility. This phenomenon can be understood, as Harmatz and Shader have suggested, by using the "social desirability response set" construct formulated by Edwards (1957). This is the set to give responses that are deemed socially desirable. Investigators must heed this problem in designing and using scales for assessing psychopathology in the elderly. Self-rating scales are at an obvious disadvantage in this respect, unless careful controls for social desirability factors are built into the scales. Observer-rating systems that involve interviews conducted by skilled clinicians who are able to recognize and supportively probe beyond surface disavowals and intrapsychic denial of symptoms may be superior to any other method of assessment for minimizing the effects of this problem.

Differentiating Overlapping Symptomatology

In psychopathology of all age groups, the problem of differential diagnosis, often in the face of overlapping symptoms, is common to both clinicians and researchers. Both, for example, continue to debate and empirically explore the question of which diagnostic criteria meaningfully differentiate schizo-affective schizophrenia from the affective psychoses (Procci, 1976). If these disorders are in fact distinct (an issue that is also a subject of considerable debate), it is critical to effective treatment and research focused upon these diagnostic entities to identify the differentiating criteria. The use of assessment procedures that fail to differentiate adequately schizo-affective patients from those suffering from affective psychoses contaminates studies that explore the effects of psychotropic agents developed to treat one or the other disorder but not both.

In like manner, overlapping symptoms of elderly patients can befuddle and mislead the clinician and researcher, introducing significant levels of error variance at both the subject-selection and dependent variable assessment phases of geriatric psychopharmacological research and interfering with the accurate evaluation of psychotropic drug efficacy. Elderly patients who say during an assessment interview that their brains are rotting may be expressing a somatic delusion associated with a late life psychotic depression, or with schizophrenia, or may be acknowledging awareness of a progressive dementia associated with a frontal lobe syndrome. The failure of a rating scale to differentiate between these overlapping symptoms will compromise the research. Overlapping symptomatology complicates the differentiation of depression and dementia in the elderly for both clinical and research purposes. The complexity of this problem is conveyed by the concept of pseudodementia in depressed elderly patients, which Post (1975) and others have discussed (cf. chapters 1, 3, and 9, this volume).

The rating scales that are reviewed here must be evaluated in terms of both the methodological problems previously discussed and the standard criteria for evaluating the adequacy of psychological assessment instruments.

OBSERVER RATING SCALES FOR ASSESSING AFFECTIVE SYMPTOMATOLOGY

Since human emotional experiences have generally been viewed as private, inner experiences, most attempts to measure mood have relied upon self-rating formats (Salzman et al., 1972). In their pioneering work, Nowlis and Nowlis (1956) generated their own scale to assess a variety of mood states. The format requires subjects to rate themselves with adjectives that have affective connotations. Many of these self-rating mood-adjective checklists have been widely used in research, ranging from studies of mood variations in normal individuals to studies of the effects of various psychotropic agents upon mood states of psychiatric patients with affective symptoms and disorders.

Despite their utility for the study of a number of mood phenomena, self-rating mood-adjective checklists have limited value for the assessment of pathological mood disorders and symptomatology because these instruments often assess only one dimension (the affective, emotional, or feeling dimension) of multidimensional disorders. Most current formulations regarding depressive disorders postulate that depressive syndromes often involve, in addition to the emotional manifestations, significant psychomotoric, cognitive, and vegetative physical signs and symptoms (Beck, 1973). As a result, researchers interested in the study of affective disorders have developed instruments, whether self- or observer-rated, that are more comprehensive.

Although rating scales that assess multiple psychopathological symptoms often include items and factors relevant to affective disorders and symptoms, this section reviews rating scales that focus exclusively on affective symptoms. Most of these selected observer-rating mood scales concentrate on depressive symptomatology, some have been designed to assess anxiety, and a few have been developed to assess multiple moods and affects. Although a few of these instruments have been used (some successfully) in geriatric psychopharmacological investigations, it is noteworthy that only one of the scales included in this review was specifically designed for the elderly population.

Depression in the Elderly

Clinical Dimensions

Busse (1975) and others (Buehler, Keith-Spiegel, & Thomas, 1973) have observed that depression is one of the most frequent psychopathological syndromes encountered in elderly populations and that "depressive episodes increase in frequency and depth in the advanced years of life" (Busse, 1975, p. 74). Depressive disorders in the elderly, as in younger populations, range from milder forms that are difficult for the clinician to detect to those characterized by extreme dejection and hopelessness and by impairment of a variety of psychological and physical functions.

Many clinicians and researchers have proposed that depression in the elderly can differ significantly from that of younger individuals with respect to precipitants, dynamic processes and clinical manifestations. This appears to be particularly true in relation to the less severe forms of depression. Busse (1975) has observed that depressive episodes in the elderly can often be "linked with the loss of so-called narcissistic supplies" (p. 74) and that depressed elderly individuals are often conscious of the factors resulting in such losses. He argues that many depressive episodes in the elderly are therefore "realistic grief response[s] to loss[es] and not primarily influenced by unconscious mechanisms" (p. 75). The elderly depressed person experiences a loss of self-esteem and feelings of inferiority. This differs from the pattern of depression relatively frequent among younger individuals characterized by guilt and the introjection of unconscious hostility or other unacceptable impulses. Other clinicians have observed, particularly in less severe depression, that apathy and disinterest are often seen in the elderly, but not in younger populations (Levin, 1965; Zung, 1973). Zung and Green (1973) proposed that this dimension may be a pathological extension of Factor 1 of his Self-Rating Depression Scale (SDS) (Zung, 1965).

In chapter 3 of this book, Salzman and Shader summarized the symptomatology of depression in the elderly. They pointed out that interpreting physical symptoms in older patients is complicated by the fact that certain physical problems (including those sometimes associated with depression processes, e.g., constipation and fatigue), frequently occur as a result of physiological changes associated with aging rather than as a result of depression. Thus, when are physical complaints to be viewed as indicators of an affective disorder? This question is most critical at the subject selection stage of psychopharmacological studies and is also important in assessing the effects of medication on the symptoms of depression. Salzman and Shader (cf. chapter 3) also discussed the problem of differentiating depressive symptomatology in the elderly from dementia associated with cerebral pathology, a task that continues to frustrate clinicians. To be effective, scales for assessing depressive symptomatology in the elderly should consist of items that focus upon those symptoms characteristic of the elderly as well as those symptoms that are not age-specific. These optimal scales should also be sensitive to the wide spectrum of depressive symptomatology in the elderly (e.g., ranging from apathy and physical complaint to severely depressed mood and major impairment of psychological functions) and have some capacity to differentiate depressive symptomatology from dementia associated with cerebral pathology.

Scales for Assessing Depressive Symptomatology

A selection of observer rating scales for assessing depressive symptomatology is presented in Table 1. This table is based, in part, upon an earlier review of rating scales for geriatric psychopharmacology research (Salzman et al., 1972).

It is important to note at the onset that none of the scales presented in Table 1 were developed specifically for the elderly. Although depressive symptomatology has been a frequent target of psychotropic drug studies of the elderly, a review of a large number of these studies revealed that depressive symptoms were, most often, assessed by means of scales unique to a given study, global in format and minimally described. Three scales are

TABLE 1 Observer Rating Scales: Depression

Name of scale	Reference	Patient type/ Rater	Description
Phenomena of Depressions	Grinker, Miller, Sabahin, Nunn, and Nunnally, 1961	Inpatients/ Psychiatrist and ward	2 checklists: a 47-item list of feelings and concerns rated by a psychiatrist and a 139-item list of current behavior rated by ward personnel
Grading Scale for Depressive Reactions	Cutler and Kurland 1961	Inpatients/ Nurse, aide	Ratings of thought and behavior (agitation, retardation)
Psychiatric Judgment of Depression Scale	Overall, Hollister, Pokorny, Casey, and Katz, 1962	Inpatients/ Clinician	Rating of depressive symptoms
NIMH Collaborative Depression Mood Scale	Raskin, 1965	Inpatients/ Nurse	Objective adjective checklist
SAD–GLAD	Simpson, Hackett, and Kline, 1966	Inpatients/ Observer	Rating of depression and elation and social participation
Hamilton Psychiatric Rating Scale for Depression[a]	Hamilton, 1967	Adult inpatients and outpatients/ Expert clinician via interview	23-item scale, drug sensitive; useful for neurotic and endogenous depressions; patient must be responsive
Verdun Depression Rating Scale[a]	Lehmann and Ban, 1967	Inpatients/ Clinician	Rating of 12 depressive symptoms
Depression Status Inventory[a]	Zung, 1972	Inpatients and outpatients/ Clinician	Professionally rated analogue of the patient-rated Zung Depression Scale; 20 items yielding a global measure of the intensity of depressive symptomatology

[a]Scale has been used in geriatric drug studies.

exceptions. The Hamilton Psychiatric Rating Scale for Depression (HAMD) (Hamilton, 1967) has been the most extensively used standard observer rating scale for assessing depressive symptomatology, having been employed in at least three psychotropic drug studies of the elderly (Burt, Gordon, Holt, & Hodern, 1962; Hodern, Holt, Burt, & Gordon, 1963; Sakalis, Gershon, & Shopsin, 1974). The Zung Depression Status Inventory (Zung DSI) (Zung, Gianturco, Pfeiffer, Wang, Whanger, Bridge, & Potkin, 1974) and the Verdun

Depression Rating Scale (Verdun DRS) (Kristof, Lehmann, & Ban, 1967) have each been used in one geriatric psychotropic drug study.

The HAMD is a 23-item scale developed by Hamilton for use with adults to quantitatively assess the severity of, and changes in, depressive symptomatology in adults. Data for ratings are obtained from a careful psychiatric interview that should be administered by a skilled, experienced clinician trained in the use of the scale. Hamilton (1967) has made available useful information for administering the interview and scoring patient responses. Scale points vary from 3 to 5. The scale items assess depressive mood, guilt, suicidal ideation and behaviors, sleep disturbances, eating disturbances (i.e., weight loss), rate of psychomotor functioning, anxiety, loss of libido, gastrointestinal and general somatic symptoms, hypochondriacal complaints (ranging from excessive preoccupations with bodily functions to somatic delusions and hallucinations), loss of insight, diurnal variation patterns, feelings of derealization and depersonalization, and paranoid and obsessional symptoms.

A recent factor analytic study of the HAMD (Cleary & Guy, Note 2; Guy, 1976) generated six factors: (1) Anxiety/Somatization, (2) Weight, (3) Cognitive Disturbance, (4) Diurnal Variation, (5) Retardation, and (6) Sleep Disturbance. Unfortunately, the HAMD has not, to the author's knowledge, been subjected to a geriatric normative study of the kind carried out by Zung and Green (1973) with respect to the Zung Self-Rating Depression Scale (Zung SDS) (Zung, 1965), the self-rating analogue of the Zung DSI. Hodern et al. (1963), however, did compare the initial symptomatology, as assessed by the HAMD, for patients of various ages hospitalized with primary depressive states and treated with antidepressant medications. They found that genital symptoms in those persons less than 50 years of age were significantly more severe than in those persons 60–70 years of age; while in the older group, agitation, delayed insomnia, loss of weight, and depressed mood were significantly more severe. Despite the need for more data of this kind, it is nevertheless possible to tentatively answer some basic questions about the utility of the HAMD for research in geriatric psychopharmacology.

A basic question that should be posed is: Does the HAMD measure depressive symptomatology as it appears in the elderly? Comparison of the clinical dimensions of depressive symptomatology in the elderly with the HAMD item composition and factor analytic data summarized above leads to an affirmative response. The HAMD does appear to assess virtually all of the major dimensions of depressive symptomatology in the elderly, and to have the potential for assessing their severity, though it may be less sensitive at the low or mild end. The HAMD also appears to have satisfactory interrater reliability as well as validity in adult populations provided the raters have been adequately trained (see Guy, 1976, p. 191 for references relevant to the reliability and validity of the HAMD). The validity of the HAMD in its sensitivity to treatment or drug effects in the elderly population also seems tentatively established. The HAMD has been used to assess antidepressant effects of amitriptyline and imipramine in women who ranged in age from 30 to 70 (Burt et al., 1962; Hodern et al., 1963). In both studies, the HAMD indicated that amitriptyline was superior to imipramine in reducing depressive symptomatology, especially in those patients over 50 years of age. Unfortunately, these early studies of amitriptyline efficacy provide a very limited test of the sensitivity of the HAMD to active drug effects, since they were not placebo-controlled studies.

The HAMD has also been employed in at least one study of the effects of Gerovital-H3 on elderly individuals. Sakalis et al. (1974) used the HAMD, as well as a behavior rating instrument and global impression measure, to assess the effects of Gerovital-H3 on 10 senile arteriosclerotic patients with depressive features. Although they concluded that Gerovital-H3 had only a mild euphoriant effect, changes on the HAMD suggestive of limited therapeutic effects became apparent (i.e., statistically significant) on the third week of drug treatment with respect to the Somatization and Anxiety/Depression clusters.

The HAMD's sensitivity to treatment effects in elderly patients has also been demonstrated in studies using treatment modalities other than chemotherapy. For example, in a recent study of the therapeutic effects of sleep deprivation on elderly depressed patients, the HAMD was again sensitive (especially on Depressed Mood and Psychomotor Retardation factors) to changes in depressive symptomatology (Cole & Miller, 1976).

The Zung DSI is the only other widely known scale, according to the author's search of the literature, that has been used in a geriatric psychopharmacology study. As reported in the ECDEU assessment manual (Guy, 1976), the Zung DSI consists of the same 20 items as its self-rating form, the Zung SDS. (Zung, 1972, reported a Pearson product moment correlation of .87 between the two scales.) The 20 items of the Zung DSI overlap considerably with those of the HAMD, but there are some important differences in the dimensions of the two scales. Both the Zung DSI and HAMD have items that assess depressive mood, diurnal variation, sleep disturbances, appetite and weight loss, decreased libido, somatic symptoms, level of psychomotor functioning, and suicide phenomena. The Zung DSI also contains items not covered by the HAMD: crying spells (an item separate from depressive mood), confusion, emptiness, hopelessness, irritability, and personal devaluation. Thus, the Zung DSI seems to focus more than the HAMD upon affective nuances of depression. However, the Zung DSI, in contrast to the HAMD, omits items that in their manifest content assess guilt feelings, hypochondriasis, insight, paranoid symptoms, and obsessive-compulsive symptoms (beyond indecisiveness). The Zung DSI also assesses only sleep disturbances occurring in the late phase of sleep (the HAMD has items relevant to initial, middle, and late insomnia) and has only two items that directly pertain to somatic complaints (constipation and tachycardia) in contrast to the HAMD, which has several. Thus, it appears that the Zung

DSI, while stressing the affective dimensions of depression (except for guilt feelings), fails to focus extensively on somatic dysfunctioning and complaints—a most important aspect of depression in the elderly.

Although the Zung DSI has been less extensively used in research than the HAMD, Zung (1972) presented data that suggest that the DSI has adequate validity and reliability. In addition to its high correlation with the Zung SDS, the DSI did differentiate depressed patients from nondepressed patients. Adequate reliability is indicated by the split-half correlation, $r = .81$.

As noted above, Zung and his colleagues (Zung & Green, 1973) have explored the self-rating analogue of the DSI with respect to elderly individuals. They have reported, for example, that their sample of normal elderly individuals had significantly higher baseline depressive symptoms, as assessed by the SDS, than normal subjects who were age 20 to 64. Factor analysis of the SDS data for those over age 65 also revealed that loss of self-esteem is a central feature of the depressive symptoms of normal elderly individuals as opposed to patients with depressive disorders.

The only geriatric psychopharmacology study that employed the Zung DSI was a double-blind, placebo-controlled study comparing Gerovital-H3 and imipramine in outpatients 60 years of age or older with at least mild depressive disorders (Zung et al., 1974). The Zung DSI (as well as the SDS) was sensitive to some limited active drug effects in this study, though it failed to differentiate among the effects of the two active drug and placebo conditions.

The final observer rating scale for assessing depressive symptomatology in the elderly is the Verdun Depression Scale (Verdun DS) (Kristof et al., 1967). The Verdun DS is not a widely known or employed scale. Data on its validity and reliability are not readily available. According to Kristof and his colleagues, the scale assesses mood, facial expression, general appearance, retardation, impaired work and social interest, agitation, depressive ideation, suicide ideation, insomnia, somatic complaints, and weight loss. All of these items are also assessed by the more widely used HAMD and Zung DSI. The Verdun DS, however, was sensitive to the effects of trimipramine in a small double-blind study without placebo control involving geriatric inpatients with depression. Active drug effects were most striking on the Total Symptomatology score and Facial Expression and Agitation items.

Conclusions

None of the available scales for assessing depressive symptomatology in the elderly is ideal. Neither the HAMD nor any of the other scales, were designed to differentiate dementia from depressive symptoms in the elderly. None of the scales reviewed, for that matter, include items that assess memory, a function that may be impaired as a result of depression in the elderly and that may improve with effective therapies for depression. Future developments in geriatric research methodology may remedy such deficiencies.

Anxiety in the Elderly

Clinical Dimensions

Anxiety is an affect that has been widely studied over the years. It has been defined in a variety of ways and a number of theories, ranging from psychoanalytic to behavioral, have been generated to enable the clinician and researcher to describe and understand conceptually various anxiety phenomena.

In general, most clinicians and researchers would agree with Zung and Green (1973) who described anxiety as "an exceedingly unpleasant feeling, . . . [or] affective state characterized by feelings of apprehension, uncertainty and helplessness which are not attached to a real external danger and frequently associated with some somatic symptoms" (p. 222). Although anxiety is a primary characteristic of the neuroses, it is by no means found only in individuals suffering from neurotic disorders. Hamilton (1959), for example, in discussing the development of his scale for assessing anxiety states, observed that "anxiety in greater or lesser degree is found in agitated depression and obsessional states particularly, and also in such states as organic dementia, hysteria and schizophrenia" (p. 50). Hamilton's list of disorders that have anxiety components, however, is far from complete.

As is the case with depressive symptoms, people of varying ages are vulnerable to anxiety (Claghorn, 1971; Zung & Green, 1973). A critical question for geriatric psychiatry and psychopharmacological research is: Does the face of anxiety in the elderly differ significantly from that in other age groups? As one might expect, the tentative answer to this question is yes.

Zung and Green (1973), for example, presented data from Zung's Self-Rating Anxiety Scale (Zung SAS) (Zung, 1971) that indicate that the normal elderly population has higher baseline values for symptoms of anxiety than do normal younger adults. In addition, Gershon (1973), in discussing antianxiety agents for the elderly, observed that "the aged have different host qualities for psychiatric disorders, and the symptomatology seen in them may not fit automatically within the established systems of classification developed for a younger age group" (p. 184).

Although anxiety in the elderly must be more extensively and intensively explored empirically, some of its features have been tentatively described. Gershon (1973) and others have described typical burdens (e.g., physical impairment, illness, poverty, and object, ability, or capacity loss) that are frequent precursors of depression and anxiety in the elderly. He also hypothesized that depressive features frequently accompany anxiety states in the elderly and that anxiety in the elderly often takes the form of a "rather primitive body focused type" associated with "pain, disability, dyspnoea, fragility, and failing bodily functions" (p. 184). Hypochondriacal symptoms, so frequently encountered in elderly patients, may also be associated with anxiety; Busse (1975) has argued that the high bodily concern of the elderly is often a "displacement of [their] anxiety" (p. 76).

One of the most comprehensive classifications of anxiety in the elderly is offered by Verwoerdt (1976) in his textbook of clinical geropsychiatry. He describes five major groupings of anxiety in the elderly: (1) depletion anxiety or insecurity about loss of external supplies and possible isolation and loneliness; (2) anxiety associated with helplessness including fears of loss of control and mastery and feelings of shame; (3) chronic neurotic anxiety, "a carry-over from earlier years; with physiological tension, motor agitation, and depressive admixtures"; (4) acute anxiety that may represent an acute stress or adjustment reaction of late life or may be associated with "a weakening of the ego's capacity to screen and ward off unwanted stimuli, as in catastrophic reactions of brain damaged patients, or informational overload"; and (5) anxiety associated with psychoses that may be linked with schizophrenic delusions, paranoid states (persecutory anxiety), or with chronic brain syndrome and senile dementia (pp. 152-158).

Scales for Assessing Anxiety Symptoms

Psychotropic drug studies focusing upon anxiety reduction in all age groups have generally relied upon a small number of self-report measures of anxiety such as the Scheier-Cattell Anxiety Battery (Scheier, Cattell, & Sullivan, 1961) or upon the anxiety factors of self-rated multiple mood inventories like the revised Psychiatric Outpatient Mood Scale (POMS) (McNair, Lorr, & Droppleman, 1971). When observer rating scales have been employed, as with the assessment of depressive symptomatology, they have frequently been nonstandard scales developed for specific studies. None of the psychiatric observer rating scales that focus exclusively upon symptoms of anxiety were designed specifically for the elderly. However, the two best known scales, the Hamilton Anxiety Scale (HAMA) (Hamilton, 1959) and the Zung Anxiety Status Inventory (Zung ASI) (Zung, 1971) may have some utility in geriatric psychopharmacology.

The HAMA, the older of the two scales, is described in the ECDEU assessment manual (Guy, 1976) as "a 14-item scale intended for use with patients already diagnosed as suffering from neurotic anxiety states—not for assessing anxiety in patients suffering from other disorders" (p. 195). The scale emphasizes the patient's subjective state and its items focus primarily upon somatic symptoms associated with anxiety. The HAMA also has items that assess affective, cognitive, and behavioral (i.e., interview behavior) dimensions. The items apparently cluster into two specific factors, Somatic Anxiety and Psychic Anxiety, in addition to a general anxiety factor (Hamilton, 1959). Although the validity and reliability of the HAMA have not been extensively explored for the elderly, Hamilton (1959, 1969) did report data that are suggestive of adequate reliability and validity for younger adults.

The HAMA has been used in at least two geriatric psychopharmacology studies with nonpsychotic senile patients (Covington, 1975; Kirven and Montero, 1973). Despite the questionable validity of the HAMA for rating nonneurotic anxiety, Kirven and Montero used an 8-item modification of the HAMA along with other scales in a double-blind study without placebo control that revealed statistically significant improvement for thioridazine on six and for diazepam on five HAMA items as well as on the global HAMA change rating.

The Zung ASI is the observer rating analogue of Zung's Self-Rating Anxiety Scale (SAS). It consists of 20 items and employs a 4-point scale. According to Zung (1971), both the ASI and SAS were designed specifically for the assessment of anxiety as a disorder rather than as a trait or feeling state. Thus, the Zung ASI, like the HAMA, is intended for adults with the diagnosis of anxiety neurosis. The Zung ASI is also similar to the HAMA in that the majority of its items assess the somatic concomitants of anxiety, while a smaller number of items focus upon affective dimensions. Although data relevant to the validity and reliability of the Zung ASI are limited, Zung has offered data that suggest his scale may have adequate validity and reliability.

The Zung ASI has been used in at least one geriatric psychopharmacological study, the Gerovital-H3 study by Zung and his colleagues previously described (Zung et al., 1974). The scale indicated that patients on Gerovital-H3 and on imipramine improved significantly, but those on placebo did not.

Conclusions

Geriatric researchers would do well to meet the methodological challenge implicit in Verwoerdt's (1976) thoughtful classification of anxiety in the elderly. Any methodologist who systematically operationalized Verwoerdt's classification through a single rating scale would provide geriatric psychopharmacologists with an age-specific, all-purpose scale that might be of considerable value for assessing anxiety in the elderly.

Multiple Affects and Moods

Before closing this section on the assessment of affective symptomatology in the elderly, it should be noted that multiple mood assessment scales, which usually rely upon adjective self-ratings with affective connotations, have at times been converted into observer rating scales. The Clyde Mood Scale (Clyde, 1960), for example, may be used as an observer- or self-rated instrument. The scale is similar to several other multiple mood rating scales in that a list of adjectives is used to assess a variety of mood factors.

The Clyde Mood Scale has been used in at least one geriatric psychopharmacological study, a double-blind comparison of tybamate and chlordiazepoxide in geriatric patients with chronic cerebral impairments associated with circulatory disturbance (Goldstein, 1967). Data from the scale indicated that the tybamate group was less sleepy (one of the six factors of the scale) than the chlordiazepoxide group, during the active drug treatment phase. Despite the economy of such multiple mood scales, their constricted scopes limit their value for assessing affective symptomatology in the elderly, especially in severely disturbed patients who may be uncooperative and experiencing impairments of a variety of psychological functions.

The Senior Apperception Test (SAT) (Bellak, 1973), a projective test based upon the standard Thematic Apperception Test for adults (Murray, 1943) but specifically designed for the clinical assessment of elderly individuals, is an interesting instrument that still remains an unknown quantity for geriatric psychopharmacological research. Although projective tests like the SAT can potentially assess a variety of moods and affects (more or less precisely, depending upon the adequacy of rating systems developed to score the projective responses), the nature of projective test formats makes it extremely difficult to achieve methodological adequacy.

OBSERVER RATING SCALES FOR ASSESSING MULTIPLE PSYCHOPATHOLOGY

In contrast to scales designed to focus upon only one realm of psychopathology (e.g., affective disorders), a number of scales have been developed to assess a wide range of symptoms simultaneously. Since these multiple psychopathology scales include factors that assess affective symptomatology, many of the issues reviewed in the preceding section are also relevant to the present discussion.

Clinical Dimensions

A comprehensive review of the complex and enormous range of psychiatric disorders and psychopathological symptoms that occur in the elderly is far beyond the scope of this chapter (see Stotsky, 1973 and Verwoerdt, 1976). For present purposes, it is important to note that age-specific patterns characterize psychopathology in the elderly including hallucinations, delusions, and psychomotor activity–a triad of psychotic symptoms highlighted by Verwoerdt (1976). He proposed that hallucinations often become less frequent and exciting in aged chronic schizophrenics, though they may be frequent and intense in late paraphrenia; delusions change in the elderly by disappearing, expanding, or consolidating; and psychomotor activity levels often decrease with aging, even in patients previously hyperactive. Optimal rating scales for use with elderly patients must reflect such age-specific patterns in addition to assessing meaningful classes of symptomatology in the elderly.

Since no single rating scale with practical utility could assess all psychopathological symptoms, a manageable number of them must be selected for any given scale. The nature of the population for which a scale is intended often determines, as it should, which symptoms are to be assessed. Among the population characteristics that are important in rating scale construction are age, patient status (i.e., inpatient versus outpatient), and kinds of psychiatric disorders.

Rating Scales

Table 2 presents a selected list of rating scales that use data derived from interviews as opposed to scales that use observer ratings of ward behavior and do not require interviews.

As Table 2 indicates, only three of the six scales have been employed in psychotropic drug studies with elderly patients. One of these scales, the Sandoz Clinical Assessment–Geriatric (SCAG) was designed specifically for assessing multiple psychopathology in elderly individuals. The other two rating scales that have been used in geriatric psychopharmacological research, the Brief Psychiatric Rating Scale (BPRS) and the Inpatient Multidimensional Psychiatric Rating Scale (IMPS) were designed primarily for assessing multiple psychopathology in inpatients. Although neither the IMPS (Lorr & Klett, 1966) nor the BPRS (Overall & Gorham, 1962) was designed for elderly patients, both have been employed extensively in geriatric psychopharmacological research. The IMPS, the older of the two scales, is, according to the ECDEU assessment manual (Guy, 1976), an 89-item scale that is rated on the basis of observations made during a psychiatric interview. It was designed for use with functionally psychotic or severely neurotic adults capable of being interviewed. A factor analysis of the scale by Guy has generated the following 10 factors: (1) Excitement, (2) Hostility and Belligerence, (3) Paranoid Projection, (4) Grandiose Expansiveness, (5) Perceptual Distortion, (6) Anxious Intropunitiveness, (7) Retardation and Apathy, (8) Disorientation, (9) Motor Disturbances, and (10) Conceptual Disorganization.

The IMPS is a widely used multiple psychopathology rating scale with apparent adequate validity and reliability when employed with populations for which the scale was originally designed, i.e., nonelderly adult patients with severe psychopathology. This scale has been employed (often in abbreviated versions) in at least five geriatric psychotropic drug studies (Honigfeld, Rosenblum, Blumenthal, Lambert, & Roberts, 1965; Judah, Murphree, & Seager, 1959; Kernohan, Chambers, Wilson, & Daugherty, 1967; Turek, Kurland, Ota, & Hanlon, 1969; Wolff, Grasberger, & Kidorf, 1962). However, the scale was sensitive to drug effects in only one of these five studies, a Veterans Administration cooperative project that compared the effects of imipramine, two phenothiazines, and placebo in geriatric chronic schizophrenic inpatients (Honigfeld et al., 1965). The three IMPS factors that reflected the change were Excitement, Motor Disturbance, and Conceptual Disorganization. It is important to note that the IMPS proved to be an inappropriate instrument for the patients selected as subjects in two of the five studies

TABLE 2 Selected Rating Scales for Multiple Psychopathology

Name of scale	Reference	Patient type/Rater	Previous use in geriatric psycho-pharmacology	Description
Wittenborn Psychiatric Scales (Short Survey (WITP)	Wittenborn, 1955	Inpatients and outpatients/ Psychiatrist, psychologist, nurse	None	17-item short form designed to ascertain rate and nature of symptomatic change; 4-point scale
Brief Psychiatric Rating Scale (BPRS)	Overall and Gorham, 1962	Primarily inpatients/Psychiatrist or psychologist	Yes	18-item scale developed from the longer Lorr Multidimensional Psychiatric Scale for Rating Psychiatric Patients and the Inpatient Multidimensional Psychiatric Scale; focus is primarily inpatient psychopathology
Inpatient Multidimensional Psychiatric Scale (IMPS)	Lorr and Klett, 1966	Functional psychotics or severe neurotics capable of being interviewed/Trained interviewers	Yes	89 items rated on basis of observations made during a psychiatric interview; has undergone extensive psychometric analysis
Physician's Outpatient Psychopathology Scale (POPS)	Free and Guthrie, 1969	Adult outpatients/Rater can be person who is not specifically a mental health professional	None	15 items clinically derived from the factors of several standard rating scales
Physician Questionnaire (PHYS)	Rickels and Howard, 1970	Neurotic outpatients/Physician	None	13 items plus a global measure of psychopathology to provide a simple measure of neurotic symptomatology
Sandoz Clinical Assessment–Geriatric (SCAG)	Shader et al., 1974	Geriatric patients/Skilled clinician	Yes	18 symptoms plus a global rating; 7 scale points

(Turek et al., 1969; Wolff et al., 1962). Apparently many of the patients in these two studies were so severely impaired that ward behavior rating scales would have been the more appropriate instruments of assessment.

The BPRS (Overall & Gorham 1962) is an 18-item multiple psychopathology rating scale that, according to the ECDEU assessment manual (Guy, 1976), was developed from the longer Lorr Multidimensional Scale for Rating Psychiatric Patients and from the IMPS. It was designed to provide a "rapid and efficient evaluation of treatment response in both clinical drug trials and routine settings" (p. 159). Although it has been used with outpatients, it was designed primarily for nonelderly adult inpatient populations. Like the IMPS, it appears to be an instrument of adequate validity and reliability (for populations for which it was designed), has been subjected to factor analytic study, and has been employed in a number of psychotropic drug studies with elderly patients. The ECDEU assessment manual reports five factors for the BPRS (based upon a large sample of subjects with a diagnosis of schizophrenia): Anxiety-Depression, Anergia, Thought Disturbance, Activation, and Hostile-Suspiciousness.

The BPRS has been used in at least six psychotropic drug studies with the elderly (Birkett & Boltuch, 1972; Goldstein & Birnbom, 1976; Kristof et al., 1967; Lu, Stotsky, & Cole, 1971; Smith, Taylor, & Linkous, 1974; Stotsky & Borozne, 1972). Despite the fact that most of these studies used severely impaired chronic geriatric patients, the BPRS was sensitive to drug effects in five of the six studies without placebo control, failing to demonstrate significant therapeutic effects of an active psychotropic drug (chlorpromazine) in only one study (Birkett & Boltuch, 1972). The drugs used in the five studies in which the BPRS was sensitive to treatment effects included antidepressant, antipsychotic, and antianxiety agents. Although most of the patients in these five studies were severely and chronically impaired, one study (Stotsky & Borozne, 1972) used nursing home patients who suffered from a variety of psychoneurotic symptoms. Significant differences between drug and placebo effects were most frequently found on the Anxiety-Depression and, to a lesser extent, Anergic clusters.

The SCAG (Shader, Harmatz, & Salzman, 1974) was developed by Sandoz Pharmaceuticals to help differentiate between early senile deterioration and depressive disorders in the elderly. It is the only standard multiple psychopathology rating scale designed specifically for geriatric patients. According to Shader et al., the SCAG is "composed of 18 symptom areas and an overall global assessment, all rated on a 7-point format (1 = not present . . . 7 = severe)" (p. 107). Since the SCAG is a rather recent rating scale, published data relevant to its validity, reliability, factorial composition, and drug sensitivity are still limited. Shader et al., however, have conducted two studies that, taken together, suggest that it is a valid and reliable instrument for assessing psychopathology in the elderly.

Inspection of the 18 symptom areas or items that comprise the SCAG suggests that the instrument assesses primarily impairments in attitude and mood (e.g., motivation initiative, mood depression, irritability); physical complaints (e.g., dizziness, appetite/anorexia); cognitive functioning (e.g., mental alertness, impairment of recent memory); and activities of daily living (e.g., self-care). All four realms are, of course, critical to the adequate adaptations of elderly individuals but are quite vulnerable to the effects of aging processes.

A few factor analytic studies of the SCAG have been undertaken, but, unfortunately, the results have not yet been published. Harmatz (Note 3), however, reported in a personal communication in 1977 that three factors emerged in preliminary analyses of data obtained in a study comparing the effects of a dihydrogenated ergot alkaloid (Hydergine), imipramine, and placebo on ambulatory elderly research volunteers with a mild degree of mood and cognitive impairments. The three factors have been tentatively labeled Mood, Bewilderment, and Aboulia.

Although several psychotropic drug studies with elderly patients in which the standard SCAG has been employed are as yet unpublished, a recent critical review by Hughes, Williams, & Currier (1976) has described eight geriatric psychopharmacological studies that employed early versions of the SCAG in investigations of the efficacy of Hydergine for the treatment of dementia. Despite some methodological and design problems in several of the studies reviewed by Hughes et al., the data derived from the early versions of the SCAG frequently indicated statistically significant improvement in several symptom areas. Most consistent and extensive improvements across the several studies were found on the cognitive functioning (mental alertness, orientation, confusion, and recent memory) and attitude or mood (depression, emotional lability, anxiety, and motivation or initiative) items. Thus, the SCAG may have considerable sensitivity to drug or other treatment effects in elderly research subjects.

Conclusions and Recommendations

Of the two rating scales originally designed primarily for adult inpatient psychopathology (the IMPS and BPRS), the BPRS appears to have the greater utility for geriatric psychopharmacological research. This conclusion is based primarily upon its brevity and apparent sensitivity to drug effects in several psychotropic drug studies with relatively severely impaired chronic geriatric inpatients and a variety of classes of psychotropic drugs. The IMPS, by contrast, is a much longer rating scale that has been relatively insensitive to drug effects (if the drugs were, in fact, therapeutic in the studies in which the IMPS was employed) and, at times, impossible to administer (though this may have been a failure in research design rather than a problem with the scale) in several geriatric psychopharmacology studies.

Clearly, rating scales like the SCAG, which have been designed for geriatric populations, hold the greatest promise for geriatric psychopharmacological research. As Shader et al. (1974) have noted, the SCAG was developed to help differentiate between early senile deterioration and depressive disorders in the elderly. The goals for the SCAG determined which psychopathological symptoms would be included in the scale. The SCAG may therefore be less sensitive to, for example, the effects of antipsychotic drugs upon elderly chronic schizophrenic patients, since it does not assess several symptoms associated with schizophrenic disturbances. Thus, rating scales should be developed that focus upon age-specific forms of symptomatology associated with a variety of psychiatric disorders of the elderly.

MENTAL STATUS EXAMINATIONS FOR ASSESSING COGNITIVE FUNCTIONING

In an excellent novel, *Memento Mori,* Muriel Spark (1960) presented a number of elderly characters who were part of the same network of friends, enemies, and lovers for a number of years, and who, one by one, were plagued by a mysterious caller who reminded each, "remember, you must die." Although they did not take the message lightly, it barely distracted them from their tragicomic obsession with the retention or deterioration of their faculties. In the novel, death, like the caller, seemed capricious, but each of the elderly characters felt some measure of satisfaction and control in the battle against mental deterioration.

This final section focuses upon the psychiatric assessment of cognitive functioning in the elderly (cf. also chapters 9, 10, and 11). As was noted in an earlier review of rating scales for geriatric psychopharmacology (Salzman et al., 1972), a wide variety of instruments and procedures have been used to assess the nature and degree of cognitive impairment in the elderly. Standard intelligence tests (for adults and, occasionally, for children) that assess a wide variety of intellectual functions (e.g., fund of general knowledge, rote memory, arithmetic reasoning, visual-motor coordination), tests that focus exclusively upon memory functioning, neuropsychological processes, and mental status have all been used to assess the cognitive functioning of elderly individuals. This section is limited to a review of mental status examinations and their utility for the assessment of cognitive functioning in geriatric psychopharmacological research.

Clinical Dimensions

Jarvik (1973), in a survey of drug effects upon cognitive activities of the aged, has observed that aging processes, when within average limits, do not result in gross impairments of cognitive functioning in late life. Despite the existence of typical speed and learning deficits and changes in perceptual and motor functioning, cognitive deficits in the normal aged individual may be relatively minimal.

However, the concerns of the characters of *Memento Mori* are not totally unrealistic. Dementia, the "global disruption of personality, affecting behavior and intelligence" (Arie, 1974, p. 94), is by no means a rare and exotic phenomenon. Although estimates of the incidence of dementia vary, Arie has proposed that 10% of the elderly are demented (half of them severely) and that the rate doubles for the population over 80 years of age (cf. also chapters 1, 2, and 3).

There are two main types of dementia, or organic brain syndromes, in the elderly: senile and arteriosclerotic. Senile dementia is associated with cerebral atrophy and neuronal loss. In arteriosclerotic dementia, "the brain substance degenerates as the result of impaired blood supply, with disseminated softenings due to infarction" (Arie, 1974, p. 95).

Although lists of the characteristic symptomatology of organic brain syndromes vary, most authorities agree with Verwoerdt (1976) that impairments of orientation, memory, intellect, and judgment are common in these conditions and that emotional lability or shallowness are not infrequent. Although Busse (1975) generally agrees with Verwoerdt's list, he has proposed that, in addition to spotty memory functioning and faulty orientation in one or more spheres, "the so-called cognitive functions which include comprehension, calculation, problem-solving, learning, and judgment are impaired" (p. 78).

Mental Status Examination in Geriatric Psychopharmacological Research

Mental status examination has played an important role in psychiatric evaluation for a number of years, since it is a procedure designed to provide a relatively rapid description of a patient's mental capacity and functioning and emotional state. As noted by Salzman et al. (1972), mental status examinations involve systems of categories that structure the reporting of clinical psychiatric findings. Appearance and behavior, speech, thought content, mood, orientation, insight, and judgment are categories frequently included in mental status examinations. However, in clinical settings, there is some variability in the categories included and in the specific questions posed by the examiner to assess the functioning relevant to each category. For example, in order to assess patients' abstract reasoning as part of a mental status evaluation, two clinicians in separate settings might ask their patients to interpret proverbs that differ in level of difficulty or other dimensions.

Clinical mental status examinations typically assess several cognitive functions (e.g., orientation, memory, and judgment) that are vulnerable to impairment with chronic brain syndromes. Thus, these examinations have been viewed as critical, in combination with other diagnostic procedures, to evaluation and assessment of organic brain syndromes. Researchers have periodically employed mental status examinations to assess the effects of psychotropic agents upon the cognitive functioning of elderly research subjects.

Table 3 presents a list of some of the more widely used mental status examinations. It is based upon a previously published list (Salzman et al., 1972) that has been expanded and updated.

There is considerable overlap among the mental status examinations presented in Table 3 with respect to the psychological functions included and the method (i.e., tasks and items) of assessment. Virtually all mental status examinations, for example, assess the patient's orientation in three spheres by asking direct questions about time, place, and person. However, several of the mental status examinations presented in Table 3 focus upon different psychological functions or attempt to measure the same functions with different tasks. For example, although the Mental Status Questionnaire (MSQ) (Kahn, Goldfarb, Pollack, & Peck, 1960), the Clifton Assessment Schedule (CAS), and the Geriatric Interpersonal Evaluation Scale (GIES) (Plutchik, Conte, & Lieberman, 1971) all assess orientation with virtually identical questions, the CAS assesses psychomotor functioning with a writing task, the GIES with a drawing task (i.e., figure reproduction) and the MSQ does not attempt to measure psychomotor functioning at all.

In 1972, my colleagues and I observed that "from the vantage point of geriatric psychopharmacology, the mental status examination is an untried area" (Salzman et al., 1972, p. 17). The present review of the relevant literature leads to the conclusion that the scales have been tried occasionally, though far from extensively or systematically, but the results have been rather disappointing.

As Table 3 indicates, only 4 of the 13 mental status examination scales included in this selection have been employed, to the author's knowledge, in published accounts of geriatric psychopharmacological research. However, several psychotropic drug studies with elderly research subjects have used nonstandard mental status examination procedures along with other scales designed to assess cognitive functioning. Frequently, a published account has referred to and vaguely described a mental status examination that seemed to be one of those listed in Table 3, but the description did not include a reference for the scale. For example, a study of the effects of cyclandelate on perception, memory, and cognition in geriatric subjects (Aderman, Giardina, & Koreniowski, 1972) used a test of general orientation and awareness that, as described, could have been the MSQ (Kahn et al., 1960). Other investigations have employed a mental status examination obviously devised for a given study, and perhaps have abandoned it when it failed to demonstrate drug effects.

Three of the four mental status examinations presented in Table 3, which have been used in geriatric psychopharmacological research, have been minimally employed. The author's search of the literature has found that the Maudsley Clinical Sensorium Test (MCST) (Shapiro, Post, Lofving, & Inglis, 1956) and Plutchik's GIES were each employed in one study and Stotsky's Mental Status Examination in two studies.

TABLE 3 Organic Mental Status

Name of scale	Reference	Patient type/Rater	Previous use in geriatric psycho-pharmacology	Description
Psychiatric Behavior Scale	Rowell, 1951	Institutionalized psychiatric patients/Nurse, psychiatrist	None	20 items, different facets of mental status; useful with psychotic individuals
Maudsley Clinical Sensorium Test (MCST)	Shapiro et al., 1956	Geriatric inpatients/Clinician	Yes	6 short subtests: orientation, immediate and delayed recall, logical memory, concentration, arithmetic, and story comprehension
Mental Status Checklist (MSCL)	Lifshitz, 1960	Geriatric inpatients/Clinician	Yes	Subtests include: orientation, successive subtractions, general information, identification of objects, abstraction, and writing performance
Mental Status Questionnaire (MSQ)	Kahn et al., 1960	Institutionalized geriatric patients/Psychologist	None	Orientation; useful in differentiating degrees of severity of chronic brain syndrome
A Brief Screening Test of Mental Status	Dixon, 1965	Normal elderly/Psychologist	None	Large number of cognitive tests each measuring a different function; useful in assessing senile impairment
Quantified Mental Status Scale	Rockland and Pollin, 1965	Normals and psychiatric patients/Psychiatrist	None	Measures various aspects of patient behavior such as appearance, affect, and thought processes; useful with normal and psychiatric populations
Mental State Rating Scale	Harris, Letemendia, & Willems, 1967	Chronic psychiatric patients/Psychiatrist, Nurse	None	Phenomenological information items and behavior items; useful in assessing therapeutic change

Patient in Nursing Home Schedule (Stotsky Mental Status Exam)	Stotsky, 1967	Nursing home residents/Psychologist	Yes	Assesses patient location, degree of mental impairment, index of change due to treatment and social functioning
Rating Scale of Psychological Function	Trier, 1968	Institutionalized elderly and psychiatric patients/Clinician	None	Measures cognitive ability and emotional aspects (perception and thought quality)
PGC Mental Status Questionnaire	Lawton, Note 4	Nursing home residents/Psychiatrist	None	Measures various aspects of cognitive functioning; specifically sensitive to very impaired patients
Mental Status Examination Record (MSER)	Spitzer and Endicott, 1971	Institutionalized psychiatric patients/Psychiatrist	None	Scale assessing attitude, mood, appearance, perception and affect of geriatric patients; useful in establishing the mental status in a wide range of psychiatric patients
Geriatric Interpersonal Evaluation Scale (GIES)	Plutchik et al., 1971	Geriatric inpatients/Clinician	Yes	Designed to assess the degree of cognitive functioning of highly regressed patients through the use of a semi-structured interview; also measures perceptual-motor ability; assesses orientation, immediate and remote memory, verbal and quantitative cognitive functions
Clifton Assessment Schedule (CAS)	Pattie and Gilleard, 1975	Elderly chronic psychiatric patients/Clinician	None	Devised to assess psychogeriatric patients in a brief reliable procedure; assesses information/orientation, mental ability, and psychomotor performance

The MCST, despite its questionable validity (Shapiro et al., 1956), was used with other psychological tests (assessing orientation, short-term memory, etc.) in a study by Ball and Taylor (1967) that explored the effects of cyclandelate on elderly geriatric inpatients. It was reported that the active drug group improved significantly on all mental functions tests except for two not part of the MCST. The Stotsky examination (Stotsky, 1967), a 20-item test (of undetermined validity and reliability) designed to assess the degree of impairment in memory, orientation, and alertness in geriatric patients, was used in a 1967 double-blind study that compared the effects of haloperidol and thioridazine upon institutionalized psychogeriatric patients (Tsuang, Lu, Stotsky, & Cole, 1971). Although the multiple psychopathology and behavioral rating scales used in the study demonstrated therapeutic drug effects for both active drugs at statistically significant levels, the Stotsky examination did not. Stotsky's examination also failed to demonstrate significant treatment effects in a study comparing Metrazol, papaverine, and niacin (Lu et al., 1971). Similarly, Plutchik's GIES (Plutchik et al., 1971), which provides a reliable and possibly valid index of various cognitive functions, did not demonstrate statistically significant differences between the effects of Gerovital-H3 and placebo in a study using samples of hospitalized geriatric patients (Zwerling, Plutchik, Hotz, Kling, Rubin, Grossman, & Siegel, 1975).

The mental status examination that has been most extensively employed in geriatric psychopharmacological research is the Mental Status Checklist (MSCL) (Lifshitz, 1960). This scale has been described by Lifshitz as a brief structured test "based on a scored, partial mental status examination" that was designed "to test varied aspects of functioning in a manner which permits the examiner to adjust to the eccentricities of the patient" (p. 302). The instrument was designed to determine which patients were suffering from psychosis of the senium (and the severity of the disease) and to be sensitive to treatment effects. Lifshitz presented data suggestive of the instrument's adequate validity, e.g., the correlation between the MSCL and an age-scaled score abbreviated, Wechsler Adult Intelligence Scale (WAIS), was .82, and reliability, e.g., a test-retest correlation of .94. However, the sensitivity of the MSCL to drug or treatment effects is still open to question, despite its relatively extensive use in geriatric psychopharmacological research.

The MSCL has been employed in at least five geriatric psychopharmacological studies; one focused upon methylphenidate and four upon Hydergine. In the methylphenidate study, the MSCL data demonstrated a statistically significant difference between the active drug and placebo groups (favoring methylphenidate) though the changes were small (Kaplitz, 1975). Of the 12 clinical trials with Hydergine that Hughes et al. (1976) critically reviewed, 4 (Jennings, 1972; Rao & Norris, 1972; Rosen, 1972; Triboletti & Ferir, 1969) employed the MSCL along with early forms of the SCAG or similar multiple psychopathology rating scales. Hughes et al. concluded that "although all of the cognitive variables improved when rated on a 7-point scale [i.e., early versions of the SCAG], none of the mental status [i.e., MSCL] variables improved" (p. 495) in at least half of the studies employing the two assessment procedures. They added the interesting observation that results were inconsistent when orientation was assessed by the two methods. One interpretation of this inconsistency is that a multiple psychopathology rating scale (like the SCAG) appears to be more sensitive than a mental status examination (like the MSCL) to the subtle and minimal cognitive improvements associated with Hydergine in the treatment of dementia. On the other hand, it is possible that cognitive items on multiple psychopathology scales, as rated on the SCAG, actually assess mood or psychological variables other than cognitive ones, while mental status examinations assess the latter.

Conclusions and Recommendations

Although several adequately reliable and valid mental status examinations developed specifically for elderly populations have been available to geriatric psychopharmacologists, their sensitivity to psychotropic drug effects has been limited. The relative insensitivity of these scales in previous geriatric psychopharmacological research appears, at least in part, to be associated with the interaction of three factors: the nature of dementia in the elderly, the questionable therapeutic efficacy of existing psychotropic agents for treating dementia, and the nature of the mental status examination format. Despite the necessary and potentially fruitful optimism of geriatric psychopharmacologists, many of the cognitive impairments of elderly individuals suffering from dementias may be refractory to drug treatments. Jarvik (1973), for example, and others have observed that motivation and mood in the elderly are more sensitive to drugs than cognitive functions, which appear to be very resistant to change or to drug effects. Thus, the problem may not lie with the insensitivity of the mental status examination but instead with the irreversibility of some forms of dementia or, more optimistically, with the relative impotence of the currently available psychotropic drugs. On the other hand, the drugs may be capable of effecting subtle and minimal but clinically significant improvements in the cognitive functioning of aged individuals that mental status examinations may be too specific and objective to detect. The pattern observed by Hughes et al. (1976) that emerged in previous research with Hydergine seems to reflect this methodological problem. Until the development of more potent agents that markedly alter the "pathophysiology of the aging process" (Jarvik, 1973, p. 130), geriatric psychopharmacological research may have to employ assessment procedures that sacrifice specificity and objectivity for flexibility and clinical perceptiveness.

REFERENCES

Aderman, M., Giardina, W. J., & Koreniowski, S. Effect of cyclandelate on perception, memory, and cognition in a group of geriatric subjects. *Journal of the American Geriatrics Society*, 1972, *20*, 268-271.

Arie, J. Dementia in the elderly: Diagnosis and assessment. In *Medicine in old age: Articles published in the British Medical Journal.* London: British Medical Association, 1974.

Ball, J., & Taylor, A. Effect of cyclandelate on mental function and cerebral blood flow in elderly patients. *British Medical Journal,* 1967, *3,* 525–528.

Beck, A. J. *The diagnosis and management of depression.* Philadelphia: University of Pennsylvania Press, 1973.

Bellak, L., & Bellak, S. S. *Manual for the Senior Apperception Test (S.A.T.).* Larchmont, N.Y.: C.P.S., 1973.

Birkett, D. P., & Boltuch, B. Chlorpromazine in geriatric psychiatry. *Journal of the American Geriatrics Society,* 1972, *20,* 403–406.

Buehler, C., Keith-Spiegel, P., & Thomas, K. Developmental psychology. In B. B. Wolman (Ed.), *Handbook of general psychology.* Englewood Cliffs, N.J.: Prentice-Hall, 1973.

Burt, C. G., Gordon, W. F., Holt, N. F., & Hodern, A. Amitriptyline in depressive states: A controlled trial. *Journal of Mental Science,* 1962, *108,* 711–730.

Busse, E. W. Aging and psychiatric diseases of late life. In M. F. Reiser (Ed.), *American handbook of psychiatry* (Vol. 4). New York: Basic Books, 1975.

Ciompi, R. *A comprehensive review of geronto-psychiatric literature in the postwar period* (U.S. Public Health Service Publication No. 1811). Washington, D.C.: National Institute of Mental Health, 1965.

Claghorn, J. The many faces of anxiety in different age groups. *New York State Journal of Medicine,* 1971, *71,* 331–334.

Clyde, D. J. Rating scales, behavior inventories, and drugs. In L. Uhr & J. G. Miller (Eds.), *Drugs and behavior.* New York: Wiley, 1960.

Cole, M. G., & Miller, H. F. Sleep deprivation in the treatment of elderly depressed patients. *Journal of the American Geriatrics Society,* 1976, *24,* 308–313.

Covington, J. S. Alleviating agitation, apprehension, and related symptoms in geriatric patients: A double-blind comparison of a phenothiazine and a benzodiazepine. *Southern Medical Journal,* 1975, *68,* 719–724.

Crampton, G. *The Little Golden Funny Book.* New York: Simon & Schuster, 1950.

Cutler, R. P., & Kurland, H. D. Clinical quantification of depressive reactions. *Archives of General Psychiatry,* 1961, *5,* 280–285.

Dixon, J. C. Cognitive structure in senile conditions with some suggestions for developing a brief screening test of mental status. *Journal of Gerontology,* 1965, *20,* 41–49.

Edwards, A. R. *The social desirability variable in personality assessment and research.* New York: Dryden, 1957.

Free, S. M., & Guthrie, M. B. A rating scale for evaluating clinical response in psychoneurotic outpatients. *Journal of Clinical Pharmacology,* 1969, *9,* 187–194.

Gershon, S. Antianxiety agents. In C. Eisdorfer & W. E. Fann (Eds.), *Psychopharmacology and Aging.* New York: Plenum Press, 1973.

Goldstein, B. Double-blind comparison of tybamate and chlordiazepoxide in geriatric patients. *Psychosomatics,* 1967, *8,* 334–337.

Goldstein, S. E., & Birnbom, F. Piperacetazine versus thioridazine in the treatment of organic brain disease: A controlled double-blind study. *Journal of the American Geriatrics Society,* 1976, *24,* 355–358.

Grinker, R. R., Sr., Miller, J., Sabahin, M., Nunn, R., & Nunnally, J. C. *The phenomena of depressions.* New York: Hoeber, 1961.

Guy, W. *ECDEU assessment manual for psychopharmacology* (Rev. ed.) (DHEW Publication No. ADM 76-338). Washington, D.C.: U.S. Department of Health, Education and Welfare, 1976.

Hamilton, M. The assessment of anxiety states by rating. *British Journal of Medical Psychology,* 1959, *32,* 50–55.

Hamilton, M. Development of a rating scale for primary depressive illness. *British Journal of Social and Clinical Psychology,* 1967, *6,* 278–296.

Hamilton, M. Diagnosis and rating of anxiety. In M. H. Lader (Ed.), *Studies of anxiety. British Journal of Psychiatry*, 1969, *3*, 76–79. (Spec. Pub.)

Harmatz, J. S., & Shader, R. I. Psychopharmacologic investigations in healthy elderly volunteers: MMPI Depression Scale. *Journal of the American Geriatrics Society*, 1975, *23*, 350–354.

Harris, A. D., Letemendia, F. J. J., & Willems, P. J. A. A rating scale of the mental state: For use in the chronic population of the psychiatric hospital. *British Journal of Psychiatry*, 1967, *113*, 941–949.

Hodern, A., Holt, N. F., Burt, C. G., & Gordon, W. F. Amitryptyline in depressive states: Phenomenology and prognostic considerations. *British Journal of Psychiatry*, 1963, *109*, 815–825.

Honigfeld, G., Rosenblum, M. P., Blumenthal, I. J., Lambert, H. K., & Roberts, A. J. Behavioral improvement in the older schizophrenic patient: Drug and social therapies. *Journal of the American Geriatrics Society*, 1965, *13*, 57–72.

Hughes, J. R., Williams, J. G., & Currier, R. D. An ergot alkaloid preparation (Hydergine) in the treatment of dementia: Critical review of the clinical literature. *Journal of the American Geriatrics Society*, 1976, *24*, 490–497.

Jarvik, L. F., & Milne, J. F. Gerovital-H3: A review of the literature. In S. Gershon & A. Raskin (Eds.), *Aging* (Vol. 2). New York: Raven Press, 1975.

Jarvik, M. A survey of drug effects upon cognitive activities of the aged. In C. Eisdorfer & W. E. Fann (Eds.), *Psychopharmacology and aging*. New York: Plenum Press, 1973.

Jennings, W. G. An ergot alkaloid preparation (Hydergine) versus placebo for treatment of cerebrovascular insufficiency: Double-blind study. *Journal of the American Geriatrics Society*, 1972, *20*, 407–412.

Judah, L., Murphree, O., & Seager, L. Psychiatric response of geriatric-psychiatric patients to Mellaril (TP-21 Sandoz). *American Journal of Psychiatry*, 1959, *115*, 1118–1119.

Kahn, R. L., Goldfarb, A. I., Pollack, M., & Peck, A. Brief objective measures for the determination of mental states in the aged. *American Journal of Psychiatry*, 1960, *117*, 326–328.

Kaplitz, S. E. Withdrawn, apathetic geriatric patients responsive to methylphenidate. *Journal of the American Geriatrics Society*, 1975, *23*, 271–276.

Kernohan, W. J., Chambers, J. L., Wilson, W. T., & Daugherty, J. F. Effects of nortriptyline on the mental status and social adjustment of geriatric patients in a mental hospital. *Journal of the American Geriatrics Society*, 1967, *15*, 196–202.

Kirven, L. E., & Montero, E. F. Comparison of thioridazine and diazepam in the control of nonpsychotic symptoms associated with senility: Double-blind study. *Journal of the American Geriatrics Society*, 1973, *21*, 546–551.

Kristof, F. H., Lehmann, H. E., & Ban, F. A. Systematic studies with trimipramine–A new antidepressive drug. *Canadian Psychiatric Association Journal*, 1967, *12*, 517–520.

Lehmann, H. E., & Ban, F. A. Central nervous system stimulants and anabolic substances in geropsychiatric therapy. In S. Gershon & A. Raskin (Eds.), *Aging* (Vol. 2). New York: Raven Press, 1975.

Levin, S. Depression in the aged. In M. A. Berezin & S. H. Cath (Eds.), *Geriatric psychiatry: Grief, loss, and emotional disorders in the aging process*. New York: International Universities Press, 1965.

Lifshitz, K. Problems in the quantitative evaluation of patients with psychoses of the senium. *The Journal of Psychology*, 1960, *49*, 295–303.

Livingston, M. C. *Poems of Lewis Carroll*. New York: Crowell, 1973.

Lorr, M., & Klett, C. J. *Inpatient Multidimensional Psychiatric Scale* (Rev. Ed.). Palo Alto, Calif.: Consulting Psychologists Press, 1966.

Lu, L., Stotsky, B. A., & Cole, J. O. A controlled study of drugs in long-term geriatric patients. *Archives of General Psychiatry*, 1971, *25*, 284–288.

McNair, D. M., Lorr, M., & Droppleman, L. F. *Psychiatric Outpatient Mood Scale* (Rev.). Boston: Psychopharmacology Laboratory, Boston University Medical Center, 1971.

Murray, H. A. *Thematic Apperception Test.* Cambridge, Mass.: Harvard University Press, 1943.

Nowlis, V., & Nowlis, H. The description and analysis of mood. *Annals of the New York Academy of Science,* 1956, *65,* 345–355.

Overall, J. E., & Gorham, D. R. The Brief Psychiatric Rating Scale. *Psychological Reports,* 1962, *10,* 799–812.

Overall, J. E., Hollister, L. E., & Meyer, F., et al. Imipramine and thioridazine in depressed and schizophrenic patients: Are there specific antidepressant drugs? *Journal of the American Medical Association,* 1964, *189,* 605–608.

Overall, J. E., Hollister, L. E., Pokorny, A. D., Casey, J. F., & Katz, G. Drug therapy in depressions. Controlled evaluation of imipramine, isocarboxazid, dextroamphetamine-amobarbital, and placebo. *Clinical Pharmacological Therapeutics,* 1962, *3,* 16–22.

Pattie, A. H., & Gilleard, C. J. A brief psychogeriatric assessment schedule: Validation against psychiatric diagnosis and discharge from hospital. *British Journal of Psychiatry,* 1975, *127,* 489–493.

Plutchik, R., Conte, H., & Lieberman, M. Development of a scale (GIES) for assessment of cognitive and perceptual functioning in geriatric patients. *Journal of the American Geriatrics Society,* 1971, *19,* 614–623.

Post, F. Dementia, depression, and pseudodementia. In D. F. Benson & D. Blumer (Eds.), *Psychiatric aspects of neurological disease.* New York: Grune & Stratton, 1975.

Procci, W. R. Schizo-affective psychosis: Fact or fiction? *Archives of General Psychiatry,* 1976, *33,* 1167–1178.

Rao, D. D., & Norris, J. R. A double-blind investigation of Hydergine in the treatment of cerebrovascular insufficiency in the elderly. *Johns Hopkins Medical Journal,* 1972, *130,* 317–324.

Raskin, A. *N.I.M.H. Collaborative Depression Mood Scale.* Rockville, Md.: National Institute of Mental Health, 1965.

Rickels, K., & Howard, K. The Physician Questionnaire: A useful tool in psychiatric drug research. *Psychopharmacologia,* 1970, *17,* 338–344.

Rockland, L. H., & Pollin, W. Quantification of psychiatric mental status: For use with psychotic patients. *Archives of General Psychiatry,* 1965, *12,* 23–28.

Rosen, H. Chronic cerebrovascular insufficiency in the elderly. *Journal of the Medical Society of New Jersey,* 1972, *69,* 445–448.

Rowell, J. T. An objective method of evaluating mental status. *Journal of Clinical Psychology,* 1951, *7,* 255–259.

Sakalis, G., Gershon, S., & Shopsin, B. A trial of Gerovital-H3 in depression during senility. *Current Therapeutic Research,* 1974, *16,* 59–63.

Salzman, C., Kochansky, G. E., & Shader, R. I. Rating scales for geriatric psychopharmacology–A review. *Psychopharmacology Bulletin,* 1972, *8,* 3–50.

Salzman, C., & Shader, R. I. Methodology for the evaluation of psychotropic agents in geriatric patients. In F. G. McMahon (Ed.), *Principles and techniques of human research and therapeutics, Vol. VIII: Psychopharmacological agents.* Mount Kisco, N.Y.: Futura, 1975.

Sathananthan, G. L., & Gershon, S. Cerebral vasodilators: A review. In S. Gershon & A. Raskin (Eds.), *Aging* (Vol. 2). New York: Raven Press, 1975.

Scheier, I. H., Cattell, R. B., & Sullivan, W. Predicting anxiety from clinical symptoms of anxiety. *Psychiatry Quarterly Supplement,* 1961, *35,* 114–126.

Shader, R. I., Harmatz, J. S., & Salzman, C. A new scale for clinical assessment in geriatric populations: Sandoz Clinical Assessment–Geriatric (SCAG). *Journal of the American Geriatrics Society,* 1974, *22,* 107–113.

Shapiro, M. B., Post, F., Lofving, B., & Inglis, J. "Memory function" in psychiatric patients over sixty, some methodological and diagnostic implications. *Journal of Mental Science*, 1956, *102*, 233–246.

Simpson, G. M., Hackett, E., & Kline, N. S. Difficulties in systematic rating of depression during outpatient drug treatment. *Canadian Psychiatric Association Journal*, 1966, *1*, 116–122. (Suppl.)

Smith, G. R., Taylor, C. W., & Linkous, P. Haloperidol versus thioridazine for the treatment of psychogeriatric patients: A double-blind clinical trial. *Psychosomatics*, 1974, *15*, 134–138.

Spark, M. *Memento mori.* New York: Meridian Books, 1960.

Spitzer, R. L., & Endicott, J. An integrated group of forms for automated psychiatric case records. *Archives of General Psychiatry*, 1971, *24*, 540–547.

Stotsky, B. A. A systematic study of therapeutic interventions in nursing homes. *Genetic Psychology Monographs*, 1967, *76*, 257–320.

Stotsky, B. A. Psychoses in the elderly. In C. Eisdorfer and W. E. Fann (Eds.), *Psychopharmacology and aging.* New York: Plenum Press, 1973.

Stotsky, B. A., & Borozne, J. Butisol sodium versus Librium among geriatric and younger outpatients and nursing home patients. *Diseases of the Nervous System*, 1972, *33*, 254–267.

Thompson, L. W. Effects of hyperbaric oxygen on behavioral functioning in elderly persons with intellectual impairment. In S. Gershon & A. Raskin (Eds.), *Aging* (Vol. 2). New York: Raven Press, 1975.

Triboletti, F., & Ferir, H. Hydergine for treatment of symptoms of cerebrovascular insufficiency. *Current Therapeutic Research*, 1969, *11*, 609–620.

Trier, T. R. A study of change among elderly psychiatric inpatients during their first year of hospitalization. *Journal of Gerontology*, 1968, *23*, 354–362.

Tsuang, M., Lu, L., Stotsky, B., & Cole, J. Haloperidol versus thioridazine for hospitalized psychogeriatric patients: Double-blind study. *Journal of the American Geriatrics Society*, 1971, *19*, 593–600.

Turek, I., Kurland, A. A., Ota, K. Y., & Hanlon, T. E. Effects of pipradrol hydrochloride on geriatric patients. *Journal of the American Geriatrics Society*, 1969, *17*, 408–413.

Verwoerdt, A. *Clinical geropsychiatry.* Baltimore: Williams & Wilkins, 1976.

Wittenborn, J. R. *Manual: Wittenborn Psychiatric Rating Scales.* New York: Psychological Corporation, 1955.

Wolff, K., Grasberger, J. C., & Kidorf, I. M. Nialamide in the treatment of schizophrenia in geriatric patients. *Journal of the American Geriatrics Society*, 1962, *10*, 148–152.

Zung, W. W. K. A self-rating depression scale. *Archives of General Psychiatry*, 1965, *12*, 63–70.

Zung, W. W. K. A rating instrument for anxiety disorders. *Psychosomatics*, 1971, *12*, 371–379.

Zung, W. W. K. The depression status inventory: An adjunct to the self-rating depression scale. *Journal of Clinical Psychology*, 1972, *28*, 539–543.

Zung, W. W. K., Gianturco, D., Pfeiffer, E., Wang, H. S., Whanger, A., Bridge, T. P., & Potkin, S. G. Pharmacology of depression in the aged: Evaluation of Gerovital-H3 as an antidepressant drug. *Psychosomatics*, 1974, *15*, 127–131.

Zung, W. W. K., & Green, R. L., Jr. Detection of affective disorders in the aged. In C. Eisdorfer & W. E. Fann (Eds.), *Psychopharmacology and aging.* New York: Plenum Press, 1973.

Zwerling, I., Plutchik, R., Hotz, M., Kling, R., Rubin, L., Grossman, J., & Siegel, B. Effects of a procaine preparation (Gerovital-H3) in hospitalized geriatric patients: A double-blind study. *Journal of the American Geriatrics Society*, 1975, *23*, 355–359.

REFERENCE NOTES

1. Harmatz, J. *Tentative approaches to testing elderly volunteers in a drug trial.* Paper presented at the Annual Meeting of the American Psychological Association, Washington, D.C., September 1976.
2. Cleary, P., & Guy, W. *Factor analyses of the Hamilton Depression Scale.* Paper presented at the International Symposium on the Evaluation of New Drugs in Clinical Psychopharmacology, Pisa, Italy, September 1975.
3. Harmatz, J. Personal communication, March 1977.
4. Lawton, M. P. *Extended Mental Status Questionnaire.* Philadelphia: Philadelphia Geriatric Center.
5. Salzman, C. *Clinical evaluation of the depressed elderly patient.* Paper presented at an NIMH Workshop in Problems in the Assessment of Psychopathology in the Elderly, Los Angeles, April 1977.

6

Self-rating Scales for Assessing Psychopathology in the Elderly

Douglas M. McNair
Boston University School of Medicine

INTRODUCTION

The major aims of this chapter are to describe and evaluate current measures, methods, and practices for obtaining self-reports of affective distress and other forms of psychiatric symptomatology from older individuals. The period covered is principally from 1970 to 1976. It is hoped this review will provide beginning answers to many questions. What measures are we asking the elderly to take? What problems are we encountering as we apply these measures? Are our scales and inventories reliable with this age group? Have we even determined that special norms are needed? How do established scales compare with scales designed for the elderly? How valid are self-report devices for detecting psychopathology in an elderly population? Are such measures useful for differential diagnosis or for evaluating the efficacy of psychotropic medicines? Are these instruments useful for evaluating nonsomatic therapeutic modalities such as psychotherapy? Are they useful for assessing the impact of physical illness upon affect and symptoms? Can meaningful comparisons be made of the relative validities of similar measures? There is precious little data pertaining to most such issues.

SEARCH PROCEDURE

A fairly routine procedure was followed to collect empirical research on the central topic. The first step was a MEDLARS search of 1970–1976 English language publications guided by an overinclusive set of key words and concepts. The next step was the identification of relevant reports and checking and cross-checking them for additional references. Then there was a scan of the contents of the 1970–1976 volumes of these journals: *Acta Psychiatrica Scandinavica, American Journal of Psychiatry, Archives of General Psychiatry, British Journal of Psychiatry, Clinical Pharmacology and Therapeutics, Current Therapeutic Research, Journal of Abnormal Psychology,*

Journal of the American Geriatrics Society, Journal of Consulting and Clinical Psychology, Journal of Gerontology, Journal of Nervous and Mental Disease, Psychopharmacologia, Psychosomatic Medicine, and *Psychosomatics.* The final step involved a search of certain recent reviews of treatment procedures for elderly psychiatric patients: antidepressant, antianxiety, and combination drug trials (Salzman & Shader, 1975; Salzman, Shader, & Van Der Kolk, 1976; Stotsky, 1975), procaine or Gerovital-H3 treatment trials (Jarvik & Milne, 1975; Ostfeld, Smith, & Stotsky, 1977), and hyperbaric oxygen studies (Thompson, 1975). A few pre-1970 reports of special interest were included.

GENERAL COMMENTS

This chapter is confined primarily to a description and a commentary on empirical findings. Particular scales and inventories were omitted if, and only if, there were no applications during the review period or there were no citations that suggested marked utility in pre-1970 research. There are no other intentional omissions. One could speculate about established scales that had no published applications and their potential usefulness with an aged population, but such inferences can and should wait for data.

Few psychopathology measures for the elderly have been designed, printed, or standardized. Most were borrowed or transferred from research with younger normals and psychiatric patients. Screening devices for the preliminary identification of psychopathology are the exceptions. Salzman, Kochansky, and Shader (1972) found a similar state of affairs when they compiled their listing of scales actually or potentially of value for geriatric psychopharmacological drug trials. Surprisingly few attempts had been made to adapt standard tests, by altering their formats or instructions, for use with the elderly.

The following parts of the chapter focus on specific scales and inventories and depict the range of applications and findings for particular measures. A few studies included more than one measure and thus receive multiple citations. In sequence, the next three sections describe (1) findings with multidimensional personality inventories; (2) measures of anxiety, depression, and other affect and symptom categories; and (3) screening devices for rapid preliminary assessment of psychopathology. Test manuals and handbooks for widely known measures are not referenced; *The Eighth Mental Measurements Yearbook* provides comprehensive information about such scales (Buros, 1978).

PERSONALITY INVENTORIES

Minnesota Multiphasic Personality Inventory

Four research groups administered the entire Minnesota Multiphasic Personality Inventory (MMPI) to elderly samples. None described patient complaints or resistance to this lengthy inventory. Only one group adapted the customary instructions or procedure. Pearson, Swenson, and Rome (1965) showed that many individual depression and anxiety items related quadratically to age in a sample of 25,000 Mayo Clinic patients. Their main point was that the endorsement rate of many such MMPI items did not increase linearly with age as is often assumed. There was, on the contrary, a rise in such symptoms to middle age, followed by a decline.

Britton and Savage (1969) factor analyzed the correlation matrix of the MMPI clinical scales for 83 randomly selected aged residents of Newcastle-upon-Tyne. Three factors were identified: General Psychopathology, Social Withdrawal, and Aggressive-Asocial. Their first factor is somewhat similar to the major factor identified in studies with younger subjects. They regarded their second and third factors as different from any identified previously. There were many problems, however, with this study. Not only was their sample size inadequate for factor analysis, but also the redundancy inherent in the scoring of the clinical scales practically guaranteed great difficulty in interpreting factors derived from the interscale correlations. The substantive findings, therefore, can not be taken too seriously. The methodological findings, however, indicate that the MMPI can be applied to a group with an average age of 75 years. The MMPI, incidentally, was read to subjects in their own homes in two sessions. Britton and Savage concluded on a moderately enthusiastic note about its potential use with the elderly.

Davis, Mosdzierz, and Macchitelli (1973) examined the discriminative power of the MMPI with young and old psychiatric patients. The task was to differentially diagnose schizophrenia from nonschizophrenia within the two age groups. The MMPI passed the test with the younger patients (the Schizophrenia and Psychoasthenia scales separated the groups) but failed with the older group. The sample sizes were small, and some limits to the applicability of the MMPI can be inferred from the exclusions from the sample. Acceptable cases were new admissions with no history of chronic hospitalization or electroconvulsive therapy, with at least an 8th grade education, and with no elevated *F/K* scale or dissimilation index.

Fracchia, Sheppard, and Merlis (1974) gave the MMPI to 90 elderly male chronic patients in a state hospital. They reported that the profiles were associated with the pattern of drug treatment. Patients currently receiving no psychotropics scored markedly and significantly higher on the Lie scale (*L*-scale) and Correction scale (*K*-scale) than did patients receiving either one drug or polypharmacy. No other profile differences among these groups were found. Fracchia et al. interpreted their results as indicating defensiveness, overcontrol, and avoidance of attention by the patients who did not receive drugs. Details of sampling, diagnosis, and other current treatments were not provided, and while their no drug group was significantly older by nearly 10 years than the other 2 groups, the authors discounted age as a biasing factor. They also did not report encountering any unusual problems in obtaining MMPIs from the people in this study.

The above findings provoke the following question: Has it occurred to anyone lately to check the MMPI's internal consistency and its test-retest stability with the elderly? These four MMPI studies can be viewed as validity trials of the test with the elderly, and, from this perspective, none provided convincing evidence of validity or high or even satisfactory reliability. It becomes incumbent on researchers who want to apply this scale with this population to produce such evidence. There were also no instances in which the entire MMPI was used to assess treatment outcome. In this regard, the MMPI and its subscales have not proven especially useful for evaluating antidepressant drug effects (McNair, 1974).

Other Personality Inventories

The Maudsley Personality Inventory (MPI) and the Sixteen Personality Factor Questionnaire (16PF) had one trial each. Bolton and Savage (1971) administered the MPI to 144 normals and inpatients over the age of 60. They found no significant differences among normals, schizophrenics, affective disorders, and brain syndromes on the MPI Extraversion factor. The organics scored significantly higher on the Neuroticism factor than normals and schizophrenics, but no other significant differences were found on the factor. The study does provide some very tentative but valuable norms for these diagnostic groups of elderly patients; their mean scores, surprisingly, differed little from Eysenck's (1959) norms for younger adults.

Costa, Fozard, McCrae, and Bosse (1976) used second-order factor scores on the 16PF to classify 969 elderly normal volunteers as anxious versus adjusted and, separately, as introverted versus extraverted. They then showed that decline in cognitive abilities with age was unrelated to these 16PF classifications.

ANXIETY, DEPRESSION, AND RELATED AFFECTS

Zung Self-Rating Depression Scale

Zung's Self-Rating Depression Scale (SDS) had more trials with the elderly than any other scale. Zung (1967, 1970) had 169 Methodist Retirement Home residents and Golden Age Club members complete the scale according to the standard instructions. He found no significant differences between these two groups, but he observed that, combined, they reported significantly higher depression scores than his younger normative group. Heidell and Kidd (1975) administered this scale, which is easy to read and comprehend, to 120 senior citizens. They found that nursing home residents judged senile by staff had significantly higher SDS scores than a group comprised of both nonsenile residents of the same home and of residents of the community. Heidell and Kidd inferred that depression in the elderly is often unrecognized and labeled as senility.

Blumenthal (1975) gave the SDS to 320 normal community residents residing in selected geographic areas. The sample apparently was a pilot trial that approximated a stratified representative sample of U.S. adults, but Blumenthal did not clarify this point. She found a modest positive correlation (.19) between the SDS and age. Particularly noteworthy is her finding that the intercluster correlations of SDS items differed markedly within her young and old subsamples. It should follow that the Zung factor structure differed with age, but Blumenthal did not test this hypothesis.

Salzman, Shader, Harmatz, and Robertson (1975) gave a battery of measures, including the SDS, to 40 normal elderly male paid volunteers before and after 2 weeks of treatment with diazepam or a placebo. The researchers implied they had recruited a mildly depressed and anxious group but provided no documentation; the Manifest Anxiety Scale (Taylor, 1955) scores for their sample, in fact, were markedly lower than college age norms. The SDS detected no treatment differences, whereas other measures did (as explained below). The same research group, Shader, Harmatz, Kochansky, and Cole (1975), compared a stimulant-vitamin elixir (Alertonic) with a placebo and with no treatment for 99 Golden Age Club members. After one week, no significant effects were identified. In spite of these nonsignificant findings, the researchers concluded that the assessment methods were readily applicable for older people.

Zung, Gianturco, Pfeiffer, Wang, Whanger, Bridge, and Potkin (1974) compared Gerovital-H3 (procaine) with imipramine and placebo in a double-blind trial with 30 depressed inpatients 60 years of age and older. The treatment groups were small, and the interpretation of results was complicated by significant baseline group differences. The Gerovital group clearly improved significantly more on the SDS than the placebo group, even allowing for baseline differences. Although Zung et al. interpreted the imipramine versus Gerovital-H3 differences as favoring the latter, I agree with Jarvik and Milne (1975) that it is impossible to draw meaningful conclusions about the relative efficacy of imipramine and Gerovital because of both baseline differences and the ordinal properties of the scale. When groups differ significantly at baseline on ordinal measures, it may be impossible to compare meaningfully group differences in magnitude of change. For example, a shift from a mean of 30 to 20 on the SDS may or may not reflect greater true change than a drop from a mean of 20 to 15. Jarvik and Milne described another comparison of Gerovital-H3 with placebo by Kurland and Hayman (Note 1). The SDS showed significant treatment differences favoring Gerovital in this trial with 63 Arizona private practice patients. Jarvik and Milne noted that the sex distribution was very different for the treatment groups and thus confounded the interpretation.

Morris, Wolf, and Klerman (1975) gave the SDS, as well as the Philadelphia Geriatric Center Morale Scale (Lawton, 1975), to 89 state hospital inpatients. They performed a factor analysis of the SDS and interpreted two varimax rotated factors as Agitation and Self-satisfaction. These factors do not correspond with previously identified factors (Guy, 1976), but no one has ever demonstrated that any SDS factors are more sensitive to change or treatment effects than the total score. The Morris et al. (1975) study is a rarity in that it reports reliability data for older people. The internal consistencies for the two factors were in the highly satisfactory .80s region. The SDS was readministered 15 weeks after the first occasion, but the authors did not report the much needed test-retest reliabilities. Instead, they provided extensive details about canonical correlations between the SDS and the Philadelphia Geriatric Center Morale Scale.

Profile of Mood States

Laforet, Sidd, and Waterman (1974) gave the Profile of Mood States (POMS) (McNair, Lorr, & Droppleman, 1971) to 13 elderly patients before and after pacemaker insertion for correction of complete heart block. The time period for rating these adjective scales was altered from the usual "past week, including today" to "right now." At presurgery, most patients had mood distress scores in the 40-50th percentile range according to college norms. The patients showed a significant decrease postsurgery on one of the six mood factors, Confusion-Bewilderment, and a trend toward reduced Tension-Anxiety. Laforet et al. found very little difficulty in applying the scale with this group, who ranged in age from 60 to 85.

Salzman et al. (1975), in their study with elderly male volunteers, found that diazepam and placebo had significantly different effects on POMS Fatigue. The diazepam group increased in Fatigue, and the placebo group showed a reduction. It is unclear from their presentation whether these differences occurred at 1 week, 2 weeks, or both. In a parallel diazepam study with men and women volunteers, Salzman and Shader (1973) observed a similar result on Fatigue. The pipradrol-vitamin elixir trial by Shader et al. (1975) showed no differences on any POMS factors among the elixir, placebo, and no treatment groups.

MMPI-Depression Scale

Three studies (all by Shader, Salzman, and associates) used the MMPI-Depression Scale. Harmatz and Shader (1975) compared the responses of young and old subjects to the measure. They found significant age differences on nearly half of the 60 items. They recommended obtaining revised norms for the elderly. They also noted that their samples of elderly people found the SDS and adjective scales easier to comprehend than MMPI-derived measures.

In a diazepam trial by Salzman et al. (1975), the MMPI-Depression Scale detected no antidepressant effects on the benzodiazepine. A modified 30-item version of this scale, however, did register such an effect, and it was highly correlated in elderly subjects with Lubin's Depression Adjective Checklist (Lubin, 1967). No description of the derivation of the modified scale was provided. In an elixir trial by Shader et al. (1975), the MMPI–Depression Scale showed no significant differences in outcome between elixir, a placebo, and no treatment.

Manifest Anxiety Scale

Taylor's (1955) Manifest Anxiety Scale (MAS) had two applications. Salzman et al. (1975) compared the distribution of scores for their elderly subjects with Taylor's norms based on younger subjects. The elderly subjects had significantly lower scores. Stotsky and Borozne (1972) found that groups treated with chlordiazepoxide and butabarbital differed significantly on the MAS after 2 weeks of double-blind treatment. An analysis of covariance showed butabarbital superior. Their group was comprised of about 50% geriatric outpatients and nursing home patients and 50% younger outpatients. There was no analysis to determine which group, if either, was more sensitive to the treatment variable. Their design involved a crossover after 2 weeks, but the results for the crossover period were essentially uninterpretable.

Hopkins Symptom Checklist

The Hopkins Symptom Checklist comes in many versions (Derogatis, Lipman, Rickels, Uhlenhuth, & Covi, 1973). The 35-item version (Guy, 1976) was applied twice in this sample of studies. Salzman et al. (1975) administered it before and during treatment in their diazepam trial, but they reported no findings. The same is true of the Shader et al. (1975) stimulant-vitamin elixir study.

Other Scales

Zung et al. (1974) administered the Zung Self-Rating Anxiety Scale (SAS) in their procaine, imipramine, and placebo trials. As with the SDS, the procaine group had significantly lower baseline SAS scores than the other two groups, but change scores on the SAS did not significantly favor procaine over placebo. Salzman et al. (1975) administered the Scheier-Cattell Anxiety Battery in their diazepam versus placebo trial and found no significant drug effects.

SCREENING DEVICES

Savage and Britton (1967) reported a MMPI-derived 15-item screening scale for the assessment of the aged. They recommended its use with a short form of the Wechsler Adult Intelligence Scale (Britton & Savage, 1966) to detect cognitive defects and psychopathology. For identifying psychiatric abnormality they reported 88% accuracy in their derivation ($N = 83$) sample and 87% accuracy in their cross-validation ($N = 30$) sample. False positives were 19% and 14%, respectively. Simon, Berkman, and Epstein (Note 2) selected 15 signs and symptoms from a longer list that best discriminated psychiatrically impaired from unimpaired elderly San Francisco institutional and community residents. Later, Simon (1970) compared the Simon-Berkman-Epstein (SBE) Index with the Cornell Medical Index, the Savage-Britton Index (SBI), and Langner's Midtown Manhattan Index (1962). The SBI had the best record for identifying true positives and the SBE was best for true negatives. The differences among the four indexes were not tested for significance, but they appeared relatively minor for true negatives. For true positives, the Cornell Medical Index and Langner's index did poorly. Lindstrom and Kahn (1976) compared the Savage-Britton and SBE Indexes as discriminators of 25 psychiatrically impaired from 25 nonimpaired nursing home residents. In this study the items were read to the subjects. The SBI had a significantly higher success rate, although neither index did as well as in the reported test construction studies. A serious problem with the SBE was that it misclassified two-thirds of the normals as psychiatrically impaired.

Another potentially useful self-rating screening device, reported by Wood, Wylie, and Sheafor (1969), is the Life Satisfaction Index in two forms, A and Z. Forms A and Z have, respectively, 20 and 13 dichotomous "agree" or "disagree" items. They reported a respectable internal consistency ($K\text{-}R_{20} = .79$) for the Z form, and correlations in the .50s with observer ratings on the Life Satisfaction Scale (Neugarten, Havighurst, & Tobin, 1961). The measure might be a practicable inverse method for assessing psychopathology. The items are direct, easy to understand, and they refer to topics many older people talk about.

Emotions Profile Index

The Emotions Profile Index (EPI) is a forced-choice scale involving 62 paired adjectives measuring 8 emotional traits (Plutchik, 1962). Plutchik and DiScipio (1974) gave the test to 60 long-term chronic schizophrenics, chronic alcoholics, and geriatric patients with chronic brain syndrome. All groups differed markedly from normals, and there were numerous significant differences between the schizophrenics and the other two groups. The authors noted that a high percentage of patients approached for the study could not complete the EPI. Fracchia et al. (1974) used the EPI and found no significant differences among their no drug, one drug, and polypharmacy treatment groups, whereas the MMPI showed some differences.

CONCLUSIONS AND RECOMMENDATIONS

There are insufficient accomplishments to provide the fundamentals of systematic psychometric knowledge about the role and value of self-measurement by elderly people. Little is known because little has been ventured.

Researchers have administered a wide range of standard rating scales and inventories to the nonpsychotic nonsenile elderly. These researchers rarely have complained in print of difficulties in testing this gerontological population, and they have exhibited sufficient confidence in their data to publish their findings. Clearly, many elderly individuals have completed lengthy self-assessment instruments such as the MMPI.

What we do not know, though, are the psychometric specifics about basic scale properties. We need to know, for instance, if test responses by the elderly are more, less, or equally reliable when compared with younger adults. Data on internal consistency and test-retest stability are essential for judging the role and value of specific tests for this population.

We have developed almost no age-appropriate norms for the elderly. We can not even state unequivocally that special age norms are needed. The proper comparisons between the young and the old have not been made. Most such available data came from studies that suffered from a confounding of age with other important influences.

When there is a choice between employing an established scale and constructing a new measure, there are enormous advantages favoring the former. The mass of accumulated data on existing scales makes them valuable, and this value should not be sacrificed lightly. There are areas of self-ratable psychopathology unique to the elderly that are missing from scales developed primarily for younger adults. The answer is to design scales aimed at such symptomatology and to add the new devices to test batteries for the elderly. It is irresponsible to claim a need to reinvent the wheel when you have nothing to add but a spoke.

Formats of existing scales can be made more appropriate to the elderly by such alterations as large print. Rating time periods can be changed, if needed, from intervals such as "past week" to "right now." Recent memory deficits in the elderly have been alleged to justify such modifications to increase or maintain scale sensitivity. Such decisions, however, should be based on data and not on the preconceptions of scale constructors.

Not one efficacy trial reviewed here included a patient global improvement rating. Such scales have proven to be very sensitive detectors of some treatment effects (McNair, 1974) and should be added to any comprehensive battery for assessing affect and symptom change in the elderly.

The state of the art is too primitive to permit sophisticated consideration of comparative choices among self-measures of the same or similar dimensions. There simply is no multimethod multitrait data of any consequence. Also, practically nonexistent are comparisons of self-ratings and observer ratings for assessing state, trait, or change. These kinds of validity data are also absolutely vital.

REFERENCES

Blumenthal, M. D. Measuring depressive symptomatology in a general population. *Archives of General Psychiatry,* 1975, *32,* 971–978.

Bolton, N., & Savage, R. D. Neuroticism and extraversion in elderly normal subjects and psychiatric patients: Some normative data. *British Journal of Psychiatry,* 1971, *118,* 473–474.

Britton, P. G., & Savage, R. D. A short form of the W.A.I.S. for use with the aged. *British Journal of Psychiatry,* 1966, *112,* 417–418.

Britton, P. G., & Savage, R. D. The factorial structure of the Minnesota Multiphasic Personality Inventory from an aged sample. *Journal of Genetic Psychology,* 1969, *114,* 13–17.

Buros, O. K. *The eighth mental measurements yearbook.* Highland Park, N.J.: Gryphon Press, 1978.

Costa, P. T., Jr., Fozard, J. L., McCrae, R. R., & Bosse, R. Relations of age and personality dimensions to cognitive ability factors. *Journal of Gerontology,* 1976, *31,* 663–669.

Davis, W. E., Mosdzierz, G. J., & Macchitelli, F. J. Loss of discriminative "power" of the MMPI with older psychiatric patients. *Journal of Personality Assessment,* 1973, *37,* 555–558.

Derogatis, L. R., Lipman, R. S., Rickels, K., Uhlenhuth, E. H., & Covi, L. The Hopkins Symptom Checklist (HSCL): A measure of primary symptom dimensions. In P. Pichot (Ed.), *Psychological measurement: Problems in psychopharmacology.* Basel: Karger, 1973.

Eysenck, H. J. *The manual of the Maudsley Personality Inventory.* London: University of London Press, 1959.

Fracchia, J., Sheppard, C., & Merlis, S. Treatment patterns in psychiatry: Clinical and personality features of elderly hospitalized patients during milieu, single-drug, and multiple-drug programs. *Journal of the American Geriatrics Society,* 1974, *22,* 212–216.

Guy, W. *ECDEU assessment manual for psychopharmacology,* (Rev. ed.) (DHEW Publication No. ADM 76-388). Washington, D.C.: U.S. Department of Health, Education and Welfare, 1976.

Harmatz, J. S., & Shader, R. I. Psychopharmacologic investigations in healthy elderly volunteers: MMPI Depression Scale. *Journal of the American Geriatrics Society,* 1975, *23,* 350–354.

Heidell, E. D., & Kidd, A. H. Depression and senility. *Journal of Clinical Psychology,* 1975, *31,* 643–645.

Jarvik, L. F., & Milne, J. F. Gerovital-H3: A review of the literature. In S. Gershon & A. Raskin (Eds.), *Aging. Volume 2. Genesis and treatment of psychological disorders in the elderly.* New York: Raven Press, 1975.

Laforet, E. G., Sidd, J. J., & Waterman, W. E. The relationship of heart rate to mood in patients with heart block: Effect of pacing. *Journal of Gerontology,* 1974, *29,* 643–644.

Langner, S. A twenty-two item screening score of psychiatric symptoms indicating impairment. *Journal of Health and Human Behavior,* 1962, *3,* 269–276.

Lawton, M. P. The Philadelphia Geriatric Center Morale Scale: A revision. *Journal of Gerontology,* 1975, *30,* 85–89.

Lindstrom, L., & Kahn, M. W. Discriminative effectiveness of two psychiatric screening instruments for a gerontological population. *Journal of Consulting and Clinical Psychology,* 1976, *44,* 151–152.

Lubin, B. *Depression adjective checklists.* San Diego: Educational and Industrial Testing Service, 1967.

McNair, D. M. Self-evaluations of antidepressants. *Psychopharmacologia,* 1974, *37,* 281–292.

McNair, D. M., Lorr, M., & Droppleman, L. F. *Profile of mood states: Manual.* San Diego: Educational and Industrial Testing Service, 1971.

Morris, J. N., Wolf, R. S., & Klerman, L. V. Common themes among morale and depression scales. *Journal of Gerontology,* 1975, *30,* 209–215.

Neugarten, B. L., Havighurst, R. J., & Tobin, S. S. The measurement of life satisfaction. *Journal of Gerontology,* 1961, *16,* 134–143.

Ostfeld, A., Smith, C. M., & Stotsky, B. A. The systematic use of procaine in the treatment of the elderly. *Journal of the American Geriatrics Society,* 1977, *25,* 1–20.

Pearson, J. S., Swenson, W. M., & Rome, H. P. Age and sex differences related to MMPI response frequency in 25,000 medical patients. *American Journal of Psychiatry,* 1965, *121,* 988–995.

Plutchik, R. *The emotions: Fact, theories and a new model.* New York: Random House, 1962.

Plutchik, R., & DiScipio, W. J. Personality patterns in chronic alcoholism (Korsakoff's syndrome), chronic schizophrenia, and geriatric patients with chronic brain syndrome. *Journal of the American Geriatrics Society,* 1974, *22,* 514–516.

Salzman, C., Kochansky, G. E., & Shader, R. I. Rating scales for geriatric psychopharmacology—A review. *Psychopharmacology Bulletin,* 1972, *8,* 3–50.

Salzman, C., & Shader, R. I. Methodology for the evaluation of psychotropic agents for geriatric patients. In F. G. McMahon (Ed.), *Principles and techniques of human research and therapeutics, Volume III. Psychopharmacological agents.* Mt. Kisco, N.Y.: Futura, 1973.

Salzman, C., & Shader, R. I. Research in geriatric psychopharmacology. *Journal of Geriatric Psychiatry,* 1975, *8,* 165–184.

Salzman, C., Shader, R. I., Harmatz, J., & Robertson, L. Psychopharmacologic investigations in elderly volunteers: Effects of diazepam in males. *Journal of the American Geriatrics Society,* 1975, *23,* 451–457.

Salzman, C., Shader, R. I., & Van Der Kolk, B. A. Clinical psychopharmacology and the elderly patient. *New York State Journal of Medicine,* 1976, *76,* 71–77.

Savage, R. D., & Britton, P. G. A short scale for the assessment of mental health in the community aged. *British Journal of Psychiatry,* 1967, *113,* 521–523.

Shader, R. I., Harmatz, J. S., Kochansky, G. E., & Cole, J. O. Psychopharmacologic investigations in healthy elderly volunteers: Effects of pipradrol-vitamin (Alertonic) elixir and placebo in relation to research design. *Journal of the American Geriatrics Society,* 1975, *23,* 277–279.

Simon, A. The psychiatric and the geriatric patient. *Journal of Geriatric Psychiatry,* 1970, *4,* 5–22.

Stotsky, B. A. Psychoactive drugs for geriatric patients with psychiatric disorders. In S. Gershon & A. Raskin (Eds.), *Aging. Volume 2. Genesis and treatment of psychological disorders in the elderly.* New York: Raven Press, 1975.

Stotsky, B. A., & Borozne, J. Butisol sodium versus Librium among geriatric and younger outpatients and nursing home patients. *Diseases of the Nervous System,* 1972, *33,* 254–267.

Taylor, J. A. A personality scale of manifest anxiety. *Journal of Abnormal and Social Psychology,* 1955, *48,* 285–290.

Thompson, L. W. Effects of hyperbaric oxygen on behavioral functioning in elderly persons with intellectual impairment. In S. Gershon & A. Raskin (Eds.), *Aging. Volume 2. Genesis and treatment of psychological disorders in the elderly.* New York: Raven Press, 1975.

Wood, V., Wylie, M. L., & Sheafor, B. An analysis of a short self-report measure of life satisfaction: Correlation with rater judgments. *Journal of Gerontology,* 1969, *24,* 465–469.

Zung, W. W. K. Depression in the normal aged. *Psychosomatics,* 1967, *8,* 287–292.

Zung, W. W. K. Mood disturbances in the elderly. *The Gerontologist,* 1970, *10,* 2–4.

Zung, W. W. K., Gianturco, D., Pfeiffer, E., Wang, H., Whanger, A., Bridge, T. P., &

Potkin, S. G. Pharmacology of depression in the aged: Evaluation of Gerovital-H3 as an antidepressant drug. *Psychosomatics,* 1974, *15,* 127–131.

REFERENCE NOTES

1. Kurland, M., & Hayman, M. *Gerovital-H3 in the treatment of depression in a private practice population: A double-blind study.* Paper presented at the meeting of the American Academy of Psychosomatic Medicine, Scottsdale, Arizona, November 1974.
2. Simon, A., Berkman, P. L., & Epstein, L. F. *Psychiatric screening of the elderly.* Paper presented at the meeting of the 7th International Congress on Mental Health, London, 1968.

7

Nurse and Psychiatric Aide Rating Scales for Assessing Psychopathology in the Elderly: A Critical Review

James M. Smith
Harlem Valley Psychiatric Center

INTRODUCTION

The usefulness of nurse and psychiatric aide ratings of ward behavior was noted early in the history of psychiatric research (Lorr, 1954; Spitzer & Endicott, 1975). Briefly, they offer several specific advantages. In mute or extremely uncooperative patients, ratings of behavior made by the nursing staff may be the only data available on a patient's response to treatment. Even for cooperative patients, nurse ratings may provide the most valid information with regard to particular aspects of behavior, for example, social functioning, assaultiveness, and performance of activities of daily living. Furthermore, one of the more convincing ways of demonstrating a therapeutic effect in psychiatry is to have that effect evident in the data obtained from multiple sources; nurse ratings often provide valuable confirmatory evidence.

A large number of behavioral rating scales have been developed for use by nurses in psychiatric research. In this chapter, no attempt has been made to be all-inclusive. Rather, the scales selected for review are those that have been widely used in studies of general psychiatric populations or that offer the promise of special value in geriatric samples. It is hoped that the considerations noted in the reviews of the scales selected will be useful in evaluating some of the less frequently used instruments. For concise information on scales not selected, there are excellent overviews by Lyerly (1973) and by Salzman, Shader, Kochansky, and Cronin (1972).

The scales selected for review are the Geriatric Rating Scale (GRS), the Physical and Mental Impairment-of-Function Evaluation (PAMIE), the Nurses' Observation Scale for Inpatient Evaluation (NOSIE), the Ward Behavior Inventory (WBI), and the Psychotic Inpatient Profile (PIP). Only two of these, the GRS and PAMIE, were developed specifically for use with geriatric patients.

GERIATRIC RATING SCALE

The Geriatric Rating Scale (GRS) is a 31-item behavioral rating scale designed to measure the physical and social functioning of geriatric patients (Plutchik, Conte, Lieberman, Bakur, Grossman, & Lehrman, 1970). It is based on the Stockton Geriatric Rating Scale (Meer & Baker, 1966) with 22 of the GRS items either verbatim or revised from this earlier scale. Although the GRS contains 31 items, only 28 are scored since 3 items relating to patient behavior at night were eliminated because the day staff complained of difficulty in obtaining this information (Plutchik et al., 1970). Items are rated on a 0-2 scale (maximum total score = 56) with the meaning of response points for each item indicated by brief phrases. For example, for the item related to friends on the ward, the response options are defined as: has several friends (0), has just one friend (1), or has no friends (2). All items are scored in the same direction with higher scores indicating increased impairment.

The interrater reliability of the GRS is satisfactory, ranging from .87 to .94 (Plutchik & Conte, 1972; Plutchik et al., 1970), and the correlations between ratings obtained approximately 1 year apart are reported to be in the mid .60s (Plutchik & Conte, 1972; Smith, Bright, & McCloskey, 1977). In terms of validity, scores on the GRS differentiate between geriatric and nongeriatric patients and between organic and functional geriatric patients (Dastoor, Norton, Boillat, Minty, Papadopoulou, & Müller, 1975; Plutchik et al., 1970). Mean GRS total scores for 9 wards were found to correlate .86 with global judgments of the overall level of functioning of the 9 wards (Plutchik et al., 1970). Finally, there is an indication that scores on the GRS may be useful in predicting discharge (Plutchik & Conte, 1972).

While the GRS was originally developed to yield only a global score of functioning, it has recently been factor analyzed (Smith, Bright, & McCloskey, 1977) and shown to be composed of 3 factors: Withdrawal/Apathy (11 items), Antisocial Disruptive Behavior (6 items), and Deficits in Activities of Daily Living (7 items). Internal consistency (alpha) coefficients for the 3 factors were .90, .75, and .78, respectively, and a 1-year follow-up of 98 of the original 370 patients yielded reliability (stability) coefficients of .65 for Withdrawal/Apathy, .32 for Antisocial Disruptive Behavior, and .63 for Deficits in Activities of Daily Living. It appears that use of these factor scores may increase the sensitivity of this scale, since these scores indicated that females were significantly more impaired than males on two factors (Antisocial Disruptive Behavior and Deficits in Activities of Daily Living), while GRS global scores failed to yield a significant sex difference (Smith et al., 1977).

The GRS has been used in several studies of treatment effectiveness in geriatric patients. In one such study (Zwerling, Plutchik, Hotz, Kling, Rubin, Grossman, & Siegel, 1975), geriatric patients selected to represent varying levels of organic brain dysfunction were involved in a double-blind study of the effects of procaine (Gerovital-H3). No significant differences in total GRS scores were found following 6 and 12 weeks of Gerovital-H3 treatment.

In another series of studies, the GRS was used as one measure of effectiveness of trazodone over a 12-week trial (Amin, Hontela, & Kussin, 1976; Derkervorkian, Ban, & Hontela, 1976; Lehmann, Ban, Hontela, Nair, & Stewart, 1976; Vergara, Ban, Lehmann, & Stewart, 1976). In summarizing the results of these studies, Stewart, Ban, and Lehmann (1976) indicated that trazodone produced statistically significant decreases (improvement) in GRS total scores by the end of the fourth week of treatment. In the reports of the individual studies, the various authors presented the results of analyses of the individual GRS items, since the factor composition of the scale had not as yet been determined. It is noteworthy that in two of these studies (Lehmann et al., 1976; Vergara et al., 1976) the investigators commented on the fact that all their patients achieved zero ratings on a few of the GRS items, most of which related to antisocial disruptive behaviors. The significance of this is discussed below in a consideration of the sensitivity of the GRS to change.

In a double-blind crossover study, the relative effectiveness of piperacetazine and thioridazine was examined in 50 geriatric patients with clinically significant manifestations of organic brain disease (Goldstein & Birnbom, 1976). Results indicated that total scores on the GRS were improved in both groups ($p < .10$) with no real differences noted between drugs. By contrast, in a double-blind crossover study of pentylenetetrazol (Metrazol) and placebo in geriatric patients with organic brain syndrome, Stotsky, Cole, Lu, and Sniffin (1972) found no reliable differences on a 27-item revised form of the GRS.

In another study, Citrin and Dixon (1977) examined the effects of a reality orientation treatment program on a small subsample of residents in a large geriatric institution. Those selected for the program were moderately disoriented without major physical disabilities. These 12 selected residents and a similar group of 13 control residents were assessed on the GRS before the program and during the seventh week of the program. Results with the GRS were inconclusive. While a significant difference in total GRS scores between groups was found at the time of posttest ($p < .05$), this appeared to be due to a slight worsening in the scores of the control group and a nonsignificant improvement in the functioning of the experimental group.

Powell (1974) contrasted the effects of exercise and social therapies using a control group in a study of institutionalized geriatric mental patients. GRS ratings as well as other outcome measures were obtained at baseline and after 8 and 12 weeks of the programs. Although there were some significant effects on cognitive measures, there were no significant effects on total GRS scores.

In overview, the GRS is brief and has a high degree of staff acceptance enhanced no doubt by the fact that many of the GRS items have high face validity and are clinically meaningful to ward staff. However, on balance, there is some question as to its sensitivity to change. An evaluation of the usefulness of the GRS as a measure of change must take two factors into account: (1) in several of the studies cited in which the GRS failed to reveal significant treatment effects, the treatments were of doubtful efficacy (e.g. procaine and exercise therapy); and (2) all treatment studies with the GRS to date have analyzed either total GRS scores or scores on the individual items; none have used scores on the recently derived factors of the GRS (Smith et al., 1977). Since these factor scores revealed significant sex differences that were masked by total GRS scores (Smith et al., 1977), there is an indication that the factor scores may be more sensitive measures, though not necessarily more sensitive to change. Factor 2 (Antisocial Disruptive Behavior), for example, one of the factors to show significant sex differences, measures a relatively high level of disturbance (physical assault, stealing, public masturbation), which is not characteristic of many patients. Consequently, baseline values on many of the items that comprise this factor tend to be low (as noted in the trazodone research already cited) with little prospect of demonstrating group change. It remains to be determined empirically whether the use of the factor scales will increase the sensitivity of the GRS to change.

PHYSICAL AND MENTAL IMPAIRMENT-OF-FUNCTION EVALUATION

The Physical and Mental Impairment-of-Function Evaluation (PAMIE) (Gurel, Linn, & Linn, 1972; Gurel, Linn, Linn, Davis, & Maroney, 1970) was developed as an instrument for the quantitative description of a wide range of behaviors relevant to chronically ill adults and institutionalized geriatric patients. The authors of the scale felt that traditional measures of psychopathological behavior inadequately covered the realm of impaired physical functioning, while scales designed for geriatric populations focused on this area to the exclusion of disturbed mental processes. By contrast, the PAMIE was designed to yield "a multifunctional assessment, one that would reflect physical, psychological, and social/interpersonal disabilities" (Gurel et al., 1972, p. 84).

The PAMIE is composed of 77 dichotomous (yes/no) items and is an outgrowth of previous work with the Self-Care Inventory (Gurel, Davis, & Stumpf, 1963; Watson & Fulton, 1967) and the Patient Evaluation Scale (Gurel, 1964; Watson & Fulton, 1968). A factor analysis of the data obtained on 845 male geriatric veterans (about evenly divided between predominantly medical/surgical and predominantly psychiatric patients) revealed that the PAMIE is composed of 10 factors: Self-Care/Dependent, Belligerent/Irritable, Mentally Disorganized/Confused, Anxious/Depressed, Bedfast/Moribund, Behaviorally Deteriorated, Paranoid/Suspicious, Sensorimotor Impaired, Withdrawn/Apathetic, and Ambulatory (Gurel et al., 1972). Internal consistency coefficients (Cronbach alpha) ranged from .703 to .914 for the 10 factors. Some special items that did not load significantly on a factor were also included, for example, whether the patient eats a regular diet or whether the patient is blind, since this information is of value in making nursing home placements.

A second order factor analysis of the matrix of factor score correlations indicated the presence of three higher order dimensions: Physically Infirm, Psychologically Deteriorated, and Psychologically Agitated (Gurel et al., 1972). It is of interest to note that the Self-Care/Dependent factor was the only factor found to load significantly on two higher order factors: Physically Infirm and Psychologically Deteriorated. This suggested to the authors that the need for assistance in self-care activities may be as important for the psychologically deteriorated patient as for the physically infirm patient. Additional analyses with the 10 factor scores revealed that several factors successfully differentiated a number of contrasting groups, for example, patients reported by nurses as needing more versus less intensive nursing care and patients judged appropriate versus not appropriate for foster home care.

In subsequent work with the PAMIE on nearly 200 inpatients in an extended care and rehabilitation center, Pablo (1976) found that several factors yielded significant differences with respect to age, sex, diagnosis (single versus multiple), or type of ward placement (long-term versus intensive rehabilitative). Furthermore, a comparison of scores of these patients with those of a group of chronic geriatric patients with psychiatric symptoms revealed statistically significant differences on six PAMIE factors. The psychogeriatric group was significantly more disturbed on five factors (Belligerent/Irritable, Anxious/Depressed, Behaviorally Deteriorated, Paranoid/Suspicious, and Withdrawn/Apathetic), while the patients in the extended care and rehabilitation facility were significantly more impaired on the Sensorimotor Impaired factor.

In a study of the effects of intrainstitutional relocation, Pablo (1977) obtained data on mortality and on the PAMIE scale 5 months prior to the move and at 6, 18, and 30 months following the move for patients involved in the relocation and for a comparison group not involved. His results indicated that mortality increased significantly for patients following a relocation in comparison with the group of nonmovers. However, scores on the 10 PAMIE factors failed to yield any significant differences attributable to the relocation. In discussing this lack of effect on the PAMIE, Pablo considered the fact that the relocation was voluntary and to similar surroundings, that the staff had well prepared both patients and relatives for the move, and that the data were obtained at points rather removed in time from the actual move (5 months before and 6 months after).

On the basis of the research with this scale to date, the PAMIE appears particularly well suited for indicating the levels of care required by different patients. Its strength appears to lie in the breadth of content areas it taps. However, more work needs to be done on determining the interrater reliability of the scale. While the original data of Gurel, Linn, and Linn (1972) indicated satisfactory levels of internal consistency for the factors, Pablo (1976) has reported that the interrater reliabilities on a subset of patients ranged from .286 to .678 for the 10 factors. Perhaps these relatively low values are the result of the restricted range of scores on some factors because of the small number of items included and the dichotomous rating format. In addition, the usefulness of the PAMIE factors as measures of change has not yet been adequately tested. This consideration is particularly important since the originators of several other nurse rating scales have specifically abandoned dichotomous ratings in favor of 4- and 5-point frequency of response formats to increase the sensitivity of their scales to change (Honigfeld & Klett, 1965; Lorr & Vestre, 1968).

NURSES' OBSERVATION SCALE FOR INPATIENT EVALUATION

Without question, the Nurses' Observation Scale for Inpatient Evaluation (NOSIE) (Honigfeld, Gillis, & Klett, 1966; Honigfeld & Klett, 1965) is by far the most widely used nurse rating scale in psychiatry. A review of the history and current status of the final version of this scale, NOSIE-30, contains summary data from over 150 studies in which this scale was used to evaluate the effects of psychotropic drug treatment (Honigfeld, 1974). The unequaled success of this scale is due to its history of empirical development (drawing many of its items from previous scales) and particularly due to the attention Honigfeld and his associates paid to deriving a measure that would be sensitive to change following psychotropic drug treatment. Its success in the latter regard resulted in the adoption of the NOSIE by the Early Clinical Drug Evaluation Units (ECDEU) of the Psychopharmacology Research Branch of NIMH as one of the six standard rating scales for use by investigators supported by ECDEU grant funds.

The NOSIE began as a 100-item scale with each item rated as to frequency of occurrence: (0) never, (1) sometimes, (2) often, (3) usually, and (4) always (Honigfeld & Klett, 1965). In assembling these items, an attempt was made to include items that measured patient assets, particularly those related to interpersonal aspects of behavior. An examination of ratings of 307 chronic male schizophrenics (aged 55-69) by pairs of ward aides led to the deletion of 20 items of low interrater reliability or markedly skewed distributions. Factor analysis of the remaining 80 items suggested that the factorial structure of the scale could be accounted for by 7 factors composed of 61 of the 80 items.

Subsequent developmental work with the NOSIE-80 centered around two aspects (Honigfeld, Gillis, & Klett, 1966). First, the original normative group was expanded to include data on younger patients, resulting in a norm group of 630 male schizophrenic patients aged 26 to 74 (mean = 52.4) with a range of continuous hospitalization of from 0 to 47 years (mean = 15.9). Second, data on the NOSIE-80 were available for the norm group before and after 24 weeks of treatment and factor analyses were performed on the change scores as well as on the pretreatment scores. Final item selection was made of items that had high factor loadings for the pretreatment factor analysis as well as for the change score factor analysis. Incorporating the results of the change score factor analysis in the item selection process resulted in the elimination of items that were not sensitive to change.

Based on these analyses, the number of items was reduced to 30 (NOSIE-30) measuring 6 factor analytically derived areas of functioning. These 6 factors are divided into positive and negative factors as follows:

Positive factors	Negative factors
Social Competence (COM)	Irritability (IRR)
Social Interest (INT)	Manifest Psychosis (PSY)
Personal Neatness (NEA)	Retardation (RET)

In addition, a Total Patient Assets score is computed by subtracting the sum of the negative factor scores from the sum of the positive factor scores and adding a constant. Since factor scores on the NOSIE are based on the sum of two raters' responses, if only one rater is used, the scores must be doubled. The median interrater reliability for the 6 NOSIE-30 factors has been reported to be .85 (Lentz, Paul, & Calhoun, 1971).

Although not designated as a geriatric rating scale, it is interesting to note that the NOSIE was originally developed "to measure therapeutic change in the older schizophrenic patient" (Honigfeld & Klett, 1965, p. 65) and the original application of the NOSIE-80 was with chronic schizophrenics aged 55 to 69. In addition, evidence for the reliability and validity of the NOSIE-80 was obtained in a VA cooperative study of the effectiveness of chemotherapy and placebo in geriatric patients with a median age of 66 years and an average length of hospitalization of over 24 years (Honigfeld, Rosenblum, Blumenthal, Lambert, & Roberts, 1965). Following 24 weeks of treatment, significant improvement due to chemotherapy ($p < .05$) was demonstrated on 4 of the NOSIE-80 factors (Social Competence, Personal Neatness, Irritability, and Manifest Psychosis), all 4 of which have been retained in the NOSIE-30. Although the investigators deliberately sought out younger samples for the further development of this scale, subsequent studies with the NOSIE have indicated that it has retained its usefulness and sensitivity for geriatric populations.

In one such double-blind study, Tsuang, Lu, Stotsky, and Cole (1971) examined the effectiveness of haloperidol and thioridazine for actively psychotic geriatric patients. Analyses of covariance on the NOSIE-30 data indicated significant improvement ($p < .05$) in both drug groups on Irritability, Manifest Psychosis, Personal Neatness, and Total Assets.

In another double-blind study, Kirven and Montero (1973) administered thioridazine or diazepam to geriatric patients with nonpsychotic symptoms associated with senility. After 4 weeks of treatment those receiving thioridazine showed significant improvement ($p < .05$) on Social Competence, Irritability, and Retardation as well as on Positive Score, Negative Score, and Total Assets. Those receiving diazepam showed significant improvement ($p < .05$) on Retardation, Negative Score, and Total Assets.

Kaplitz (1975) studied the effects of methylphenidate on withdrawn senile geriatric patients. Following 6 weeks of double-blind treatment, the methylphenidate group showed significant improvement ($p < .01$) over the placebo group on the Total Assets score and on all NOSIE factors except Personal Neatness.

After 4 weeks of double-blind treatment with thioridazine or placebo in geriatric patients with chronic organic brain syndrome, Rada and Kellner (1976) found a significant ($p < .05$) drug/placebo difference on the Manifest Psychosis factor.

The NOSIE has also been used in geriatric samples to evaluate the effects of exercise therapy (Powell, 1974), intrahospital transfer (Raasoch, Willmuth, Thomson, & Hyde, 1977), anticoagulant therapy for senile dementia (Ratner, Rosenberg, Kral, & Engelsmann, 1972), pentylenetetrazol for organic brain syndrome (Stotsky et al., 1972), piperacetazine versus thioridazine in organic brain disease (Goldstein & Birnbom, 1976) and inpatient versus community treatment (Watson, 1976). In none of these studies were significant treatment effects found on the NOSIE. However, at least in some of these studies the treatments were of doubtful efficacy.

WARD BEHAVIOR INVENTORY

The Ward Behavior Inventory (WBI) is composed of 138 dichotomous items descriptive of ward behavior, such as "acts afraid" and "soils bed or clothing with excrement" (Burdock & Hardesty, 1968). Almost one-third of the items relate to the patient's verbal behavior, for example, "says he hates people" and "complains of insomnia." Each item of the WBI is rated yes or no and the score on the WBI is the number of maladaptive behaviors characteristic of the patient (range: 0–138). The immediate forerunner of the WBI was the 150-item Ward Behavior Rating Scale (WBRS) (Burdock, Hakerem, Hardesty, & Zubin, 1960) and some of the data cited in the WBI manual were actually obtained with that scale. An early version of the WBRS (Burdock, Elliot, Hardesty, O'Neill & Sklar, 1960) was very similar to the Albany Behavioral Rating Scale (ABRS) developed by Shatin and Freed (1955) that, in turn, drew heavily on the Hospital Adjustment Scale (HAS) (Ferguson, McReynolds, & Ballachey, 1953).

There have been two factor analytic studies of the WBRS involving data on young acute schizophrenics. In one (Raskin & Clyde, 1963), 11 factors were identified: Self-Care, Social Participation, Extraversion, Irritability, Anxiety, Guilt Feelings, Depression, Feelings of Unreality, Slowed Speech and Movements, Paranoid Projections, and Excitement. In the other study (Goldberg, Cole, & Clyde, 1963) 7 factors emerged: Social Participation, Irritability, Self-Care, Appearance of Sadness, Feelings of Unreality, Resistive, and Confused. In both studies, ratings were also obtained on the Inpatient Multidimensional Psychiatric Scale (IMPS) (Lorr, Klett, McNair, & Lasky, 1963), an interview instrument, and significant relationships were found between several of the WBRS factors and IMPS factors. It is interesting to note that in both of these factor analytic studies fewer than half of the WBRS items had significant factor loadings. In the study by Raskin and Clyde (1963) 67 of the 150 WBRS items had factor loadings high enough to be included in 1 of the identified factors and in the study by Goldberg, Cole, and Clyde (1963) 45 were so included. Subsequent factor analyses of WBRS ratings obtained on depressed patients (Raskin & McKeon, 1971; Raskin, Schulterbrandt, Reatig, & McKeon, 1969; Raskin, Schulterbrandt, Reatig, & Rice, 1967) yielded some of the same factors as those identified above and others quite distinct (e.g., hypochondriasis, sleep disturbance, and denial of illness).

Several studies have demonstrated the sensitivity of the WBI (WBRS) to treatment effects. In a study by the NIMH Psychopharmacology Service Center Collaborative Study Group (1964) (Goldberg, Klerman, & Cole, 1965) following 6 weeks of double-blind treatment with either chlorpromazine, fluphenazine, thioridazine, or placebo, 344 acute schizophrenics showed significant drug/placebo differences on 4 WBI factors: Social Participation, Irritability, Self-Care, and Confusion. In another large study comparing the sensitivity of various outcome measures to drug treatments of patients with symptoms of depression, Raskin and Crook (1976) found the WBRS to be most helpful for detecting the sedative-hypnotic effects of the study drugs.

There have also been reports of its value when used with geriatric patients. Burdock, Hakerem, Hardesty, and Zubin (1960) noted that the WBRS distinguished a group of female geriatric patients treated with drugs from a matched placebo group ($p < .05$). In another study, a preliminary 112-item form of the WBRS was used to evaluate the effectiveness of an intensive treatment program for female geriatric patients admitted to a state hospital (Burdock, Elliot, Hardesty, O'Neill, & Sklar, 1960). Analyses revealed that while there were no significant differences between the intensive treatment and control groups on admission, after 1 month the intensive treatment group had significantly better scores on the WBRS than the control group ($p < .001$).

However, there are several problems with the WBI. First, it is quite lengthy and tedious to complete and thus has relatively poor staff acceptability for all but the most highly motivated staff (especially when used as a frequently repeated measure). Staff often complain of the inappropriateness of many of the items for a particular patient. In addition, the factor analytic studies demonstrate that fewer than half of the items can be grouped into any meaningful factors. This necessitates the inclusion of the data on the remaining items into a global score, which lacks the specificity required in many research and clinical situations. The final problem, perhaps more relevant to geriatric samples than to others, is that almost one-third of the WBI items relate to patients' verbal reports. Thus, mute patients and geriatric patients who are often reluctant to discuss their feelings tend to score low on the WBI. At least for some of these patients, improvement in clinical condition may be indicated by a worsening of WBI scores (i.e., patients may become more willing to discuss their problems).

The latter effect is illustrated in the data of Loew and Silverstone (1971) who studied the value of increased social, psychological, and physical stimulation on the cognitive, affective, and social functioning of 14 males in a geriatric center ward. As one of their outcome measures, the WBI was completed before implementation and at a 6-month follow-up. Results indicated that the experimental group changed significantly more on the WBI than the control group at the time of follow-up but in the direction of increased psychopathology. In explanation of this unexpected finding, the investigators noted that one of the effects of the increased stimulation was to make patients more critical, demanding, and challenging.

In overview, the WBI appears to be of limited usefulness in geriatric research although some investigators may choose to use subsets of items based on the factor analytic results.

PSYCHOTIC INPATIENT PROFILE

The Psychotic Inpatient Profile (PIP) (Lorr & Vestre, 1968) is a 96-item scale that is a major revision and extension of the earlier Psychotic Reaction Profile (PRP) (Lorr, 1961) based on the results of several factor analyses. The first section of this scale consists of 74 statements descriptive of manifest ward behavior and is rated on the following frequency-of-occurrence scale: not at all (0), occasionally (1), fairly often (2), and nearly always (3). Ratings on these items yield scores on 8 factors: Excitement (EXC), Hostile Belligerence (HOS), Paranoid Projection (PAR), Anxious Depression (ANX), Retardation (RTD), Seclusiveness (SEC), Care Needed (CAR), and Psychotic Disorganization (PSY). The second section consists of 17 statements descriptive of patient self-reports and requires the rater to talk to the patient. On these items, the patient is given a rating of 3 if the item is true and 0 if it is not true. This section yields scores on Grandiosity (GRN), Perceptual Distortion (PCP), and Depressive Mood (DPR). The final section has 5 additional statements descriptive of patient reports related to orientation. They are rated 0 if true and 3 if not true (the reverse of the rating of the previous section) and yield a score on a Disorientation (DIS) factor. Extensive norms on the PIP on drug-free and drug-treated samples are presented, though these appear to be based on relatively young samples.

Interrater reliabilities for the PIP (intraclass correlations) are satisfactory, ranging from .74 for Perceptual Distortion to .99 for Grandiosity (Lorr & Vestre, 1968). Concurrent validity and treatment sensitivity of the PIP also appear satisfactory at least in nongeriatric samples. Lorr and Vestre (1968) noted that 10 of the PIP scales are essentially equivalent to those measured by the Inpatient Multidimensional Psychiatric Scale (Lorr et al., 1963), an interview schedule. Vestre and Zimmerman (1970) found that many of the PIP scales differentiated between patients on open and closed wards and between patients recently admitted and others near discharge. Two other studies (Dehnel, Vestre, & Schiele, 1968; Hall, Vestre, Schiele, & Zimmerman, 1968) demonstrated that the PIP is sensitive to the effects of psychotherapeutic drugs. Similar validating data are available for the original PRP (Caffey, Diamond, Frank, Grasberger, Herman, Klett, & Rothstein, 1964; Casey, Hollister, Klett, Lasky, & Caffey, 1961; Hanlon, Nussbaum, Wittig, Hanlon, & Kurland, 1964; Lasky, Klett, Caffey, Bennett, Rosenblum, & Hollister, 1962; Vestre, 1966).

The PIP has not been used extensively in studies with geriatric samples. Sugerman, Williams, and Alderstein (1964) used the PRP to study the effects of haloperidol on geriatric patients diagnosed as chronic brain syndrome associated with senile brain disease or cerebral arteriosclerosis. Although significant differences between placebo-treated and haloperidol-treated patients were found on some of the outcome measures employed, no significant changes were found on the PRP. In discussing this, the authors noted that the PRP did not appear apprορriate for use with geriatric patients.

An examination of the content of the items comprising the 12 PIP scales suggest that normative data on most, if not all, of the scales would be greatly different if obtained on geriatric samples. With regard to the appropriateness of specific scales, seven scales seem to offer no problem for use with geriatric samples: Excitement, Hostile Belligerence, Retardation, Seclusiveness, Care Needed, Grandiosity, and Disorientation. The remaining five scales (Paranoid Projection, Anxious Depression, Psychotic Disorganization, Perceptual Distortion, and Depressive Mood) are of questionable value both because the clustering of the items appears to be of doubtful validity in geriatric samples and because of questions concerning the frequency (in geriatric samples) of the types of symptomatology represented by the items. For example, an item such as "Looks tired and all worn out," which is scored in the Anxious Depression scale, may not be an appropriate item in this scale for geriatric patients. Similarly, while the items "Says he feels tired and lacks energy to do things" and "Reports he cannot concentrate or remember things" may be indicative of Depressive Mood in younger patients, these items may reflect valid somatic complaints in the elderly and have relatively little to do with depression. As a final example, the item "Makes unusual movements of mouth, eyebrow or other parts of face" would not appear appropriate for inclusion in the Psychotic Disorganization factor for geriatric patients since it describes the cardinal features of a neuroleptic-induced motor disorder known as tardive dyskinesia, which has a high prevalence in chronic geriatric patients treated with these drugs (Crane, 1973; Kazamatsuri, Chien, & Cole, 1972).

Additional problems with the PIP are that it is somewhat long (96 items) and that the response categories change for all 3 sections. Particularly confusing is the reversal of response weights for the true/not true categories for the last 2 sections.

If this scale is to be of value in geriatric research, a determination must be made of its factor analytic composition in geriatric samples, and further studies must be conducted on its usefulness as a measure of change in these groups. Until that time, the value of the PIP in this area remains questionable.

CONCLUSIONS

Two of the most common uses of nurse rating scales in the elderly are to differentiate patients in terms of functioning (especially concerning appropriate placement) and to evaluate the effectiveness of various forms of treatment. These functions correspond to Honigfeld's (1974) distinction between status-descriptive and change-sensitive scales. As indicated in the discussion of the development of the NOSIE, this scale was designed to be useful for both functions. As a result, items were eliminated that had a low frequency of occurrence and/or that were insensitive to change.

The elimination of items with a low frequency of occurrence (e.g., physical assault) in favor of those assessing a more prevalent, albeit less severely disturbed, behavior (e.g., irritability) will undoubtedly yield a scale more sensitive to group change in the general psychiatric population. However, this may mean sacrificing valuable descriptive information. Furthermore, it is not necessarily true in all instances that the scale assessing the lower level of psychopathology is more sensitive to change. For example, if a ward is set up to admit only physically assaultive patients, one may find that physical assaults decline significantly following successful treatment, while measures of irritability remain relatively unchanged.

Items that measure relatively permanent and unchangeable aspects of behavior (e.g., due to physical disability) seem unnecessary in a rating scale for younger patients. By contrast, some of the most critical information about geriatric patients may relate to these disabilities; thus, a good descriptive scale for geriatric patients should include such items. Of course, measures on this subset of items are not expected to be sensitive to change.

The preceding discussion leads to several general observations regarding nurse rating scales in geropsychiatry. The first observation, which relates to the use of such scales in psychiatry at large, is that a scale must be selected that measures a level of severity of dysfunction that is appropriate for the sample under consideration. A comparison of the factors of the GRS and the NOSIE-30 helps to illustrate the differences between scales in this regard. The Social Interest factor of the NOSIE-30 is very similar to the Withdrawal/

Apathy factor of the GRS. However, the Antisocial Disruptive Behavior factor of the GRS taps much more severe forms of behavior disturbance (such as exhibitionism, destructiveness, and assaultiveness) than does the NOSIE-30 Irritability factor, which essentially measures how easily a patient becomes upset. Similarly, the GRS Deficits in Activities of Daily Living factor taps severe forms of disturbance such as incontinence, visual impairment, loss of ambulation, and the inability to feed oneself, while the NOSIE-30 Personal Neatness and Social Competence factors appear to assess lesser degrees of disturbance in Activities of Daily Living.

To use these scales in geriatrics it is necessary to understand the relative importance of the status-descriptive and change-sensitive functions of the evaluation and to select a scale accordingly. Based on the reviews of the specific scales, no one scale has demonstrated optimal usefulness in geriatric patients both for evaluating the effectiveness of treatment and for indicating the type of placement most suitable for a given patient. While the NOSIE is the best currently available change-sensitive scale for geriatric patients, it does not appear to be the best status-descriptive scale for this population. On the other hand, while the PAMIE appears to be a good status-descriptive scale for this population, there is some question as to its sensitivity to change. Hence, one must make a choice between scales based on the goals of each specific project.

Another observation emerging from the discussion of the specific scales is that caution should be used with behavior rating scales not devised specifically for geriatric samples. Since factor analytic techniques have been employed in the development of many of these scales, it is perhaps useful to indicate briefly some of the limitations of this technique. First, and perhaps so obvious that it is sometimes forgotten, is the fact that factor analysis is a data-dependent technique. In other words, it will indicate only the nature of obtained data (in terms of the interrelationships among items or variables) and is therefore limited in its generalizability to the parameters of such data. Consequently, the number and types of factors found will be limited both by the specific types of items (variables) on which data have been obtained and by the characteristics of the samples tested. Several of the scales discussed were originally developed with a large pool of items thought to be descriptive of the behavior of young psychiatric patients. Perhaps a different item pool would have resulted if items thought to be descriptive of the behavior of geriatric patients had been selected. It is possible that the factor composition may differ with different types of patient samples even when the same pool of original items is used. Recall that the factor solution for the WBRS was not the same when based on the data obtained on schizophrenic and depressed patients. Similarly, the factor composition of the various scales discussed may be different in geriatric samples from that found in younger samples. The need for a reevaluation of the factor composition on geriatric samples has already been noted in connection with the PIP. Furthermore, even if some factors are found to be the same for geriatric and younger samples, one cannot assume that the factors are measuring identical underlying pathologies. One example may be the Retardation factor often found in younger samples reflecting the presence or absence of psychopathological motor retardation; a similar factor in geriatric samples may reflect a predominantly physical disability (e.g., Parkinson's disease or arthritis).

In relation to the latter point, there appears to be some value in developing scales for geriatric patients that allow for a differentiation to be made between impairment of function due to physical or due to psychiatric/psychosocial factors. Recall in this connection that the Self-Care Dependent factor of the PAMIE scale loaded significantly on the higher order factors of Physically Infirm and Psychologically Deteriorated (Gurel et al., 1972). A ward of geriatric patients with poor Activities of Daily Living functions due to serious arthritic complaints is quite different from a ward of geriatric patients with similar Activities of Daily Living deficits due primarily to chronic institutionalization with its resulting apathy and indifference. The inclusion of patients with physical impairments in a remotivation program would make the demonstration of significant change less likely than using a sample limited to patients with psychiatric/psychosocial impairments.

A final point about factor analysis is that often a strategy is adopted whereby items that fail to load significantly on a factor are eliminated. However, a good status-descriptive scale for geriatric use should probably include items that are unlikely to load highly on any single factor. This has been acknowledged by Gurel et al., (1972) in their development of the PAMIE scale. They retained several items in their scale (e.g., blindness, deafness, drunkeness, diet restriction, physical assaultiveness, and desire to leave the hospital), because they were clearly important considerations for nursing home placements, even though they failed to meet the .30 cutoff loading for inclusion in a specific factor.

Another relevant consideration is that in the scales cited no attempt has been made to include items that might load on an Unpredictability factor. Since geriatric patients are often labile in their mood and behavior, such a measure may prove useful. It is not unusual for a geriatric patient to score very well on one of the scales reviewed, and when staff is questioned about why the patient remains in the institution, they will respond that the patient happened to be rated during a good week. However, such patients have periodic episodes of severe behavioral disorganization that make them unlikely candidates for successful community placement.

Finally, a word should be mentioned about evaluating the sensitivity to change of the various behavioral rating scales in geriatric research. Since much needs to be learned about the effective treatment of the psychopathologies of old age, a variety of substances of unknown value are currently under investigation. In these studies, one must be careful not to attribute lack of effect to the lack of sensitivity of the scale, when instead the treatment may be of no value. For example, as noted in connection with the GRS, the failure to demonstrate a significant change on the GRS following Gerovital-H3 may reveal more about the lack of effect of Gerovital-H3 than about the lack of sensitivity of the GRS. Until much more is known about the measurement and treatment of psychopathology in the elderly, this determination continues to be a difficult one to make.

REFERENCES

Amin, M., Hontela, S., & Kussin, D. New research on the use of trazodone in old age. A placebo-controlled clinical trial. *Psychopharmacology Bulletin,* 1976, *12,* 45-46.

Burdock, E. I., Elliot, H. E., Hardesty, A. S., O'Neill, F. J., & Sklar, J. Biometric evaluation of an intensive treatment program in a state mental hospital. *Journal of Nervous and Mental Disease,* 1960, *130,* 271-277.

Burdock, E. I., Hakerem, G., Hardesty, A. S., & Zubin, J. A ward behavior rating scale for mental hospital patients. *Journal of Clinical Psychology,* 1960, *16,* 246-247.

Burdock, E. I., & Hardesty, A. S. *Ward Behavior Inventory Manual.* New York: Springer, 1968.

Caffey, E. M., Jr., Diamond, L. S., Frank, T. V., Grasberger, J. C., Herman, L., Klett, C. J., & Rothstein, C. Discontinuation or reduction of chemotherapy in chronic schizophrenics. *Journal of Chronic Diseases,* 1964, *17,* 347-358.

Casey, J. F., Hollister, L. E., Klett, C. J., Lasky, J. J., & Caffey, E. M., Jr. Combined drug therapy of chronic schizophrenics: Controlled evaluation of placebo, dextro-amphetamine, imipramine, isocarboxazid and trifluoperazine added to maintenance doses of chlorpromazine. *American Journal of Psychiatry,* 1961, *117,* 997-1003.

Citrin, R. S., & Dixon, D. N. Reality orientation: A milieu therapy used in an institution for the aged. *The Gerontologist,* 1977, *17,* 39-43.

Crane, G. E. Persistent dyskinesia. *British Journal of Psychiatry,* 1973, *122,* 395-405.

Dastoor, D. P., Norton, S., Boillat, J., Minty, J., Papadopoulou, F., & Müller, H. F. A psychogeriatric assessment program. I. Social functioning and ward behavior. *Journal of the American Geriatrics Society,* 1975, *23,* 465-471.

Dehnel, L. L., Vestre, N. D., & Schiele, B. C. A controlled comparison of clopenthixol and perphenazine in a chronic schizophrenic population. *Current Therapeutic Research,* 1968, *10,* 169-176.

Derkervorkian, K., Ban, T. A., & Hontela, S. New research on the use of trazodone in old age. A standard-controlled clinical trial. *Psychopharmacology Bulletin,* 1976, *12,* 46-47.

Ferguson, J. T., McReynolds, P., & Ballachey, E. L. *Hospital Adjustment Scale.* Palo Alto, Calif.: Consulting Psychologists Press, 1953.

Goldberg, S. C., Cole, J. O., & Clyde, D. J. Factor analyses of ratings of schizophrenic behavior. *NIMH Psychopharmacology Service Center Bulletin,* 1963, *2,* 23-28.

Goldberg, S. C., Klerman, G. L., & Cole, J. O. Changes in schizophrenic psychopathology and ward behaviour as a function of phenothiazine treatment. *British Journal of Psychiatry,* 1965, *111,* 120-133.

Goldstein, S. E., & Birnbom, F. Piperacetazine versus thioridazine in the treatment of organic brain disease: A controlled double-blind study. *Journal of the American Geriatrics Society,* 1976, *24,* 355-358.

Gurel, L. *Patient evaluation scale.* (Mimeographed report). Washington, D.C.: Veterans Administration, 1964.

Gurel, L., Davis, J. E., & Stumpf, J. C. *Survey of the self-care dependent in VA hospitals* (Psychiatric Evaluation Project). Washington, D.C.: Veterans Administration, 1963.

Gurel, L., Linn, M. W., & Linn, B. S. Physical and mental impairment-of-function evaluation in the aged: The PAMIE scale. *Journal of Gerontology,* 1972, *27,* 83–90.

Gurel, L., Linn, M. W., Linn, B. S., Davis, J. E., Jr., & Maroney, R. J. Patients in nursing homes: Multidisciplinary characteristics and outcomes. *Journal of the American Medical Association,* 1970, *213,* 73–77.

Hall, W. B., Vestre, N. D., Schiele, B. C., & Zimmerman, R. A controlled comparison of haloperidol and fluphenazine in chronic treatment-resistant schizophrenics. *Diseases of the Nervous System,* 1968, *29,* 405–408.

Hanlon, T. E., Nussbaum, K., Wittig, B., Hanlon, D. D., & Kurland, A. A. The comparative effectiveness of amitriptyline, perphenazine, and their combination in the treatment of chronic psychotic female patients. *The Journal of New Drugs,* 1964, *4,* 52–60.

Honigfeld, G. NOSIE-30: History and current status of its use in pharmacopsychiatric research. *Modern Problems in Pharmacopsychiatry,* 1974, *7,* 238–263.

Honigfeld, G., Gillis, R. D., & Klett, C. J. NOSIE-30: A treatment-sensitive ward behavior scale. *Psychological Reports,* 1966, *19,* 180–182.

Honigfeld, G., & Klett, C. J. The Nurses' Observation Scale for Inpatient Evaluation: A new scale for measuring improvement in chronic schizophrenia. *Journal of Clinical Psychology,* 1965, *21,* 65–71.

Honigfeld, G., Rosenblum, M. P., Blumenthal, I. J., Lambert, H. L., & Roberts, A. J. Behavioral improvement in the older schizophrenic patient: Drug and social therapies. *Journal of the American Geriatrics Society,* 1965, *13,* 57–72.

Kaplitz, S. E. Withdrawn, apathetic geriatric patients responsive to methylphenidate. *Journal of the American Geriatrics Society,* 1975, *23,* 271–276.

Kazamatsuri, H., Chien, C.-P., & Cole, J. O. Therapeutic approaches to tardive dyskinesia. *Archives of General Psychiatry,* 1972, *27,* 491–499.

Kirven, L. E., & Montero, E. F. Comparison of thioridazine and diazepam in the control of nonpsychotic symptoms associated with senility: Double-blind study. *Journal of the American Geriatrics Society,* 1973, *21,* 546–551.

Lasky, J. J., Klett, C. J., Caffey, E. M., Bennett, J. L., Rosenblum, M. P., & Hollister, L. E. Drug treatment of schizophrenic patients: A comparative evaluation of chlorpromazine, chlorprothixene, fluphenazine, reserpine, thioridazine and triflupromazine. *Diseases of the Nervous System,* 1962, *23,* 698–706.

Lehmann, H. E., Ban, T. A., Hontela, S., Nair, N. V. P., & Stewart, J. A. New research on the use of trazodone in old age. An uncontrolled clinical trial carried out in Verdun, Quebec, Canada. *Psychopharmacology Bulletin,* 1976, *12,* 42–44.

Lentz, R. J., Paul, G. L., & Calhoun, J. F. Reliability and validity of three measures of functioning with "hard-core" chronic mental patients. *Journal of Abnormal Psychology,* 1971, *78,* 69–76.

Loew, C. A., & Silverstone, B. M. A program of intensified stimulation and response facilitation for the senile aged. *The Gerontologist,* 1971, *11,* 341–347.

Lorr, M. *Manual: The Psychotic Reaction Profile.* Beverly Hills: Western Psychological Services, 1961.

Lorr, M. Rating scales and check lists for the evaluation of psychopathology. *Psychological Bulletin,* 1954, *51,* 119–127.

Lorr, M., Klett, C. J., McNair, D. M., & Lasky, J. J. *Manual: Inpatient Multidimensional Psychiatric Scale.* Palo Alto, Calif.: Consulting Psychologists Press, 1963.

Lorr, M., & Vestre, N. D. *Psychotic Inpatient Profile Manual.* Los Angeles: Western Psychological Services, 1968.

Lyerly, S. B. *Handbook of psychiatric rating scales* (2nd ed.). Rockville, Md.: NIMH, 1973.

Meer, B., & Baker, J. A. The Stockton Geriatric Rating Scale. *Journal of Gerontology,* 1966, *21,* 392–403.

NIMH Psychopharmacology Service Center Collaborative Study Group. Phenothiazine treatment in acute schizophrenia. *Archives of General Psychiatry*, 1964, *10*, 246–261.

Pablo, R. Y. The evaluation of the physical and mental impairments of a long-term and rehabilitation hospital patient population. *Canadian Journal of Public Health*, 1976, *67*, 305–313.

Pablo, R. Y. Intra-institutional relocation: Its impact on long-term care patients. *The Gerontologist*, 1977, *17*, 426–435.

Plutchik, R., & Conte, H. Change in social and physical functioning of geriatric patients over a one-year period. *The Gerontologist*, 1972, *12*, 181–184.

Plutchik, R., Conte, H., Lieberman, M., Bakur, M., Grossman, J., & Lehrman, N. Reliability and validity of a scale for assessing the functioning of geriatric patients. *Journal of the American Geriatrics Society*, 1970, *18*, 491–500.

Powell, R. R. Psychological effects of exercise therapy upon institutionalized geriatric mental patients. *Journal of Gerontology*, 1974, *29*, 157–161.

Raasoch, J., Willmuth, R., Thomson, L., & Hyde, R. Intra-hospital transfer: Effects on chronically ill psychogeriatric patients. *Journal of the American Geriatrics Society*, 1977, *25*, 281–284.

Rada, R. T., & Kellner, R. Thiothixene in the treatment of geriatric patients with chronic organic brain syndrome. *Journal of the American Geriatrics Society*, 1976, *24*, 105–107.

Raskin, A., & Clyde, D. J. Factors of psychopathology in the ward behavior of acute schizophrenics. *Journal of Consulting Psychology*, 1963, *27*, 420–425.

Raskin, A., & Crook, T. H. Sensitivity of rating scales completed by psychiatrists, nurses and patients to antidepressant drug effects. *Journal of Psychiatric Research*, 1976, *13*, 31–41.

Raskin, A., & McKeon, J. J. Super factors of psychopathology in hospitalized depressed patients. *Journal of Psychiatric Research*, 1971, *9*, 11–19.

Raskin, A., Schulterbrandt, J., Reatig, N., & McKeon, J. J. Replication of factors of psychopathology in interview, ward behavior and self-report ratings of hospitalized depressives. *Journal of Nervous and Mental Disease*, 1969, *148*, 87–98.

Raskin, A., Schulterbrandt, J., Reatig, N., & Rice, C. E. Factors of psychopathology in interview, ward behavior, and self-report ratings of hospitalized depressives. *Journal of Consulting Psychology*, 1967, *31*, 270–278.

Ratner, J., Rosenberg, G., Kral, V. A., & Engelsmann, F. Anticoagulant therapy for senile dementia. *Journal of the American Geriatrics Society*, 1972, *20*, 556–559.

Salzman, C., Shader, R. I., Kochansky, G. E., & Cronin, D. M. Rating scales for psychotropic drug research with geriatric patients. I. Behavior ratings. *Journal of the American Geriatrics Society*, 1972, *20*, 209–214.

Shatin, L., & Freed, E. X. A behavioral rating scale for mental patients. *Journal of Mental Science*, 1955, *101*, 644–653.

Smith, J. M., Bright, B., & McCloskey, J. Factor analytic composition of the Geriatric Rating Scale (GRS). *Journal of Gerontology*, 1977, *32*, 58–62.

Spitzer, R. L., & Endicott, J. Psychiatric rating scales. In A. M. Freedman, H. I. Kaplan, & B. J. Sadock (Eds.), *Comprehensive textbook of psychiatry* (Vol. 2). Baltimore: Williams & Wilkins, 1975.

Stewart, J. A., Ban, T. A., & Lehmann, H. E. New research on the use of trazodone in old age. A summary of systematic studies. *Psychopharmacology Bulletin*, 1976, *12*, 47–48.

Stotsky, B. A., Cole, J. O., Lu, L.-M., & Sniffin, C. M. A controlled study of the efficacy of pentylenetetrazol (Metrazol) with hard-core hospitalized psychogeriatric patients. *American Journal of Psychiatry*, 1972, *129*, 387–391.

Sugerman, A. A., Williams, B. H., & Alderstein, A. M. Haloperidol in the psychiatric disorders of old age. *American Journal of Psychiatry*, 1964, *120*, 1190–1192.

Tsuang, M.-M., Lu, L.-M., Stotsky, B. A., & Cole, J. O. Haloperidol versus thioridazine for hospitalized psychogeriatric patients: Double-blind study. *Journal of the American Geriatrics Society*, 1971, *19*, 593–600.

Vergara, L. E., Ban, T. A., Lehmann, H. E., & Stewart, J. A. New research on the use of trazodone in old age. An uncontrolled clinical trial carried out in Panama City, Panama. *Psychopharmacology Bulletin,* 1976, *12,* 41–42.

Vestre, N. D. Validity data on the Psychotic Reaction Profile. *Journal of Consulting Psychology,* 1966, *30,* 84–85.

Vestre, N. D., & Zimmerman, R. Validation study of the Psychotic Inpatient Profile. *Psychological Reports,* 1970, *27,* 3–7.

Watson, C. G. Inpatient care or outplacement: Which is better for the psychiatric medically infirm patient? *Journal of Gerontology,* 1976, *31,* 611–616.

Watson, C. G., & Fulton, J. R. Treatment potential of the psychiatric-medically infirm. I. Self-care independence. *Journal of Gerontology,* 1967, *22,* 449–455.

Watson, C. G., & Fulton, J. R. Treatment potential of the psychiatric-medically infirm. II. Psychiatric symptomatology. *Journal of Gerontology,* 1968, *23,* 226–230.

Zwerling, I., Plutchik, R., Hotz, M., Kling, R., Rubin, L., Grossman, J., & Siegel, B. Effects of a procaine preparation (Gerovital-H3) in hospitalized geriatric patients: A double-blind study. *Journal of the American Geriatrics Society,* 1975, *23,* 355–359.

8

Assessing Community Adjustment in the Elderly

Margaret W. Linn
Veterans Administration Hospital
and University of Miami School of Medicine

At least two events have highlighted the need for measuring community adjustment in older patients. The deinstitutionalization movement, responsible for partially emptying and sometimes closing large mental hospitals, has sent many older patients back into the community or to some other form of care. In addition, the mandate to community mental health centers to provide a treatment component for geriatric patients has emphasized the need for evaluating treatment within a community setting.

Although there are no geriatric community adjustment scales, two routes are currently possible for evaluating adjustment in elderly psychiatric subjects. One can select an adjustment scale from a number of existing ones developed for and, for the most part, tested on younger subjects. Or, one can assemble a battery of scales, each of which measures one dimension (such as life satisfaction or morale) appropriate for older subjects but none of which are comprehensive enough to stand along as a measure of community adjustment. Both of these approaches are covered in this chapter. Several existing scales of adjustment are described and critiqued according to their adaptability for the elderly. Also, an example is given of the smorgasbord approach commonly used to measure specific areas of adjustment that seem especially important for older individuals.

Other issues such as professional versus nonprofessional raters, mailed versus in-person assessments, and informant versus self-reports have been covered extensively by others (Ellsworth, 1975; Hogarty, 1973; Weissman, 1974) and will not be repeated here.

A DEFINITION OF ADJUSTMENT

Most definitions of adjustment deal with the concept of equilibrium. As such, adjustment is defined as a state. This state of equilibrium can describe a balance in the person's interaction with the external environment or a balance within the person's own internal system. The equilibrium concept is related to the idea of tension reduction and leads to the definition of adjustment as a process rather than a state. The process of adjustment describes how a person achieves satisfaction of needs, thereby reducing tensions, particularly when the usual ways of meeting needs are blocked. The latter notion has received considerable attention in describing adaptability or coping behaviors that are adequate or inadequate in old age. Some of the developmental tasks for the elderly have been described by Havighurst and Albrecht (1953). Many of these concern adjustment to losses such as decreasing strength and health, retirement and loss of usual level of income, death of spouse or friends, and decreasing social status. Pushed to a Darwinian level, the process of adjustment might be defined as successfully meeting the challenges of a threatening environment.

Adjustment, for purposes of measurement, is generally divided into social and personal spheres of reference. In a social context, a person might be judged as poorly adjusted when compared with some cultural norm. Value judgments are often made by reference to behaviors in one of several major role areas such as work, marriage, leisure, or family activities. Social adjustment may include how the person interacts with others or, in a more narrow sense, how the person conforms to social expectations. Informant ratings of a subject's behavior can be used to determine social deviance or to describe interpersonal interactions.

The personal aspects of adjustment can be determined only by asking the individual about his or her feelings; only the individual can assess the degree of satisfaction experienced. Kuhlen (1959) suggested three major determinants of personal adjustment: (1) subjective happiness and contentment, (2) relative freedom from handicapping anxiety, and (3) sufficient frustration tolerance and flexibility to meet and deal with stress without undue anxiety. Kuhlen implied that frustration tolerance and flexibility are extremely important for older subjects not only for how happy they are now but also for how well they can maintain this state of affairs as they meet the inevitable crises of aging.

PROBLEMS IN MEASURING ADJUSTMENT IN THE ELDERLY

Several authors of adjustment rating scales have stressed the need for considering and rating the positive aspects of adjustment or mental health and not just the negative or maladaptive patterns of behavior. The concept of normality, particularly for the aged, is an illusive one. Rosow (1963) pointed out that normality is based on three notions: (1) ideal standards epitomizing the models of what behaviors ought to be, and these vary by moral compulsions; (2) statistical norms describing what is, regardless of its approximation to ideal standards, and these reflect current cultural practices; and (3) clinical norms representing acceptable mental health according to standards of practice. There are insufficient statistical norms on older subjects' behavior, and even if there were more, Rosow has wondered to what extent normative standards can be inferred from modal distributions. What meaning can be given to deviant patterns of behavior? If the culture fails to generate preference for one style of adjustment over another (active versus inactive elderly, for example), then additional statistical data will not solve the problem. Therefore, cultural norms and role definitions for the aged are serious problems in the measure of adjustment. Cattell (1950) also concluded that adjustment should describe the goodness of the internal arrangements by which adaptation is maintained, but added, "Until mental energy and goodness of adaptation can be measured, it is thus not possible to measure, except in theory, the *goodness* of adjustment" (p. 263).

The absence of clear social roles and expectations of the aged are a central issue in selection of community adjustment instruments. Not only do the retired and widowed present special problems for most scales, but preconceived ideas about the desirability of a high level of activity and social participation may either be unfounded or, at the least, confusing. Often it is assumed that more activity means more interaction with the environment and, therefore, better adjustment. Kutner, Fanshel, Togo, and Langner (1956) were perhaps the first to point out that only activities that are meaningful to the individual contribute to morale. Data on activities are commonly used in rating an older person's social role performance in relation to family, groups, or community. Most scales reward the active and involved, so that individuals who withdraw from some roles receive lower adjustment scores. Is this as it should be for the elderly? Many sedentary older people have good adjustment when judged clinically by standards other than activity.

Although some studies (Graney, 1975; Havighurst and Albrecht, 1953) have shown positive relationships between voluntary participation and morale or activity and life satisfaction, others have reported conflicting findings (Bell, 1974; Bull & Aucoin, 1975). Cutler (1973) reported that older persons with higher levels of participation were generally in better health and had higher socioeconomic status. When health and social status were held constant, the significant positive association between degree of participation and life satisfaction disappeared, in line with the significant relationship between health, social status, and life satisfaction.

Assumptions such as the ones made about activity are likely to be the result of building and norming scales in one age group and then applying them to persons in other age groups. Many questions do not have the same response equivalency. For example, avoiding crowds may be considered maladaptive behavior for youth but adaptive for elderly persons.

Undoubtedly, some of the dilemmas posed by scales that reflect inappropriate social roles for the elderly, or overemphasize activity or participation, have lead many gerontologists to take the route of constructing or using existing scales that measure such areas as well-being, self-esteem, morale, and life satisfaction. Justification for this approach lies in the fact that the personal adjustment of older people depends largely upon their present happiness, much more so than it does for younger people. In fact, feelings of inner satisfaction are perhaps a better index of adjustment than role performance in the aged.

In the section that follows, a selected group of community adjustment scales are reviewed. They are presented in chronological order, according to their development, since this also reflects something about the state of the art in this field of measurement.

A SELECTION OF ADJUSTMENT RATING SCALES

Normative Social Adjustment Scale

The Normative Social Adjustment Scale (Barrabee, Barrabee, & Finesinger, 1955) is included because it is one of the first published rating scales of social adjustment and has a well-written conceptual framework for evaluation of adjustment. It was designed to measure outcome of psychotherapy. It is based on the premise that social adjustment is the degree to which individuals fulfill the normative social expectations of behavior constituting their roles. The authors defined adjustment as a process that involves doing and feeling. They suggested that evaluation of the process should take into account existing norms and standards of performance. Complete evaluation is seen as encompassing performance and affect. Performance is judged objectively through observation of the person's role activities. Affect is judged subjectively and covers the person's attitudes about his or her performance. The authors outline four subsystems to be rated: employment, economics, family life, and community. There are 27 items measured on 5-point scales, with scale points defined by such statements as 1 = not employed to 5 = full-time employment. A semistructured interview conducted by a professional with the subject takes about 1 hour. Some items are given more weight than others.

Comments

The theoretical foundation for measuring adjustment is described fully. It has probably inspired other investigators who subsequently developed rating scales. Unfortunately, the scale itself is incomplete and does not match the conceptual framework set forth in the first part of the article. For example, employment is the only area of the scale that is provided for the reader. There are no reliability data reported and validity rests predominantly on content. No rationale is given for the system of weights. With the particular emphasis on employment, many of the items are not relevant for the older retired person. Because of the problems cited, it cannot be recommended for use with the elderly.

Social Adjustment Rating Scale

The Social Adjustment Rating Scale (Mandel, 1959) is based on evaluation of role performance and attitudes. Seven areas of adjustment are covered: occupational, family, health, economics, religion, residence, and community/social. Ratings are made on 5-point scales for 37 items and the score for each area is the average of the items rated; a total score consists of the mean of the 7 subscales. A semistructured interview by a professional is required. No specific time frame for assessments is given. The occupational and family life areas are the most fully developed. The occupational area is divided into employed and retired; employed persons are scored for hours per week, regularity, stability, interpersonal relationships, and attitudes toward work; retired persons are scored for daily activity schedule or adequacy of self-care. The content area is similar to the Barrabee Scale reviewed above except for the added section on retirement. The family life area covers agreement with spouse, relationship with children, and relationship with family of orientation (parents and siblings). The economic area covers level of financial independence, management of funds, and solutions of problems. Health is rated on its effect on functioning in life roles and on the person's attitude about health. Frequency of participation in religious activities and attitudes about religion are also rated, as are stability and adequacy of living arrangements. Participation in organized activity, recreation, number of friends, degree of socialization with friends and relatives, degree of enjoyment, and heterosexual adjustment are measured under the community/social area.

Comments

This scale, an extended and better developed version of the Normative Social Adjustment Scale (Barrabee et al. 1955), has much to recommend it, even though there is no information on its validity. It is predominantly role oriented, and yet it allows for some deviations from young or middle age norms of behavior and provides considerable emphasis on personal satisfaction. The scale has been used with subjects over age 55 (Gilderstadt, Aberwald, Crosbie, Schuell, & Jimenez, 1968) with high reliability ($r = .87$) as measured by comparing patients' and informants' ratings. The fact that a retired person can be rated in terms of activities of daily living and adequacy of self-care is an attractive feature of the scale, and the health, economic, and residence areas are important ones for the elderly. Most widowed or single elderly, however, could not be rated on any of the seven items under family life, and one might argue with the emphasis placed on frequency of participation in religious and other organized activities as favorable signs of adjustment, unless these activities were meaningful for the individual. The scale might be worth consideration where a brief role-oriented assessment of adjustment, which takes into account some personal viewpoints of the patient, is needed.

Personal Adjustment and Role Skills Scale

The fourth revision of the Personal Adjustment and Role Skills Scale (PARS) (Ellsworth, 1959) has been completed. The original plan was to have a series of statements reflecting instrumental role performance that could be rated by relatives or significant others. The PARS-I consisted of 39 items describing 4 areas of personal adjustment and 2 role skills and was tested on male schizophrenics. PARS-II was an expanded version with 115 items for males and 120 items for females. PARS-III was reduced to 57 items based on a series of factor analyses. Statements were rated on 5-point scales from "never" to "always," describing the subject's behavior. Two forms, male and female, were used. Because the PARS-III was sex-role stereotyped, too long, could not be keypunched directly, and relatives rarely used the "never" and "always" categories, the author developed PARS-IV. This latest version contains 36 items for males and 30 for females. There is provision for the informant to estimate the extent to which each area represents a problem for the person being rated. An example of the type of item rated is: "How often would you say that he has said that life is not worth living?" Seven factors were described by factor analysis of PARS-IV for males: Interpersonal Relationships, Agitation-Depression, Confusion, Alcohol-Drugs, Household Management, Outside Social, and Employment. Six factors were described for females, which were the same as for males except that Agitation was dropped from the Agitation-Depression factor and the Confusion factor was combined with Depression. PARS-IV has pre- and posttest treatment norms established. Standard and residual scores can be computed for analysis.

Comments

This scale has stood the test of time, although it keeps shifting and changing with the years. This is frustrating when one attempts to compare factor scores with those cited in published works based on earlier versions of the scale. In many ways, the PARS-III seems superior to the PARS-IV, since it contains more scale points and a more comprehensive item content. One advantage of the latest version is that relatives can specify what they think is the most serious problem for the patient and that area can be given additional weight. This is valuable only if the relative can accurately define the key problem for the patient. The question of who is to provide ratings for the elderly is an important one. Job satisfactions were often rated by relatives when the patient did not work; thus, the items related to job satisfaction were eliminated in the fourth revision. The fact that the Employment factor accounts for much of the variance in outcome leads to the question of applicability for elderly subjects. The scale is somewhat symptom-oriented for an adjustment rating scale. Extensive reliability and validity data have been reported. It is one of the first adjustment scales with reported factor structure. The scale has generally been used as a mail questionnaire. Unanswered items can present a problem. The descriptive material that is frequently written in the margin and at the bottom of the scales by relatives is often as revealing as the scale scores themselves. The Katz Adjustment Scale (KAS) is far more comprehensive than the PARS. However, if a shorter mail questionnaire for relatives is desired, the PARS-III and IV are certainly acceptable substitutes for the KAS.

Social Adjustment Inventory

The Social Adjustment Inventory (Berger, Rice, Sewall, & Lemkau, 1964) was developed to assess the impact of the hospital on the patient's adaptation to the community. The authors contended that community adjustment is only meaningful when it is compared with the pretreatment condition of the patient. They also stated that adjustment can be assessed by information provided from the patient's social group members. They quoted Mead (1936) as suggesting that "the individual experiences himself as such, not directly, but only indirectly, from the particular standpoint of the social group as a whole to which he belongs" (p. 26). Their scale provides four scores related to family/social adjustment, social productivity, self-maintenance, and antisocial behavior. Ratings are made on 33 items scored mostly on 6-point scales. There are separate forms for males and females. The scale has been used most frequently as a mail questionnaire.

Comments

The scale is an acceptable gauge of social behaviors as viewed by some person close to the patient. It lacks the dimension of personal satisfaction supplied by the subject and shares with many other scales the problems inherent in a relative's ratings of a patient's adjustment. The scale has good reliability correlations between different informants ranging in the low .80s. Since personal satisfaction is such an important area of adjustment in old age, the scale is recommended only if it is used in combination with some other instrument that taps the personal satisfaction dimension.

Katz Adjustment Scale

The Katz Adjustment Scale (Katz & Lyerly, 1963) is perhaps the best known and most widely used community adjustment rating scale. The scale was developed to reflect treatment outcome. Adjustment is seen as agreement between self and one's environment. The authors pointed out that a minimal goal of adjustment is absence of gross signs of psychopathology; however, they stressed that symptom rating scales alone are not able to measure deeper change related to follow-up in the community. Adjustment is seen by the authors as a positive concept in addition to the absence of negative behaviors. They envisioned adjustment as having a personal and social reference that separates out behaviors from attitudes. They pointed out that patients, if highly disturbed, are not the best sources of information about their own behavior. They acknowledged, however, that patients are the only source of information about their own comfort and satisfaction. The KAS provides five subscores, each considered a separate scale. One set of the five scales is answered by the patient (S1-S5). Another set is completed by the relative (R1-R5). With the exception of the first scale, items are identical for the patient and relative. The S1 has 55 items taken from the Hopkins Symptom Checklist (Parloff, Kelman, & Frank, 1954). The R1 is a more extensive list of 127 symptoms and behaviors. The R2 and S2 describe level of performance in 16 socially expected activities, such as helping with household chores. The R3 and S3 repeat these 16 items and ask that the relative and patient indicate whether these activities are expected in terms of performance. The R4 and S4 are adapted from another scale (Cavan, Burgess, Havighurst, & Goldhamer, 1949) and measure involvement in 22 free-time activities. The R5 and S5 repeat these 22 leisure activities but ask for the relative and patient to judge degree of satisfaction the patient receives from these activities.

Comments

The scale has an excellent theoretical foundation. It also permits comparisons between actual performance with expected levels of performance and between the patient's assessment of performance with that of the relative's. It has demonstrated good reliability and validity. Data from the original publication of the scale (Katz & Lyerly, 1963) showed that the scale differentiated between patients with good and poor adjustment defined by global ratings of social workers and psychiatrists at the Manhattan Aftercare Clinic. The authors also reported intercorrelations for the R1 form, and those with phi coefficients greater than .40 were grouped into 13 clusters. These clusters were observed to have a high degree of consistency and stability in 242 ratings of state hospital and other samples in an NIMH Collaborative Study (1963). Factor analysis of the clusters identified three factors that accounted for 57% of the variance: Socially Obstreperous, Acute Psychotism, and Withdrawal/Depression. Six patient types have been identified from ratings of patient profiles (Katz, 1968). The validity of relatives' reports has been confirmed by symptom ratings of psychiatrists, which also corresponded with patient types identified by the relatives' ratings (Katz, 1966). Predictive validity of the R form has been demonstrated by Michaux, Katz, and Kurland (1969) in a study of adjustment and status of patients 1 year after hospital discharge. Out of 26 variables 16 had predictive weight in that study, and 11 of the 16 scores were derived from the KAS. Hogarty and Katz (1971) have shown that the scale effectively discriminated between levels of social behavior and performance by age, sex, marital status, and social class of persons in the general population. Norms have been developed by Hogarty and Katz.

Only a few minor limitations seem worth mentioning. Although the background cites the need for inclusion of positive evaluations of adjustment, only 15 of the 127 items on the R1 are stated in what might be considered positive wording, and none of these form part of the 85 items comprising the 13 clusters or 3 factors. Thus, as in other scales, it is mostly the negative aspects of adjustment that are scored. The scale is quite lengthy, even though it is stated to take between 45 minutes and 1 hour. Over the years the part of the scale that has received the most attention and use is the R form, particularly the R1 form, which highlights symptoms, and the use of this form alone de-emphasizes the importance of the subject's own response. The 55 items of the S1 are not directly comparable to those of the R1 and are, in fact, heavily weighted toward physiological symptoms or neurotic behaviors, which might not be entirely bad from the viewpoint of rating older subjects. Just as with the PARS, there may be a problem in finding suitable raters for the R forms when it comes to older subjects. Although the scale has the advantage of not requiring behavior evaluation in terms of specific role performance, it is highly oriented toward activity levels and attitudes about activities, which for the older patient, may be less valid than direct measures of life satisfaction.

Social Dysfunction Rating Scale

The Social Dysfunction Rating Scale (Linn, Sculthorpe, Evje, Slater, & Goodman, 1969) was developed as a measure for adults of all ages and for both men and women. It stresses role-free assessments that may be needed for the elderly and can be applied to subjects in any setting, community as well as hospital. Dysfunction implies discontent and unhappiness accompanied by negative self-regarding attitudes. Adjustment is seen as a process of coping, problem solving, and adapting as a way of achieving one's goals or as self-actualization in a role one considers significant. There are 21 items that are rated according to degree of severity on 6-point scales organized under self, interpersonal, and performance systems. Items call for a combination of subjective and objective evaluations involving the rater's opinion and the subject's self-evaluation. The ratings draw heavily on personal satisfaction and self-fulfillment. For example, the rater makes a judgment about the individual's use of leisure time. Also, the rater compares the person with others of the same age in the general population. This item is followed by a rating of whether the patient feels the need for more activity. Therefore, the person who has few activities and is dissatisfied with the situation receives a higher dysfunction score than a person who feels content with things as they are. The same is true for the item dealing with friends. In this regard, the happy isolate is not penalized as much as the person who feels lonely and unfulfilled. A semistructured interview guide has been developed. Reliability, validity, and factor structure of the scale have been reported (Linn et al., 1969). Intraclass item reliabilities ranged from .54 for Manipulation to .86 for Lack of Friends. Validity was gauged by the scale's ability to distinguish psychiatric from nonpsychiatric patients ($F = 4.20$; $p < .01$) and the product moment correlation between total scores and global judgments of improvement by social workers ($r = 0.89$). Five factors were identified following a principal components analysis and a normal varimax rotation. These were labeled Apathetic-Detachment, Dissatisfaction, Hostility, Health-Finance Concern, and Manipulative-Dependency. The SDRS has been used with elderly patients, alcoholics, drug addicts, normals, and psychiatric patients. It has demonstrated sensitivity to change in two large-scale follow-up studies of mental hospital patients (Linn, Caffey, Klett, & Hogarty, 1977; Linn, Note 1).

Comments

The scale was designed for research purposes as a brief assessment tool sensitive to change. It requires a professional rater and an interview of about half an hour. Its item definitions have the most consensual validity to clinical social workers, and the scale is seen as a way of quantifying their observations. The author has a self-report version of the scale that has not yet been published, but data are available on the reliability, validity, and factor structure of this scale. The original version of the scale provides a better assessment of adjustment when there are no serious limitations on staff and patient time. The scale is applicable to older patients, particularly in regard to meaningfulness of their life, their goals, and their satisfactions. It does not provide descriptive assessments of different kinds of activities. Lack of work is rated whether the person has a job or not, since it is based on a level of productive work activity (such as chores, hospital assignments, and housework) insufficient to generate feelings of usefulness. Factor scores reflect Apathetic-Detachment, Dissatisfaction, Hostility, Health-Finance Concern, and Manipulative-Dependency.

The Structured and Scaled Interview to Assess Maladjustment

The Structured and Scaled Interview to Assess Maladjustment (SSIAM) (Gurland, Yorkston, Stone, Frank, & Fleiss, 1972) is an extension and elaboration of the Social Ineffectiveness Scale (Parloff et al., 1954) with some overlap in authors. It defines social maladjustment as ineffective performance in roles and tasks for which the individual is socialized. It covers objective behavior as well as subjective reactions of interest to clinicians. It assumes that the goals of treatment are to reduce stress and to return subjects to normal behaviors and interactions with others. Three types of maladjustment are measured: distress, deviant behavior, and friction. Five areas of adjustment (work, social, family, marriage, and sex) are rated by means of a structured interview with probing questions. There are 60 items rated; 45 cover maladaptive behaviors and 15 relate to evaluation of stress, prognosis, and positive mental health. There is also an opportunity to measure and report environmental constraints. Items concerning maladaptive behaviors are rated on 10-inch lines with scale points placed every inch, and 4 of these scale points are defined by statements. For example, the most maladjusted rating under marriage is: "marriage is breaking up: grossly incompatible." The factor structure, reliability, and validity data were reported in a separate article (Gurland, Yorkston, Goldberg, Fleiss, Sloane, & Cristol, 1972).

Comments

Though this scale is relatively new, a considerable amount of data on its reliability and validity is available. In one study, 12 items were rated as not applicable by 20% of the sample (most of these were from the marriage and sexual adjustment factor). An additional 12 items were excluded from the 45 because of low intraclass correlations between raters or because of high correlations with other factors. The remaining 21 items accounted for over 40% of the variance in factor analysis. From the 21 items describing social isolation, 6 factors emerged: Work Adequacy, Family Friction, Sexual Dissatisfaction, and Friction Outside the Family. Comparison of interviewers' scores with informants' ratings on 89 subjects showed statistically significant product moment correlations (.35 to .70) for all factors except the one describing sexual adjustment (r = .20). One feature that seems unique, and perhaps particularly desirable for older patients, is the opportunity for rating the environment as being either favorable or not. The areas of distress and friction seem relevant to the elderly, and the opportunity to provide a relatively precise measurement through a structured interview and the use of 10 scale points has some advantages. The major disadvantage is that for older subjects some of the five areas of role performance may often be absent. Furthermore, some items are highly value laden. For example, "marriage breaking up" may not always be the most negative kind of adjustment. In general, the scale offers some new elements to the assessment of adjustment.

The Social Adjustment Scale

The Social Adjustment Scale (SAS) (Paykel, Weissman, Prusoff, & Tonks, 1971) was published one year before the SSIAM, but it is reportedly based on a variation of the SSIAM then available in mimeograph form. The scale was developed to measure social adjustment in depressed women. The authors reported that in planning a study of maintenance treatment for depressed patients, they were impressed with the paucity of available empirical data on components of social maladjustment in this patient group. They were also impressed with the need for more scales developed through factor analytic techniques, and they noted that adjustment scales lagged far behind other types of rating scales in this respect. In the SAS, a semistructured interview is used to rate 48 items covering detailed aspects of functioning. Two systems of scoring are used: items grouped by six role areas such as Work, Social and Leisure, Extended Family, Marital, Parental, and Family Unit; and items grouped without regard to roles, into the categories of Satisfactions and Feelings as well as Global Judgments and ratings of actual behaviors subdivided into Performance, Interpersonal Relationships, and Friction. A factor analysis was done, since neither system produced adequately homogeneous rating dimensions. A 6-factor solution was obtained describing Work Performance, Interpersonal Friction, Inhibited Communication, Submissive Dependency, Family Attachment, and Anxious Rumination. The factor scores are recommended for observing patterns of change and measuring the effects of psychotherapy or other treatments.

Comments

Since depression is an important symptom in many elderly patients, this scale may have some usefulness for elderly subjects. Weissman and Bothwell (1976) have reported a self-report version of this scale in which responses by 76 depressed outpatients were comparable to those obtained from relatives, as well as by a rater who interviewed the patients directly. The SAS has some of the same problems as the SSIAM in its concentration on role performance, which could be troublesome in rating older patients. Both the original SAS and the self-report version are quite recent, but look promising in terms of scale construction.

Other Adjustment Scales

Several other scales were reviewed but not included in the above descriptions. The Social Ineffectiveness Scale (Parloff et al., 1954) requires such a complicated system of observations that the SSIAM is preferable. The Personality and Social Network Scale (Clark, 1968) has only 17 items, and global assessments are made. It was designed for evaluating effectiveness of therapeutic communities. Scale points are limited to a yes or no format. The Community Adaptation Schedule (Roen & Burnes, 1968) is a self-report of adjustment on 217 items. In reading the items, only 3 of the first 43 could be answered by elderly retired persons. The origin of the scale is unclear and items mix lifelong patterns with current functional status. The Social Disability Scale (Ruesch, 1969) has 196 items with weights that rate impact of health on behavior. The emphasis is more physical than social, and it seems to provide an assessment of illness at one point in time rather than a measure that would be sensitive to change. The Psychiatric Status Schedule (Spitzer, Endicott, & Fleiss, 1970), the Psychiatric Evaluation Form (Endicott & Spitzer, 1972b), and the Current and Past Psychopathology Scales (Endicott & Spitzer, 1972a) are all very good scales with considerable development through psychometric techniques, but in general seem too symptom oriented, history related, or role bound to be particularly useful for elderly patients.

PROXY MEASURES OF ADJUSTMENT

In the absence of geriatric social adjustment scales, many investigators have turned to established rating scales that measure specific aspects of adjustment. The rationale behind this approach is that if the byproducts of adjustment can be defined, it may be possible to use these as indicators of a person's equilibrium with the environment. For example, if well-adjusted people are happy and content, then scales that measure life satisfaction, morale, and well-being are appropriate avenues for exploration. If a positive attitude toward self is part of good adjustment, self-esteem or self-rewarding attitudes might be considered important correlates. Along these same lines, a lack of a feeling of alienation and evidence of self-directed inner control could be considered essential to interaction with the environment. Although these concepts approach a quality-of-life assessment so important to the elderly, they measure only the affective part of adjustment. What is still needed is a way of describing the coping behaviors that are maladaptive and that lead to the person's inability to function effectively. A few comments follow on proxy measures of adjustment, with at least one scale selected and described for each of the major areas.

Subjective Happiness

The criteria of happiness have dominated the thoughts of those working in the field of gerontology. An abundance of research has been done in the past few years that examines correlates of such factors as Life Satisfaction, Morale, and Well-being. It is difficult to untangle the definitions of life satisfaction and morale. They become even less clear when items on two scales purported to measure them are compared, since many of the items on the two scales sound almost identical. For example, the following two items are taken from a well-known life satisfaction scale (Neugarten, Havighurst, & Tobin, 1961): "As I grow older, things seem better than I thought they would be." "I am just as happy as when I was younger." For comparison, these two items are taken from a well-known morale scale (Lawton, 1975): "As I get older, things are (better, worse, same) than I thought they would be" and "I am as happy now as I was when I was younger." The general consensus is that well-being is a multidimensional concept. Although some investigators have assumed that morale was unidimensional, (Kutner et al., 1956), others such as Lawton (1972) have not. In fact, Lawton has pointed out that morale has been linked to optimistic ideology, acceptance of status quo, lack of self-perceived negative change, rejection of stereotypes about the aged, and positive evaluation of the environment. Life satisfaction has also been shown to be multidimensional. It has been generally accepted that life satisfaction decreases with age; however, since it is also significantly related to marital status, differences by age largely disappear when corrections are made for older unmarried and widowed subjects. The value of life satisfaction as an indicator of adjustment has been questioned, because happiness is culture bound and has been shown to favor the higher socioeconomic classes. The question also arises concerning the relationship between professed contentment and actual behavior. If one looks for the ultimate manifestation of unhappiness, it is suicide. Robinson (1973) has pointed out that despite the lack of studies providing data measuring life satisfaction prior to suicide, the correlates of life satisfaction and suicide are strikingly similar and include other variables such as age, marital status, sex, and race.

The two scales selected for review were developed by gerontologists. Since the recommended scales are quite similar, they will be discussed together. The Life Satisfaction Index (LSI) (Neugarten et al., 1961) and the Philadelphia Geriatric Center Morale Scale (PGC) (Lawton, 1975) are both multidimensional, even though many investigators continue to derive a single global index from them. The PGC is a self-report scale constructed on very old subjects in institutions. It has been reduced from 50 to 22 items; reliability and validity data are encouraging. Six factors have been extracted to explain: Surgency (quickness and cleverness), Attitude Toward Aging, Acceptance of Status Quo, Agitation, Easygoing Optimism, and Lonely Dissatisfaction. The LSI has been used much more extensively than the PGC, although the latter is gaining in popularity. The LSI was also developed on elderly subjects. It is a self-report instrument, taking only a few minutes to administer and score. Form A contains 25 attitude items requiring an agree or disagree response. Form B has 12 open-ended questions and checklist items scored on 3-point scales. The LSI was based on five theoretical components of well-being: Zest Versus Apathy, Resolution and Fortitude, Congruence Between Desired and Achieved Goals, Positive Self-Concept, and Mood Tone. Most investigators have simply summed the various scales; however, factor analyses done by Adams (1969) show at least four factors of Mood Tone, Zest for Life, Congruence, and Resolution.

Either of the above scales can be recommended as a good measure of well-being in older subjects. Also, they correlate reasonably well with each other ($r = .57$) when used on the same subjects (Lawton, 1972).

Self-Concept

It seems apparent that the well-adjusted person has attitudes of positive self-regard with feelings of satisfaction and self-confidence. Data seem to indicate that as people age, they develop a less positive attitude toward themselves. Some studies have shown that older persons who preserve a younger self-concept tend to function better than those who see themselves as old. Rosow (1963) pointed out that older self-image was tantamount to acceptance or at least resignation to an old status. New self-images are normally associated with good adjustment and effective functioning in new roles. In fact, he pointed out that no role transition can take place without the emergence of a new self-image. Yet, acceptance of a new image for the elderly may be related to poor adjustment, or it may be due to the lack of clear role definitions carrying respect and worth for the elderly in our culture. The Self-Esteem Scale (Rosenberg, 1965) has been used with the elderly in numerous studies, even though it was developed on high school students. It has the virtue of being short (only 10 items) and measuring the self-acceptance aspect of self-esteem. It has been found to correlate well with similar measures and clinical assessments and to have a test-retest reliability of .85.

Alienation

Although the concept of alienation has not been used frequently to measure any aspect of adjustment, it seems likely that it would have considerable relevance for assessing feelings of social isolation, social malintegration, or self-to-others alienation that are often expressed by the elderly. The Anomie Scale (Srole, 1956) seems to be an appropriate measure of this dimension.

Locus of Control

Another measure that may be useful in describing adaptation or adjustment is Rotter's (1966) concept of locus of control. "Internals" believe that some control resides within themselves as opposed to "Externals" who believe that their lives are determined by factors extrinsic to themselves. Rotter has contended that people are handicapped by external locus of control orientations. It is considered desirable to change persons who are not doing well in our society in the direction of internality. Most of the literature on locus of control can be summarized by saying that Internals and Externals differ in instrumental and expressive behaviors. Internals engage in more instrumental goal-directed activity, whereas Externals more often manifest emotional non-goal-directed responses. Buhler (1951) has pointed out the need for the elderly to continue to grow and expand as goals and life-styles change. With the increasing years, there is a shift from more active direct gratification of needs to indirect vicarious gratification. For example, starting in the teens, the following pattern usually develops: romance, marriage, birth of children, work, satisfaction with children's success. The identification with one's own children provides an avenue for growth and expansion. In very old age, there may be increased interest in genealogy, religion, and immortality. Thus, goal-directed acitivity and orientation toward the future can be essential elements of good adjustment. The Internal-External Locus of Control Scale (Rotter, 1966) has been used extensively. The scale consists of 23 paired statements with a forced choice format. Scores range from 0, the most internal, to 23, the most external. The scale can be administered in about 15 minutes. There is an 11-item version of the scale that might be preferable for use with the elderly because it is brief.

SUMMARY AND FUTURE DIRECTIONS

In this chapter adjustment has been defined as a process or a state with both an instrumental and an affective component. The dilemma faced by those who wish to measure community adjustment in the elderly is that most of the existing scales have been developed for use with younger subjects and focus on role behaviors that are not appropriate for older subjects. Two commonly used approaches, neither of which is perfect, have been reviewed. One approach is to select a scale from those that are available, knowing that some of the items will probably be inappropriate; the other approach is to select a combination of scales that, used together, might form a proxy measure of the personal sphere of adjustment. Scales developed or appropriate for the elderly in measuring such areas as life satisfaction, morale, self-concept, alienation, and locus of control have been suggested. The problem with the latter approach is that the instrumental component of adjustment is missed.

In the proxy measures, it is evident that there is considerable overlap in the concepts and items that describe the affective or personal domain of functioning. This is undoubtedly true for the larger areas of functioning as well. What seems to be needed is a comprehensive scale that assesses physical, mental, and social function together. This idea has been expressed in more detail elsewhere (Linn, 1976). Statistical techniques are available that could eliminate the redundancy in items across these areas, and thereby produce a comprehensive but not too lengthy set of variables that uniquely measure overall functioning in the elderly.

REFERENCES

Adams, D. L. Analysis of Life Satisfaction Index. *Journal of Gerontology,* 1969, *24,* 470–474.

Barrabee, R., Barrabee, E. L., & Finesinger, J. F. A Normative Social Adjustment Scale. *American Journal of Psychiatry,* 1955, *112,* 252–259.

Bell, B. D. Cognitive dissonance and life satisfaction of older adults. *Journal of Gerontology,* 1974, *29,* 564–571.

Berger, D. G., Rice, C. E., Sewall, L. G., & Lemkau, P. V. The posthospital evaluation of psychiatric patients: The Social Adjustment Inventory method. *Psychiatric Studies and Projects,* 1964, *2,* 1–30.

Buhler, C. Maturation and motivation. *Personality,* 1951, *1,* 184–211.

Bull, C. N., & Aucoin, J. B. Voluntary association participation and life satisfaction: A replication note. *Journal of Gerontology,* 1975, *30,* 73–76.

Cattell, R. B. *Personality.* New York: McGraw-Hill, 1950.

Cavan, R. S., Burgess, E. W., Havighurst, R. J., & Goldhamer, H. *Personal adjustment in old age.* Chicago: Science Research Association, 1949.

Clark, A. W. The Personality and Social Network Adjustment Scale. *Human Relations*, 1968, *21*, 85–95.

Cutler, S. J. Voluntary association, participation, and life satisfaction. *Journal of Gerontology*, 1973, *28*, 96–100.

Ellsworth, R. B. Measurement of improvement in mental illness. *Journal of Consulting Psychology*, 1959, *23*, 15–20.

Ellsworth, R. B. Consumer feedback in measuring the effectiveness of mental health programs. In M. Guttentag & M. Streuning (Eds.), *Handbook of evaluation research*. Beverly Hills: Sage Publications, 1975.

Endicott, J., & Spitzer, R. L. Current and Past Psychopathology Scales (CAPPS). *Archives of General Psychiatry*, 1972, *27*, 678–687. (a)

Endicott, J., & Spitzer, R. L. What! Another rating scale? The Psychiatric Evaluation Form. *Journal of Nervous and Mental Disease*, 1972, *154*, 88–104. (b)

Gilderstadt, H., Aberwald, R., Crosbie, S., Schuell, H., & Jimenez, E. Effect of surgery on psychological and social functioning in elderly patients. *Archives of Internal Medicine*, 1968, *122*, 109–115.

Graney, M. J. Happiness and social participation. *Journal of Gerontology*, 1975, *30*, 701–706.

Gurland, B. J., Yorkston, N. J., Goldberg, K., Fleiss, J., Sloane, R. B., & Cristol, A. H. The Structured and Scaled Interview to Assess Maladjustment (SSIAM) II. *Archives of General Psychiatry*, 1972, *27*, 264–267.

Gurland, B. J., Yorkston, N. J., Stone, A. R., Frank, J. D., & Fleiss, J. L. The Structured and Scaled Interview to Assess Maladjustment (SSIAM) I. *Archives of General Psychiatry*, 1972, *27*, 259–263.

Havighurst, R. J., & Albrecht, R. *Older people*. New York: Longmans Green, 1953.

Hogarty, G. Informant ratings of community adjustment. In I. E. Waskow & M. B. Parloff (Eds.), *Psychotherapy change measures: Report of Clinical Research Branch, NIMH*. Washington, D.C.: U.S. Government Printing Office, 1973.

Hogarty, G. E., & Katz, M. M. Norms of adjustment and social behavior. *Archives of General Psychiatry*, 1971, *25*, 470–480.

Katz, M. M. A phenomenological typology of schizophrenia. In M. M. Katz, J. O. Cole, & W. E. Barton (Eds.), *The role and methodology of classification in psychiatry and psychopathology* (U.S. Public Health Service Publication No. 1584). Washington, D.C.: U.S. Government Printing Office, 1968.

Katz, M. M., Lowery, H. A., & Cole, J. O. Behavior patterns of schizophrenics in the community. In M. Lorr (Ed.), *Explorations in typing psychotics*. Oxford: Pergamon Press, 1966.

Katz, M. M., & Lyerly, S. B. Methods of measuring adjustment and social behavior in the community. *Psychological Reports*, 1963, *13*, 503–535.

Kuhlen, R. G. Aging and life adjustment. In J. E. Birren (Ed.), *Handbook of aging and the individual*. Chicago: University of Chicago Press, 1959.

Kutner, B., Fanshel, D., Togo, A. M., & Langner, T. S. *Five hundred over sixty*. New York: Russel Sage Foundation, 1956.

Lawton, P. The dimensions of morale. In D. P. Kent, R. Kastenbaum, & S. Sherwood (Eds.), *Research planning and action for the elderly*. New York: Behavioral Publications, 1972.

Lawton, P. The Philadelphia Geriatric Center Morale Scale: A revision. *Journal of Gerontology*, 1975, *30*, 85–89.

Linn, M. W. Studies in rating the physical, mental, and social dysfunction in the chronically ill aged. *Medical Care*, 1976, *14*, 119–125. (Suppl.)

Linn, M. W., Caffey, E. M., Klett, C. J., & Hogarty, G. Hospital versus community (foster) care for psychiatric patients: A V.A. cooperative study. *Archives of General Psychiatry*, 1977, *34*, 78–83.

Linn, M. W., Sculthorpe, W. B., Evje, M., Slater, P. H., & Goodman, B. P. A social dysfunction rating scale. *Journal of Psychiatric Research,* 1969, *6,* 299–316.

Mandel, N. G. *Mandel Social Adjustment Scale.* Minneapolis: University of Minnesota, 1959.

Mead, B. H. *Mind, self, and society.* Chicago: University of Chicago Press, 1936.

Michaux, W. W., Katz, M. M., Kurland, A. A., & Ganserit, K. H. The first year out: Mental patients after hospitalization. Baltimore: Johns Hopkins University, 1969.

Neugarten, B. L., Havighurst, R. J., & Tobin, S. S. The measurement of life satisfaction. *Journal of Gerontology,* 1961, *16,* 134–143.

Parloff, M. B., Kelman, H. C., & Frank, J. D. Comfort, effectiveness, and self-awareness as criteria of improvement in psychotherapy. *American Journal of Psychiatry,* 1954, *3,* 343–351.

Paykel, E. S., Weissman, M., Prusoff, B., & Tonks, M. B. Dimensions of social adjustment in depressed women. *Journal of Nervous and Mental Disease,* 1971, *152,* 158–172.

Robinson, J. P. Life satisfaction and happiness. In J. P. Robinson & P. R. Shaver (Eds.), *Measures of social psychological attitudes.* Ann Arbor: University of Michigan, 1973.

Roen, S. R., & Burnes, A. J. *Community Adaptation Schedule: Preliminary manual.* New York: Behavioral Publications, 1968.

Rosenberg, M. *Society and the adolescent self image.* Princeton: Princeton University Press, 1965.

Rosow, I. Adjustment of the normal aged. In R. H. Williams, C. Tibbetts, & W. Donahue (Eds.), *Processes of aging II.* London: Atherton Press, 1963.

Rotter, J. B. Generalized expectancies for internal versus external control of reinforcement. *Psychological Monographs,* 1966, *80* (Whole No. 609).

Ruesch, J. The assessment of social disability. *Archives of General Psychiatry,* 1969, *21,* 655–664.

Spitzer, R. L., Endicott, J., & Fleiss, J. L. The Psychiatric Status Schedule. *Archives of General Psychiatry,* 1970, *23,* 41–55.

Srole, L. Anomie. *American Sociological Review,* 1956, *21,* 709-716.

Weissman, M. M. The assessment of social adjustment. *Archives of General Psychiatry,* 1974, *32,* 357-365.

Weissman, M. M., & Bothwell, S. Assessment of social adjustment by patient self-report. *Archives of General Psychiatry,* 1976, *33,* 1111–1115.

REFERENCE NOTE

1. Linn, M. W., Caffey, E. M., Klett, C. J., Hogarty, G., & Lamb, R. Day treatment and psychotropic drugs in the aftercare of schizophrenic patients. *Archives of General Psychiatry* (in press).

II

ASSESSING COGNITIVE DISTURBANCES

9

Psychometric Assessment in the Elderly

Thomas H. Crook
National Institute of Mental Health

Most psychometric performance tests employed to assess cognitive abilities were constructed for use with children or young adults. These tests may have limited utility in an aged population where a number of unique problems characterize psychometric assessment. The objective of this chapter is to review a series of issues that merit consideration by the investigator who wishes to develop or employ psychometric tests for assessing cognitive abilities in aged subjects. Emphasis is placed on issues that arise when tests are employed in the clinical research setting to assess the effects of an experimental treatment on cognitive status.

FACE VALIDITY

Since most standard tests of cognitive abilities were constructed for children or young adults, tasks or stimulus materials employed frequently appear unrelated to the cognitive tasks faced by aged individuals in daily life. It is generally recognized that tests used with adults must possess face validity (i.e., appear to measure the ability being assessed) in order to function effectively in practical situations (Anastasi, 1961, p. 138). Face validity may be more important in tests for older subjects, since aged persons tend to be quite selective about what they choose to learn (Fozard & Thomas, 1975). Both behavioral studies (e.g., Hulicka, 1967) and psychophysiologic investigations (e.g., Shmavonian & Busse, 1963) have suggested that personally relevant stimuli are of greater importance in maintaining appropriate task involvement in aged than in young subjects.

CRITERION-RELATED VALIDITY

Application of tests developed for younger individuals to the aged is likely to involve problems of even greater significance than the motivational deficit associated with inadequate face validity. The principal problem may concern criterion-related validities, i.e., what can be inferred from a subject's test performance about his or her present standing (concurrent validity) or future standing (predictive validity) on another variable (the criterion). In applied research the criterion should be chosen with reference to the problem at hand and the test chosen with reference to the criterion (American Psychological Association, 1974). In the context of research concerning assessment of treatment for cognitive deficits, the criterion is assumed to be some direct measure of the subject's efficiency in dealing with cognitive tasks encountered in daily life. Unfortunately, few measures of cognitive abilities have been validated against performance outside the laboratory in everyday tasks involving those same abilities. The logic of criterion-related validity assumes that the criterion possesses validity and yet, in those few instances where validity coefficients have been calculated for an aged sample, investigators have employed criteria such as neurologic or psychiatric diagnosis or scores on other unvalidated psychometric tests.

The problem is particularly serious, since some evidence has suggested that scores of aged persons on standard psychological tests do not reflect the ability of the subjects to deal with the ecologically valid problems of later life. For example, Demming and Pressey (1957) have demonstrated in one group of subjects that a decline with age in performance on traditional psychometric tasks was actually accompanied by improved performance on tests composed of problems and tasks "indigenous" to adult life. Similarly, Welford (1969) has suggested that the same age-related changes in functioning that reduce scores on standardized tests could produce improvements in executive abilities.

Over 40 years ago, David Wechsler recognized that the Stanford-Binet and other tests developed to measure intelligence in children had certain drawbacks when applied to adults. It was Wechsler's intention in developing the Wechsler-Bellevue Intelligence Scale (which was later modified and restandardized as the Wechsler Adult Intelligence Scale [WAIS] in 1955) to develop a measure appropriate for adults in both content and scoring procedure (Wechsler, 1939). Wechsler recognized some years later that standard tests, including his scales, developed for young adults were probably not appropriate for use with aged individuals. He argued, for example, that "we ought to have special tests of intelligence for older individuals just as we now have them for young children . . . because the thing we call intelligence at different ages is evaluated in terms of quite different criteria" (Wechsler, 1955, p. 276). Unfortunately, little progress seems to have been made in that direction and inferences concerning learning, memory, and other cognitive processes in the aged continue to be based on psychometric measures standardized on middle-aged or younger adults.

CONTEXTUAL VALIDITY AND RESPONSE INHIBITION

Not only are specific psychometric tests frequently unrelated to the ecologically valid problems of later life, but also the physical and psychological context in which assessment occurs may be so different from that in which cognitive tasks are faced in daily life that performance under the two conditions may be quite different (Jenkins, 1974). Tests used with children are generally validated against performance in a context similar to that in which assessment occurs (i.e., the school), whereas tests used with adults and aged persons are employed to measure performance capacity in the diverse and unstructured tasks of daily life.

Test taking is a familiar experience for most children and young adults but often an alien and threatening experience for aged individuals. Older persons are more cautious than their juniors, and in situations perceived as threatening or uncertain they will simply fail to act (response inhibition) unless confident they are correct (Botwinick, 1973, pp. 94–120). The result may be spuriously low scores on many performance tests due to errors of omission. The formal laboratory test setting is particularly likely to be threatening, to arouse anxiety, and to induce errors of omission in the aged (Eisdorfer, 1967).

Anxiety can be mitigated, however, and errors of omission decreased if an attempt is made to familiarize subjects with the setting and the procedures prior to testing (Troyer, Eisdorfer, Bogdonoff, & Wilkie, 1967). Uncertainty can also be reduced and performance facilitated if explicit statements and perhaps a demonstration of task requirements are given to the subjects (Brinley, 1965). Also, artifacts of response inhibition can be avoided if instructions are supportive rather than challenging and are aimed at disassociating performance from personal worth or functional capacity (Ross, 1968). Instructions that increase the subject's feeling of competence and reduce anxiety are particularly important in the organically impaired aged (Parsons & Stewart, 1966).

Structuring psychometric assessment to avoid a series of failures is also useful. For example, rather than ending a task at the point at which a subject fails, that failure might be followed by several trials known to be within the person's capacity, thus engendering a feeling of successful accomplishment. Particular caution should be taken to avoid the effects of response inhibition when testing procedures are rapidly paced (Eisdorfer, Axelrod, & Wilkie, 1963) or involve stimuli that are novel, unexpected, rapidly changing, and productive of fatigue (Appley & Trumbull, 1967).

PERFORMANCE SPEED

Another issue to be considered in the application of standard psychometric measures to the elderly is the adequacy of specified stimulus presentation and response time intervals. The behavioral change that has been found to occur most consistently with advanced age is a decline in performance on fast-paced tasks (Jarvik & Cohen, 1973). The performance decrement persists when response inhibition artifacts are controlled and probably reflects an age-related increase in central information processing time (Birren, 1965). If an investigator wishes to assess the effect of treatment on performance within a time limit considered reasonable for younger persons, then specified time limits on standard measures are justified. Since rapid processing and responding are required for successful completion of many tasks in a fast-paced urban environment, such an outcome measure is, of course, quite reasonable. However, if an investigator wishes to assess the effect of treatment on performance capacity without regard to speed, time limits may be inappropriate. Some data, although quite limited, are available concerning the adequacy for aged subjects of response time limits imposed in a few specific psychometric tests. Doppelt and Wallace (1955), for example, found standard time limits for the WAIS appropriate for all ages, although one quarter of the aged subjects did not complete one or more of the timed subtests. Storandt (1977) recently confirmed the finding that WAIS time limits are adequate for aged subjects. She also found that bonus points for speed differentially aided the young and therefore recommended against their use where speed of performance is not of interest. Unfortunately, the effect of standard time limits on performance by aged subjects is unknown for most measures.

DISTRACTIBILITY AND INTERFERENCE

Aged persons are more easily distracted than their juniors by irrelevant stimuli presented simultaneously with stimuli relevant to a cognitive task (Rabbitt, 1965). The problem is particularly severe in brain damaged subjects where the ticking of a clock or a muffled street noise may completely disrupt performance (Lezak, 1976, pp. 109–110). Distraction by irrelevant stimuli would of course impair the ability of the individual to deal with tasks ranging from conducting a conversation to driving an automobile, and an investigator may well choose to systematically introduce irrelevant with relevant stimuli and assess distractibility as a dependent measure. At least one standard psychometric test that provides such a measure has been shown to reliably distinguish healthy from senile aged subjects (Canter & Straumanis, 1969). A problem arises, however, when test materials or procedures introduce unintended distractions that diminish performance on measures of other cognitive abilities. In memory assessment, for example, irrelevant information introduced after stimulus material has been presented but before it is recalled is unlikely to have greater effects on the performance of healthy aged subjects than on that of young subjects. However, if the interpolated material resembles that in storage, aged subjects are likely to suffer a relatively greater decline in recall ability (Suci, Davidoff, & Braun, 1962). The disruptive effects of this retroactive interference are minimized when to-be-recalled material is well learned, when performance is slowly paced, and when interfering material is presented soon after learning (Botwinick, 1973, pp. 240–241). Again, in the organically impaired elderly the disruptive effects of interference are far more dramatic than in the healthy aged, indeed, susceptibility to interference is a hallmark of organic brain syndrome (Goldfarb, 1967).

Interference resulting from the process of recalling and responding also appears to exert a differential effect on retention in young and old subjects (Talland, 1965) and should be givén attention in psychometric assessment. For example, many standard tests that purport to measure nonverbal information require subjects to draw a geometric figure from memory following visual presentation. The process of drawing the figure introduces response interference. Verbal recall immediately following the presentation of verbal information introduces considerably less response interference and, consequently, fewer errors. This difference in response interference under the two conditions of recall may account for the findings of many early investigators (e.g., Gilbert, 1941) that retention of verbal information is superior to retention of nonverbal information.

FATIGUE

The effects of fatigue may diminish the validity of psychometric assessment, particularly in a sample of impaired aged subjects. Even casual observation suggests that aged subjects become fatigued more easily on most physical and mental tasks than do young adults. Furry and Schaie (1973) have demonstrated that mental and physical fatigue in the aged exert significant and complex effects on test performance. The effects of mental fatigue at any age include various sensory and perceptual changes, slowed and disorganized performance, and, perhaps, short-term memory impairment (Welford, 1965, pp. 438–449). Although the acceptable duration of testing varies with several factors, including physical health and degree of cognitive deterioration, it is likely that after some relatively brief period (perhaps 30 minutes in mild to moderately impaired subjects), the effects of fatigue will diminish performance. Together with poor memory, fatigue is the most common symptom of chronic brain damage, and the acceptable duration of testing in such patients may be 10 minutes or less (Lezak, 1976, p. 160). To detect the possible influence of fatigue on performance, it is recommended, therefore, to routinely examine data for order effects.

SENSORY FUNCTION AND PHYSICAL IMPAIRMENT

Advanced age is generally accompanied by a decline in visual acuity (Chapanis, 1960) and visual accommodation (Hofstetler, 1954) such that performance on many standard cognitive tests involving visual stimuli may be dramatically affected. Increased levels of illumination are required by the aged for maximum visual acuity (Wetson, 1949), and adaptation to the dark is generally poorer in old than in young subjects (Birren & Shock, 1950). Vision should be examined routinely prior to psychometric assessment, and measures that involve small visual stimuli, particularly where rapid response is required, should be modified or avoided. Measures that involve differential response based on color discrimination may also yield invalid estimates of cognitive ability, particularly if fine discriminations are required in the blue portion of the spectrum (Gilbert, 1957).

A hearing loss, particularly for high-pitched sounds, also occurs in advanced age (Spoor, 1967) and should be considered in auditory stimulus presentation. Recently Granick, Kleban, and Weiss (1976) demonstrated a substantial association between hearing loss and cognitive test performance in both healthy and physically impaired aged subjects whose hearing was within normal limits. The association was particularly striking for several verbal subtests of the WAIS. The authors concluded that "findings imply that aged subjects may be more intellectually capable than their test performances suggest and that hearing is an important variable to be considered in the assessment of their cognitive functioning" (p. 434).

In addition to sensory changes that occur in healthy elderly individuals, there are sometimes dramatic alterations in sensory capacity associated with a broad range of disease states common in the aged. Similarly, motor impairments or communication difficulties resulting from disease processes may significantly alter test performance, although they may be unrelated to the ability being assessed. The utility of many visuopractic measures that provide correlates of cognitive abilities in the young is, of course, quite limited in a population where arthritis, stroke, and other diseases associated with motor impairment are common. Of course, even minor subclinical variations in general health adversely affect test performance in the aged (Botwinick & Birren, 1963), and confusional states psychometrically indistinguishable from organic brain syndrome may result from nutritional deficiency, kidney disorder, drug intoxication, and a variety of infections (Prien, 1972; cf. also chapters 2 and 3).

DEPRESSION

The relationship between depression and cognitive test performance merits consideration in view of the apparently high prevalence of affective disorder in later life (Kay, Beamish, & Roth, 1964). In young and middle-aged adults, depression appears to exert a minimal influence on psychometric performance (Friedman, 1964), although depressed patients tend to report difficulty in performing tasks and tend to underestimate their performance capacities (Beck, 1971, pp. 154–164). Subtle effects on performance do occur and appear to include increased errors of omission on serial learning tasks, perhaps resulting from brain biogenic amine depletion rather than clinical aspects of depressive disorder (Henry, Weingartner, & Murphy, 1973).

In aged subjects depression may exert a considerably more dramatic effect on performance. Depression may develop as an early secondary symptom of organic brain syndrome, reflecting the individual's reaction to diminished cognitive abilities, and may exacerbate the performance decrement associated with impaired brain function (Lezak, 1976, pp. 171-172). Alternatively, and of greater concern in treatment assessment, depression in the intact aged individual may result in a performance decrement clinically and psychometrically similar to that associated with organic impairment (Post, 1976). Differentiation between cognitively impaired individuals who are depressed and cases of so-called depressive pseudodementia is essential in treatment assessment, since cognitive function in the latter group would be expected to improve regardless of treatment intervention as depression remits (Madden, Luban, Kaplan, & Manfredi, 1952). Clinical differentiation is quite imprecise, unless one waits to observe the patient when depressive symptomatology is in remission, and it is based primarily on a history of sudden onset of organic symptomatology, low premorbid intelligence, and apathy during interview (Langley, 1975). A number of attempts have been made by British investigators (e.g., Hemsi, Whitehead, & Post, 1968) to distinguish organically impaired aged subjects from pseudodemented depressives on the basis of psychometric performance. Unfortunately, most of these investigations have involved rather crude measures, principally a digit copying test and a synonym learning test. As in the case of clinical interview, adequate discrimination between demented and pseudodemented subjects with such measures seems to require that an investigator reexamine a subject 6 weeks or so after an initial assessment (Kendrick, 1972). Thus, to assess the effect of a treatment in organically impaired individuals, one may be forced to exclude depressed individuals from the sample or employ an extended pretreatment observational period during which cognitive performance can be assessed under different affective states (cf. also chapters 1 and 3 for a discussion of depressive pseudodementia).

PERFORMANCE VARIABILITY

Increases with age in intraindividual variability pose another series of problems in psychometric assessment involving the elderly (Heron & Chown, 1967). Test-retest reliability coefficients may not reflect the magnitude of the problem since interindividual variability may also be high (Botwinick, 1973, pp. 309-310). Intraindividual variability is particularly extreme in chronic organic brain syndrome associated with arteriosclerosis, where cognitive test performance may fluctuate sharply within a period of several hours, perhaps as a function of circulatory changes (Prien, 1972). Such individual variability raises several issues in psychometric assessment of treatment effects. It is hazardous to rely on a single test performance as a measure of pre- or posttreatment level of function. Repeated daily test sessions may be required prior to treatment in order to establish baseline performance, and, similarly, evaluation of treatment effects may require repeated assessment both during and after treatment. In order to control item-specific practice effects, repeated assessment of some abilities will require the use of several equivalent test forms. While as many as 20 alternate forms are available for tests in the repetitive psychometric battery developed by Moran and Mefferd (1959), few standard measures have more than two equivalent forms and many have none. Repeated baseline testing may also allow the investigator to confine to pretreatment the sometimes large initial practice effects that result from factors other than familiarity with the items of a particular test. Repeated testing not only provides the investigator with a more reliable estimate of ability than a single test result, but also provides a measure of variability in performance. Performance variability may actually be of interest as a dependent variable in treatment assessment rather than regarded simply as a source of error.

Increases with age in intersubject variability are of such magnitude that one must dramatically restrict the range of individual variability in which treatment is to be assessed, if psychometric devices are to be of any use. Persons of advanced age who present for treatment of cognitive dysfunction range from the corporate executive who complains of having to work 9 hours to complete tasks he could once complete in 8, to the nursing home resident who no longer recognizes visiting family members. While these individuals might occupy opposite ends on a symptom rating scale, it is difficult to imagine any cognitive task equally relevant to both individuals or any test that would measure the same ability at such widely divergent levels of competence.

COGNITIVE LOSS WITH AGE

A fundamental problem in assessing the effects of treatment on cognitive function in the aged relates to selection of appropriate subjects for study. Presumably, an appropriate sample is composed of individuals who have experienced significant cognitive loss. Complaints of diminished cognitive abilities are likely to be quite unreliable. For example, Kahn, Zarit, Hilbert, and Niederehe (1975) have demonstrated that complaints of memory impairment by an aged individual are likely to reflect depression rather than an actual performance decrement. Several attempts have been made to develop psychometric techniques that would allow identification of elderly individuals who have experienced a decline in cognitive abilities greater than that expected at their age. Of course, in order to establish extent of decline, one must have an index of the individual's cognitive ability during earlier life. The psychometric index most often employed is vocabulary level, since it has been shown repeatedly to be well maintained in healthy aged individuals, and since it represents the best single index of general intellectual ability during early adulthood (Botwinick, 1967, pp. 1-27). Any attempt to estimate prior ability on the basis of current behavior is likely to be hazardous. For example, Foulds and Raven (1948) demonstrated some time ago that verbal abilities remain relatively constant with age only when initial ability is high. With vocabulary score as a crude index of initial ability, an investigator may select aged subjects who have experienced cognitive decline by comparing the performance of the individual on an appropriate measure with that of healthy individuals of the same age and vocabulary level. A significant decrement relative to the comparison group may then be taken as an indication of abnormal decline. Few psychometric measures, however, provide any normative data for aged subjects, let alone norms for various levels of vocabulary function. The Guild Memory Test (Gilbert, 1968), which is intended as a supplement to the WAIS, is the only test for which normative data have been gathered for several levels of WAIS Vocabulary function within several age ranges above 65. The test has been employed in subject selection for several treatment assessment studies (Crook, Ferris, Sathananthan, Raskin, & Gershon, 1977; Raskin, Gershon, Crook, Sathananthan, & Ferris, 1978). To be admitted to those studies subjects were required to obtain scores of at least 1 standard deviation below the mean established for their age group and vocabulary level on at least 3 of the 6 Guild subtests.

A number of indexes of cognitive impairment have been suggested based on the well-documented differential effect of age on WAIS subtest scores. Most of these involve some variation on Wechsler's (1938) Deterioration Quotient (DQ). The DQ is calculated by summing the age-corrected scaled scores for the WAIS or Wechsler-Bellevue I (WB-I) verbal and performance subtests that "hold" with age and those that "don't hold," i.e., are markedly affected by the aging process. The quotient is expressed as: hold-don't hold/hold. While each of the five performance tests declines with age more than each of the six verbal measures, the "hold" and "don't hold" categories contain equal numbers of verbal and performance tests so that some functional similarity exists between the contrasted categories. The "hold" subtests of the WAIS are Vocabulary, Information, Object Assembly, and Picture Completion; the "don't hold" subtests are Digit Span, Similarities, Digit Symbol, and Block Design. Since the raw score on each subtest is converted to a scaled score for the individual's age group, the DQ expresses the amount of deterioration in excess of that expected in the normal aging process. Wechsler has provided means and standard deviations of WAIS DQs for each of 11 age groups (Wechsler, 1958). Unfortunately, Botwinick and Birren (1951), as well as other investigators, have found that the DQ is an inadequate index of cognitive decline.

The Digit Symbol subtest of the WAIS has consistently shown the most age sensitive (Botwinick, 1967, pp. 1-27), and investigators have occasionally employed entrance criteria based on some specified disparity between an individual's age-corrected Vocabulary and age-corrected Digit Symbol scores. Unfortunately, motor persistence, sustained attention, response speed, and visual-motor coordination play significant roles in Digit Symbol performance (Lezak, 1976, pp. 213-214), and performance is relatively unaffected by intellectual prowess, memory, or learning (Murstein and Leipold, 1961).

ORGANIC IMPAIRMENT VERSUS NORMAL AGING

The Digit Symbol subtest not only discriminates clearly between young and old individuals, but, like many other age-sensitive measures, it also distinguishes between brain-damaged and non-brain-damaged patients (Gonen, 1970). The similarity between psychometric performance decrements associated with advanced age and those associated with diffuse brain damage has led a number of investigators to assume that cognitive decline in the aged results from otherwise unrecognized cerebral pathology and that dysfunction associated with clinically recognized organic brain syndrome is simply an extreme form of that seen in normal aging. The DQ and related indexes reflect the same assumption. Reed and Reitan (1963) have compared the psychometric performance of young brain-damaged and old normal subjects and concluded that differences in test performance associated with aging could, in fact, be partially explained on the basis of changes in the organic condition of the brain. On the other hand, Hallenbeck (1964) has argued that old age is a poor prototype of deterioration associated with organic injury and that one must excercise caution in employing psychometric instruments based on that assumption. In a compromise position, Goldstein and Shelly (1975) have suggested that age and diffuse brain damage exert similar effects on motor abilities but largely dissimilar effects on language abilities, nonverbal memory, and psychomotor problem solving.

Overall and Gorham (1972) have also suggested that the performance of aged subjects differs from the performance of young subjects along a continuum quite different from the one that separates chronic brain syndrome patients from the normal aged. Multiple discriminant analysis involving WAIS subtest scores have suggested that in normal aging, Similarities, Digit Symbol, Picture Arrangement, and Object Assembly decline relative to Vocabulary. On the other hand, organic brain syndrome patients can be distinguished from normal aged subjects by a contrast between Similarities, Vocabulary, and Object Assembly, on the one hand, and Comprehension, Arithmetic, and Picture Completion on the other. The three former measures were much more significantly affected by organic brain disease than by age. Other evidence (e.g., Botwinick & Birren, 1951) is also available that suggests that the WAIS performance patterns that distinguish young from old individuals are not identical to those that distinguish the organically impaired from the healthy aged. The conclusion of Overall and Gorham (1972) has clear implications for the selection of treatment outcome measures. According to the authors:

> The results clearly reveal that the pattern of changes associated with old age is different from the pattern of changes associated with chronic brain syndrome. The difference between old age and chronic brain syndrome was evident in both objective and projective test-score profiles. This is not to say that there *may* not be an organic basis for the

> poor performance of old persons, but the nature of the organic component is surely different from that in patients with clinical chronic brain syndrome. We conclude that normally aging individuals are not marching along the road to chronic brain syndrome. (pp. 104–105)

If this view is correct, appropriate dependent measures for assessment of treatment effects in the impaired aged may be those that are sensitive to the effects of organic impairment but insensitive to the effects of age. As noted previously, the WAIS Digit Symbol subtest is frequently used as an outcome measure on the basis of its demonstrated sensitivity to the effects of age and organic impairment. However, if one assumes that the goal of treatment is restoration of the impaired individual's cognitive capacity to what is normal for that age, then such a measure may be relatively insensitive to treatment effects.

CONCLUSION

A number of issues have been discussed that may limit the utility of standard performance tests in providing measures of cognitive abilities in aged subjects. It does not necessarily follow, however, that the widespread criticism of measures presently used with the elderly is entirely valid.

As Fozard and Thomas (1975) have suggested, tests are often attacked for failing to accomplish tasks for which they were never intended. It is not surprising that tests constructed to predict educational success in children may be inappropriate for measuring treatment response in the elderly.

The widespread criticism that existing measures are insensitive to treatment effects may also be misleading. For example, in the study by Kahn et al. (1975), complaints of memory impairment by aged individuals were found to reflect depression rather than an actual performance decrement. Memory complaints may affect ratings of impairment by other observers as well. Thus, a drug or other treatment that exerts mild antidepressant effects may appear on the basis of self-report or behavioral rating to improve cognitive function. In an uncontrolled study, the treatment need exert no effect, and apparent improvement might occur as a function of the natural course of an affective disorder. One might speculate that such factors partly account for frequent reports in the psychopharmacology literature of improved ratings of memory function following treatment, without a corresponding improvement in psychometric test performance. In discussing such a finding an investigator is not unlikely to suggest that the treatment induced a change in cognitive function, but the psychometric tests employed were not sensitive enough to detect it.

Attempts have been made to develop measures of cognitive function appropriate for impaired aged individuals (e.g., Dana, White, & Merlis, 1970), but most of the tests produced have been technically inadequate. Several groups around the country are now involved in efforts to develop cognitive performance measures for aged subjects that take into account issues such as those raised in this chapter. Several of these projects are described in chapters 10 and 11.

REFERENCES

American Psychological Association. *Standards for educational and psychological tests* (Rev. ed.). Washington, D.C.: American Psychological Association, 1974.

Anastasi, A. *Psychological testing* (2nd ed.). New York: Macmillan, 1961.

Appley, M. H., & Trumbull, R. (Eds.). *Psychological stress.* New York: Appleton-Century-Crofts, 1967.

Beck, A. T. *Depression: Clinical, experimental and theoretical aspects.* New York: Hoeber, 1971.

Birren, J. E. Age changes in speed of behavior: Its central nature and physiological correlates. In A. T. Welford & J. E. Birren (Eds.), *Behavior, aging and the nervous system.* Springfield, Ill.: Charles C Thomas, 1965.

Birren, J. E., & Shock, N. W. Age changes in rate and level of visual dark adaptation. *Journal of Applied Physiology,* 1950, *5,* 216–221.

Botwinick, J. *Cognitive processes in maturity and old age.* New York: Springer, 1967.

Botwinick, J. *Aging and behavior.* New York: Springer, 1973.

Botwinick, J., & Birren, J. E. The measurement of intellectual decline in the senile psychoses. *Journal of Consulting Psychology,* 1951, *15,* 145–150.

Botwinick, J., & Birren, J. E. Cognitive processes: Mental abilities and psychomotor responses in healthy aged men. In J. E. Birren, R. N. Butler, S. W. Greenhouse, L. Sokoloff, & M. R. Yarrow (Eds.), *Human aging: A biological and behavioral study.* Washington, D.C.: U.S. Government Printing Office, 1963.

Brinley, J. F. Cognitive sets and accuracy of performance in the elderly. In A. T. Welford and J. E. Birren (Eds.), *Behavior, aging and the nervous system.* Springfield, Ill.: Charles C Thomas, 1965.

Canter, A., & Straumanis, J. J. Performance of senile and healthy aged persons on the BIP Bender test. *Perceptual and Motor Skills,* 1969, *28,* 695–698.

Chapanis, A. Relationships between age, visual acuity and color vision. *Human Biology,* 1950, *22,* 1–33.

Crook, T. H., Ferris, S., Sathananthan, G., Raskin, A., & Gerson, S. The effect of methylphenidate on test performance in the cognitively impaired aged. *Psychopharmacology,* 1977, *52,* 251–255.

Dana, L. A., White, L., & Merlis, S. A new approach to measuring short-term memory in geriatric subjects: A pilot study. *Psychological Reports,* 1970, *27,* 8–10.

Demming, J. A., & Pressey, S. L. Tests "indigenous" to the adult and older years. *Journal of Counseling Psychology,* 1957, *2,* 144–148.

Doppelt, J. E., & Wallace, W. L. Standardization of the Wechsler Adult Intelligence Scale for older persons. *Journal of Abnormal and Social Psychology,* 1955, *51,* 312–330.

Eisdorfer, C. New dimensions and a tentative theory. *Gerontologist,* 1967, *7,* 14–18.

Eisdorfer, C., Axelrod, S., & Wilkie, F. Stimulus exposure time as a factor in serial learning in an aged sample. *Journal of Abnormal and Social Psychology,* 1963, *67,* 594–600.

Foulds, G. A., & Raven, J. C. Normal changes in the mental abilities of adults as age advances. *Journal of Mental Science,* 1948, *94,* 133–142.

Fozard, J. L., & Thomas, J. C. Psychology of aging: Basic findings and some psychiatric applications: In J. G. Howells (Ed.), *Modern perspectives in the psychiatry of old age.* New York: Brunner/Mazel, 1975.

Friedman, A. S. Minimal effects of severe depression on cognitive functioning. *Journal of Abnormal and Social Psychology,* 1964, *69,* 237-243.

Furry, C. A., & Schaie, K. W. Fatigue and intellectual performance in the aged. *Gerontologist,* 1973, *13,* (3, Pt. 2), 80.

Gilbert, J. G. Memory loss in senescence. *Journal of Abnormal and Social Psychology,* 1941, *36,* 73-86.

Gilbert, J. G. Age changes in color matching. *Journal of Gerontology,* 1957, *12,* 210-215.

Gilbert, J. G., Levee, R. F., & Catalano, F. L. A preliminary report on a new memory scale. *Perceptual and Motor Skills,* 1968, *27,* 277-278.

Goldfarb, A. I. Geriatric psychiatry. In A. M. Freedman & H. I. Kaplan (Eds.), *Comprehensive textbook of psychiatry.* Baltimore: Williams & Wilkins, 1967.

Goldstein, G., & Shelly, C. H. Similarities and differences between psychological deficit in aging and brain damage. *Journal of Gerontology,* 1975, *30,* 448-455.

Gonen, J. Y. The use of Wechsler's deterioration quotient in cases of diffuse and symmetrical cerebral atrophy. *Journal of Clinical Psychology,* 1970, *26,* 174-177.

Granick, S., Kleban, M. H., & Weiss, A. D. Relationships between hearing loss and cognition in normally hearing aged persons. *Journal of Gerontology,* 1976, *31,* 434-440.

Hallenbeck, C. E. Evidence for a multiple process view of mental deterioration. *Journal of Gerontology,* 1964, *19,* 357-363.

Hemsi, L. K., Whitehead, A., & Post, F. Cognitive functioning and cerebral arousal in elderly depressives and dements. *Journal of Psychosomatic Research,* 1968, *12,* 145-156.

Henry, G. M., Weingartner, H., & Murphy, D. L. Influence of affective states and psychoactive drugs on verbal learning and memory. *American Journal of Psychiatry,* 1973, *130,* 966-971.

Heron, A., & Chown, S. *Age and function.* London: J. A. Churchill, 1967.

Hofstetler, H. W. Some interrelationships of age, refraction, and rate of refractive changes. *American Journal of Optometry and Archives of the American Academy of Optometry,* 1954, *31,* 161-169.

Hulicka, I. M. Age differences in retention as a function of interference. *Journal of Gerontology,* 1967, *22,* 180-184.

Jarvik, L. F., & Cohen, D. A biobehavioral approach to intellectual changes with aging. In C. Eisdorfer and M. P. Lawton (Eds.), *The psychology of adult development and aging.* Washington, D.C.: American Psychological Association, 1973.

Jenkins, J. J. Remember that old theory of memory? Well forget it! *American Psychologist,* 1974, *29,* 785-795.

Kahn, R. L., Zarit, S. H., Hilbert, N. M., & Niederehe, G. M. Memory complaint and impairment in the aged. *Archives of General Psychiatry,* 1975, *32,* 1569-1573.

Kay, D. W. K., Beamish, P., & Roth, M. Old age mental disorders in Newcastle upon Tyne. Part 1: A study of prevalence. *British Journal of Psychiatry,* 1964, *110,* 146-158.

Kendrick, D. C. The Kendrick battery of tests: Theoretical assumptions and clinical uses. *British Journal of Social and Clinical Psychology,* 1972, *11,* 373-386.

Langley, G. E. Functional psychoses. In J. G. Howells (Ed.), *Modern perspectives in the psychiatry of old age.* New York: Brunner/Mazel, 1975.

Lezak, M. D. *Neuropsychological assessment.* New York: Oxford University Press, 1976.

Madden, J. J., Luban, J. A., Kaplan, L. A., & Manfredi, H. M. Nondementing psychoses in older persons. *Journal of the American Medical Association,* 1952, *150,* 1567-1573.

Moran, L. J., & Mefferd, R. B. Repetitive psychometric measures. *Psychological Reports,* 1959, *5,* 269-275.

Murstein, B. I., & Leipold, W. D. The role of learning and motor abilities in the Wechsler-Bellevue digit symbol test. *Educational and Psychological Measurement,* 1961, *21,* 103–112.

Overall, J. E., & Gorham, D. R. Organicity versus old age in objective and projective test performance. *Journal of Consulting and Clinical Psychology,* 1972, *39,* 98–105.

Parsons, O. A., & Stewart, K. D. Effects of supportive versus disinterested interviews on perceptual-motor performance in brain-damaged and neurotic patients. *Journal of Consulting Psychology,* 1966, *30,* 260–266.

Post, F. Geriatric depression. In D. M. Gallant & G. M. Simpson (Eds.), *Depression: Behavioral, biochemical, diagnostic and treatment concepts.* New York: Halsted Press, 1976.

Prien, R. F. *Chronic organic brain syndrome.* Washington, D.C. Veterans Administration Department of Medicine and Surgery, 1972.

Rabbitt, P. An age-decrement in the ability to ignore irrelevant information. *Journal of Gerontology,* 1965, *20,* 233–238.

Raskin, A., Gershon, S., Crook, T. H., Sathananthan, G., & Ferris, S. The effects of hyper- and normobaric oxygen on cognitive impairment in the elderly. *Archives of General Psychiatry,* 1978, *35,* 50–60.

Reed, H. B. C., & Reitan, R. M. Comparison of the effects of the normal aging process with the effects of organic brain damage in adaptive abilities. *Journal of Gerontology,* 1963, *18,* 177–179.

Ross, E. Effects of challenging and supportive instructions in verbal learning in older persons. *Journal of Educational Psychology,* 1968, *59,* 261–266.

Shmavonian, B. M., & Busse, E. W. The utilization of psychophysiological techniques in the study of the aged. In R. H. Williams, C. Tibbitts, & W. Donahue (Eds.), *Process of aging: Social and psychological perspectives.* New York: Atherton Press, 1963.

Spoor, A. Presbycusis values in relation to noise induced hearing loss. *International Audiology,* 1967, *6,* 48–57.

Storandt, M. Age, ability level, and method of administering and scoring the WAIS. *Journal of Gerontology,* 1977, *32,* 175–178.

Suci, G. H., Davidoff, M. D., & Braun, J. C. Interference in short-term retention as a function of age. In C. Tibbitts & W. Donahue (Eds.), *Social and psychological aspects of aging.* New York: Columbia University Press, 1962.

Talland, G. A. Three estimates of the word span and their stability over the adult years. *Quarterly Journal of Experimental Psychology,* 1965, *17,* 301–307.

Troyer, W. G., Eisdorfer, C., Bogdonoff, M. D., & Wilkie, F. Experimental stress and learning in the aged. *Journal of Abnormal Psychology,* 1967, *72,* 65–70.

Wechsler, D. Mental deterioration; its measurement and significance. *Journal of Nervous and Mental Disease,* 1938, *87,* 89–97.

Wechsler, D. *Measurement of adult intelligence.* Baltimore: Williams & Wilkins, 1939.

Wechsler, D. The measurement and evaluation of intelligence of older persons. In *Old age in the modern world.* Edinburgh and London: E. & S. Livingstone, 1955.

Wechsler, D. *The measurement and appraisal of adult intelligence* (4th ed.). Baltimore: Williams & Wilkins, 1958.

Welford, A. T. Fatigue and monotony. In O. G. Edholm and A. L. Bacharach (Eds.), *The physiology of human survival.* New York and London: Academic Press, 1965.

Welford, A. T. Age and skill: Motor, intellectual and social. *Interdisciplinary topics in gerontology,* 1969, *4,* 1–22.

Weston, H. C. On age and illumination in relation to visual performance. *Transactions of the Illuminating Engineering Society.* London, 1949, *14,* 281–297.

10

Assessment of Intellectual Changes in the Elderly

Nanette A. Kramer
University of Southern California

Lissy F. Jarvik
Veterans Administration Hospital, Brentwood and University of California, Los Angeles

INTRODUCTION

The major purpose of this chapter is to provide a critical review of instruments used to assess cognitive changes in intact and cognitively impaired elderly. The term *cognitively impaired* is used to describe those persons whose intellectual functioning has diminished or is atypically low. It is preferred over the term *brain damaged* because cognitive impairment may be present without brain damage. In the landmark study on the interrelation between antemortem functioning and postmortem pathology, some persons with minimal post-mortem manifestations of neuropathology had displayed cognitive impairment on psychological testing, while other individuals with extensive brain damage had not given notable indications of cognitive impairment (Blessed, Tomlinson, & Roth, 1968). These authors remind us of the possibility that "in a proportion of severely demented subjects there are qualitatively distinct pathological changes inaccessible to available techniques of examination" (p. 805). The term *brain damaged* is used when a study refers to subjects as brain damaged on the basis of clinicians' ratings, psychophysiological measures, surgical procedures, and other diagnostic tests. The term *intact* is used to refer to persons whose test scores fell into or above the normal or average range, or, if longitudinally studied, whose scores did not decline significantly upon retesting.

Investigations of cognitive functioning have been carried out by means of neuropsychodiagnostic testing, psychiatric ratings, and psychometrics, but rarely have these three approaches been combined in the assessment of any single group, and comparison of the results obtained by these different methods in the same individuals are practically nonexistent. Clinical and developmental psychologists rely mainly on psychometrics, psychiatrists generally favor rating scales and qualitative clinical evaluations, while neurologists and experimental psychologists tend to restrict themselves to neuropsychodiagnostic measures. Moreover, the trend has been to use the same instruments for the old as for the young, and usually these instruments were standardized on young rather than old persons. Finally, even within any of these three approaches, there is little data available on the validity of the various instruments. Inconsistencies between studies in recognizing and dealing with extraneous influences on test performance constitute a major obstacle to the integration of available information. The review by Goldstein and Shelly (1975) has illustrated the conflicting conclusions that can be explained on the basis of methodological differences. Clearly, the three major approaches to functional assessment differ in methodology as well as subject populations.

Psychometric procedures (i.e., quantifiable measures of behavioral or functional output without regard to cerebral localization) monopolize the literature on presumably intact normally aging subjects. They are often administered to representative population groups, and norms are then published for these groups. An individual's intactness of functioning is judged on the basis of these norms. There are several problems with these studies, among them the following:

1. The marked variability among persons, especially the aged, throws into question the representativeness of any one group for any other group.
2. Cohort effects are not controlled or accounted for so that factors other than the aging of the individual may be contributing to the outcome scores. For example, the same items or questions may have different meanings for groups of subjects from different social classes and ethnic backgrounds.
3. When norms exist, they usually give a handicap for being older. Increasing age presumes decreasing ability.
4. Even though psychometric tests are used, on occasion, to detect organic mental disturbances in persons considered intact by other means, individuals diagnosed as brain damaged on other grounds have been known to perform within the normal range on psychometric tests, and thus false negatives commonly occur.

Although psychometric tests generally do not provide a qualitative analysis of the psychological abnormalities on which the subjects' defects are based (Luria, 1966), they do produce a descriptive pattern of an individual's strengths and weaknesses of specific functions at the time of testing. Therefore, despite their limitations, they are widely used by psychologists working with the elderly. Neuropsychological tests, by contrast, are employed by relatively few clinical psychologists although their usage with older populations is growing. They tend to be employed by neurologists and experimental psychologists in attempts to localize specific organic lesions and/or functional changes in individuals who are often already exhibiting overt signs of organic impairment. It appears that these tests have been underutilized. For example, Hans-Lucas Teuber (Note 1) reported that two-thirds of an unselected group of brain-injured men improved their psychometric scores from test to retest despite an intervening brain injury. By contrast, neuropsychological measures would, according to Teuber, have shown a significant decline in performance and, therefore, indicated the presence of brain damage. The division between neuropsychological and psychometric instruments is not absolute. The Wechsler Adult Intelligence Scale (WAIS), for example, has been incorporated into both types of batteries (e.g., psychometric, when examining differences between young and old intact subjects and neuropsychological, when comparing persons with left or right hemiplegia). The division between these instruments and psychiatric rating scales, however, tends to be much firmer with little or no overlap.

Psychiatric rating scales tend to be impressionistic, whether based on observer ratings or on self-reports, and do not rely on formal standardized measurements. Assessment of ability or behavior is indirect since it depends on the subjective report or opinion of the respondent. These tests far surpass in popularity any other type of measure when it comes to the assessment of drug effects on geriatric populations.

TESTS OF ATTENTION AND RELATED AREAS

Testing cognitive performance, regardless of the instrument used, rests on the assumption that the individual being tested is attentive to the task and cognizant of its requirements. For cognitively impaired individuals, this assumption may be invalid; therefore, it is often desirable to specifically examine performance on tasks of attention and orientation before testing higher order cognitive functioning. Tests of attention are generally simple, presumably demanding only immediate reproduction or recall with a bare minimum of processing. On many attentional tests, the items tend to be easy and of little inherent interest. Vulnerability to distraction is therefore high, and poor performance cannot be taken as definitive of cerebral damage. As pointed out by Talland (1968), older persons tend to do better on tests of meaningful items and consequently might be penalized on the usual attentional tests. The following tests, commonly employed in cognitive assessment of the elderly, have a large attentional component.

Digit Span Forward

Performance on Digit Span Forward (DSF) can be predicted with more certainty than almost any other measure of cognitive performance, for it is unusual for anyone to exhibit severe impairment of performance on this test. Most individuals will recall six or seven digits regardless of age or diagnosis.

Numerous studies have given evidence of the stability of performance on this measure. Kahn, Zarit, Hilbert, and Niederehe (1975) showed stability for intact and brain-damaged persons to age 91; Whitehead (1973) for intact, depressed, and brain-damaged persons to over 73 years; Granick and Friedman (1967) for intact and psychotic persons to over 60 years; Reed and Reitan (1963) for intact persons into their mid-50s; Kaszniak, Garron, and Fox (Note 2) for intact and brain-damaged persons to 89 years; Bromley (1958) for intact persons through 82 years; and Sterne (1969) for brain-damaged patients and hospitalized controls to 80 years.

Hulicka (1966) did find a decline in DSF with age. However, the differences in background factors between the young subjects (high school students or dropouts, ages 15-17) and the old subjects (residents of hospitals or nursing homes or members of senior citizens clubs, ages 60-99) may have contributed to differential attention spans. Educational differences were not significant, at least in Granick and Friedman's (1967) study. Blum, Jarvik, and Clark (1970) also found a significant though small decline on DSF for persons 65-73 years and a more marked decline for persons 73-85 years.

Decline has also been noted in the presence of organic impairment. Persons with Korsakoff's syndrome, whose memory dysfunctions are often far worse than other cognitive impairments, do considerably less well on DSF, and Digit Span Backward (DSB), than on tests of long-stored memory or new learning and abstraction (Horenstein, 1971).

According to McFie (1975), perseveration errors may indicate general impairment, while transpositions, omissions, and inclusions of new digits are often observed in the performance of dysphasics. Finally, the mean digit score has been noted as lowest in patients with left frontal lesions, who often demonstrate impaired memory for verbally presented material and impaired verbal fluency. Therefore, if a person does poorly on DSF, and attentional conflicts are ruled out, other tests of verbal functioning should be administered to investigate the extent of the problem. Tests should also be given in other modalities to determine whether short-term recall is impaired diffusely or only in conjunction with verbal processing (cf. subsection on Block Tapping for a nonverbal analogue).

One's ability to retain meaningless, serially presented information appears to be better with auditory than with visual presentation (Murdoch, 1966), suggesting that acoustical properties are more memorable than semantic properties of such items (McFie, 1975). In one group (ages 18-80) this modality difference was even more apparent with old than with young subjects in that a decline in visual retention was found to increase with age (McGhie, Chapman, & Lawson, 1965).

Not surprisingly, therefore, on DSF a greater difference was observed between old and young on visual than auditory presentation (Taub, 1975). Also, Bromley (1958) attributed his subjects' relatively better performance on DSF than on a test of immediate memory for geometric shapes to the different sensory modalities in which the materials were presented (auditory versus visual).

Although the DSF test should not be the sole instrument used to assess an individual's cognitive functioning, it is a good test to administer first in a battery, since the high success rate tends to set a tone of achievement. Such a tone is particularly desirable among the aged, who generally feel less confident about their judgments than do the young (Wallach & Kogan, 1961). Since a positive relationship between correct responses on one trial and success on subsequent trials has been reported (Arenberg & Robertson-Tchado, 1977), beginning the testing session with DSF may alleviate the anxieties older persons have about their own inadequacies and may improve subsequent performance.

Finally, if an individual does poorly on DSF, it may be unwise to continue testing other functions unless the cause of the poor performance is clarified. If the problem is one of distraction, testing should not proceed until the distracting agent or situation has been remedied. If no distractions can be ascertained in the testing situation or in the person's daily life, other reasons for impairment should be sought.

Continuous Performance Test

In explanation of the stability on DSF performance, even in brain-damaged individuals, it has been said that the test requires only short intermittent bursts of attention to the stimulus and response time is unlimited (Rosvold, Mirsky, Sarason, Bransome, & Beck, 1956). In effect, testees may reorganize their attention between momentary lapses of stimulus presentation, an opportunity that organically impaired persons often are capable and desirous of utilizing to conceal or deny pending problems. Since the conventional digit span test does not require prolonged attentions, the lapses would then not affect their scores to any measurable degree.

In order to account for the ceiling effects produced by tests as undemanding as the DSF, Rosvold et al. (1956) developed the Continuous Performance Test (CPT), which requires lengthy sustained performance (usually over 10 or 20 minutes with 12 responses required per minute), and timing of response that is not chosen by the person being tested. Letters of the alphabet are presented at 1-second intervals and the subject must press a key when predetermined single letters or particular sequences of letters are displayed. The test begins on a level of demand similar to that of conventional digit span tests, and most brain-damaged persons do as well as do intact individuals. However, the demand for sustained attention becomes increasingly difficult, and a point is usually reached where the performance of older brain-damaged persons becomes markedly less correct than that of older intact persons (Davies & Davies, 1975; Canestrari, Note 3). Canestrari's study is particularly interesting in that older subjects tended to make more errors of both commission and omission than younger subjects when required to detect the appearance of an X or a T, but more errors of only omission when the task difficulty was increased, e.g., detect an X immediately preceded by an A. In line with Botwinick's (1966, 1969, 1973) findings of increased cautiousness with age, the elderly tended to give fewer answers rather than increasing the number of incorrect answers as the task became more difficult. In an auditory continuous performance task, older subjects tended to make more errors of omission than younger subjects but not more errors of commission. In that study (Griew & Davies, 1962), subjects were asked to press a key after hearing 3 consecutive odd numbers occurring randomly in a series of numbers presented at 1-second intervals over a 40-minute period.

In a study (Thompson, Optin, & Cohen, 1963) in which subjects had to attend to combinations of odd and even numbers, no age differences showed up at speeds of either 4 or 2 seconds (auditory or visual presentation, respectively), but the older were notably slower than the younger subjects in both modalities when presented with the information for only 1 second. These authors have suggested that "the 'vigilance' aspect of this task becomes increasingly less important as speed is increased, while perceptual-motor speed becomes more important" (p. 368). That is, seemingly identical tasks administered at varying speeds may tap different abilities. Although the findings are not definitive, it is clear that attention can be highly situational. It is important to determine whether an individual's poor score is due to situational variables that could be manipulated and rendered uninfluential, or whether the inattention is pervasive and irremediable. If the former is the case, valid cognitive testing can be done once the appropriate controls for distractive influences have been introduced. If the latter is the case, testing of specific cognitive skills will be difficult, since inattentiveness is likely to underlie the testee's performance deficit throughout the testing situation.

Number Ability

The Number Ability subtest of the Primary Mental Abilities Test (PMA) also falls into the attention category, because its relatively undemanding nature (elementary addition) allows for assessment of attention and concentration.

In a cross-sectional study, Number Ability subtest scores for college graduates ages 70–84 were comparable to those for a reference population of persons age 17 (Strother, Schaie, & Horst, 1957). In a later cross-sectional study (Birkhill & Schaie, 1975), stability of performance on this subtest was confirmed under a variety of test-taking instructions, again sampling highly educated older subjects. The authors themselves, however, warned against overgeneralizing their findings, since the cross-sectional approach may miss some influential variables. In a cross-sequential investigation, Schaie and associates nonetheless found individuals whose performances were resistant to age change on the Number Ability subtest, although persons born in different generations who were tested when they reached the same age showed some performance differences (Schaie & Labouvie-Vief, 1974; Schaie & Strother, 1968). These authors suggested that cohort differences are greater than individual changes over time for this ability.

In general, then, scores on the Number Ability subtest appear to remain stable for most individuals. As with DSF, poor performance on this subtest may indicate attentional problems as well as organic disturbance. For persons who are uneasy in the test situation, but who appear to function well, administration of the Number Ability subtest may help to reduce anxiety.

Arithmetic Subtest–WAIS

Because the WAIS Arithmetic subtest (Wechsler, 1958) includes increasingly demanding questions, it is difficult to sort out the influence of mathematical skill from that of attention and concentration. Bromley (1966) has stated that it tests a "relatively simple cognitive skill, well-practiced in childhood and used from time to time throughout life, so that it tends not to fall into disuse . . . [and] it requires little arithmetical skill or reasoning" (p. 187). It has been shown to remain stable with age (Reed & Reitan, 1963) and brain damage (Overall & Gorham, 1972) and even rise with age (Goldstein & Shelly, 1975). Nevertheless, the test questions demand progressively greater reasoning ability independent of mathematical skill. Therefore, persons who do worse on the first few items compared to the later ones, or have equal difficulties with all of them, are most likely to suffer from inability to attend to the material and/or to process numerical information.

McFie's (1975) factor analysis of WAIS subtests found Arithmetic to load highly on a Freedom from Distractibility factor, although it also had another small but exclusive loading suggesting that it measures a separate numerical ability. The numerical ability factor emerged even more clearly in other studies where the verbal presentation was simplified to make comprehension as easy as possible (Hine, 1970; McFie, 1966). McFie suggested that if an individual's verbal comprehension is in question, the simplified verbal modification should be used to determine more accurately the extent of any deficit in numerical ability. If a person performs well on the modified but not on the conventional version, other tests of verbal comprehension should be administered to explore the deficit.

Subtracting Serial Sevens Test

The Subtracting Serial Sevens Test (Smith, 1967) is frequently used in neurological and psychiatric examinations of patients suspected of having brain lesions, although in the original study only intact older persons were included. Sequentially subtracting seven, beginning with 100, requires only the most basic knowledge of arithmetic but demands considerable attention to the task at hand. Only 56 of 132 subjects (ages 18–65) with above average education and socioeconomic status performed all subtractions without errors. Some subjects displayed patterns of performance previously described as indicative of psychiatric disorders (Hayman, 1942) and frontal lobe lesions (Luria, 1966), e.g., simplification, fragmentation, stereotyped responses, miscellaneous error patterns, and conversion of the task into a series of consecutive operations in which all the actions are constantly denoted aloud (Luria, cited in Smith, 1967). Those who were more highly educated, male, and less than 45-years-old, did significantly better than less educated women over the age of 45. It is not known why the older women did less well than the younger women, nor has performance on this test been directly related to performance on other cognitive measures.

Mental Status and Orientation

In general, the currently available tests of mental status and orientation represent attempts to quantify and render more objective the usual clinical mental status examination. However, two cautions need to be mentioned regarding their use: (1) the diagnosis of organic brain damage cannot be ruled out solely on the basis of good performance on this type of examination, and (2) poor performance, though usually indicative of an organic mental disorder, may, on occasion, result from attentional deficits, particularly those seen in affective disorders (cf. chapter 5).

There is no need to go into a discussion of the expanding array of mental status and orientation tests, as other authors have described the current ones quite adequately. Salzman, Kochansky, and Shader (1972) have covered those most commonly used and designed specifically for older persons. Lezak's (1976) section on tests of orientation, while not geared specifically to older persons, may provide the creative examiner with ideas readily adaptable for use with older persons. The tests she has described are more interesting, both to administer and receive, than the typical mental status questions. For example, Lezak asks for an estimation of the time just taken for the testing session.

TEST BATTERIES

With the realization that no one test can provide an overall assessment of an individual's ability to function cognitively, one popular approach has been to administer a battery of tests, thus taking advantage of the cumulative validity of a well-balanced battery. The purpose of administering more than one test is not only to observe performance on a number of tests but also to compare meaningful interrelationships, trends, and discrepancies among the tests. In this way one can focus on patterns of scores achieved at one time (as in cross-sectional studies), or on patterns that emerge on the basis of retest performance (as in longitudinal studies). The number of batteries that have been employed is extensive. The subsequent discussion highlights a number of the more popular test batteries as a sampling of the kinds of information multiple complementary tests can elicit.

The Wechsler Adult Intelligence Scale (WAIS)

The WAIS (Wechsler, 1955) is one of the most widely used clinical instruments, and it is age adjusted for adults. In addition to giving an overall full-scale IQ score, the WAIS provides subtest scores that can be examined separately or in various groupings; the most common one separates abilities into performance and verbal components (Botwinick, 1967; Cohen, 1957; Eisdorfer, Busse, & Cohen, 1959; Maxwell, 1960; McFie, 1961; Russell, 1972; Wechsler, 1958). The classical pattern in intact older persons is maintenance of, or even increase in, verbal scores (especially Vocabulary and Information) and decline in performance scores (especially Block Design, Picture Arrangement, and Digit Symbol) (Birren & Morrison, 1961; Botwinick, 1967, 1977; Corsini & Fassett, 1953; Doppelt & Wallace, 1955; Eisdorfer & Cohen, 1961; Eisdorfer et al., 1959; Green, 1969; Harwood & Naylor, 1971; Jarvik, 1973).

In one study Harwood and Naylor (1971) have shown that even when young and old subjects are matched on total WAIS score, the performance-verbal discrepancy remains more marked for the older persons. Old subjects did significantly better than young subjects on verbal tests (Information, Comprehension, and Vocabulary), whereas the young subjects did better than the old subjects on performance tests (Digit Symbol, Picture Completion, and Picture Arrangement, and to some degree, Object Assembly).

The longitudinal studies suggest that overall intelligence as measured by the WAIS is more or less maintained into the eighth decade of life, although individual differences in the rate and direction of change are considerable (Berkowitz & Green, 1963; Blum et al., 1970; Eisdorfer, 1963; Eisdorfer & Wilkie, 1973; Jarvik, 1967; Jarvik, Kallman, Falek, & Klaber, 1957; Kallmann & Jarvik, 1959; Kleemeier, 1962; Kleemeier, Note 4).

One problem, however, is that similar subtest patterns have been observed in the aged and in persons with organic impairment (Horenstein, 1971). Digit Symbol, Similarities, and Block Design (and sometimes Digit Span) are referred to as "don't hold" subtests because they tend to show decline with organicity, regardless of the type of organic disturbance or background factors of the individual. The "don't hold" subtests are generally considered to be tests of new learning or abstracting from prior learning, in contrast to the "hold" subtests (Vocabulary, Picture Completion, Information, and sometimes Object Assembly), which require primarily recognition or recall of stored information. The latter subtests appear to be relatively resistant to organic changes and have, therefore, been used as indicators of premorbid levels of functioning.

Although the subtests should not be used singly for diagnostic purposes, intertest scatter or profile may highlight relative deficits and associated sites of organic damage and aid in the discrimination of different types of brain damage (Horenstein, 1971). Others, too, have reported on the relationship between WAIS performance and brain damage (Crookes, 1974; Perez, Rivera, Meyer, Gay, Taylor, & Mathew, 1975). Perez et al., for example, have tested patients diagnosed as having Alzheimer's disease, vertebrobasilar insufficiency, or multi-infarct dementia; 74% of the subjects were correctly classified by discriminant function analysis of the individual WAIS scores.

Analysis of intertest patterns, when examined longitudinally, have revealed other relationships as well. At the 12-year analysis of one longitudinal study (Blum et al., 1970), subjects who had shown a critical loss on Vocabulary, Digit Symbol, and/or Similarities had significantly higher rates of mortality than those without such loss. Clearly, cognizance of earlier test performance helps to determine whether a given score reflects the normal ability of an individual or a critically aberrant one. The relationship between cognitive decline and mortality has been noted in numerous other reports as well (Jarvik & Falek, 1963; Lieberman, 1965; Palmore, 1969; Kleemeier, Note 4; Granick & Birren, Note 5). It appears from the above that longitudinal studies become increasingly loaded with those who are most fit and mentally intact (Riegel, 1969; Riegel, Riegel, & Meyer, 1967) and that the sample characteristics are constantly changing in a self-selective fashion (Siegler, 1975).

A variety of factors other than intellectual ability are also claimed to affect performance on the WAIS. These include educational background (Birren & Morrison, 1961; Granick & Friedman, 1967), physical health (Birren, Butler, Greenhouse, Sokoloff, & Yarrow, 1963; Birren & Spieth, 1962; Spieth, 1964, 1965; Thompon, Eisdorfer, & Estes, 1966; Wang & Busse, 1974; Wilkie & Eisdorfer, 1971), and the speed component of the test (Botwinick, 1977; Botwinick & Storandt, 1973; Klodin, 1975). In a longitudinal study of aging twins (Jarvik, 1967; Jarvik & Blum, 1971; Jarvik & Falek, 1963; Jarvik, Kallmann, & Falek, 1962), stability characterized performance on nontimed tasks, while decline predominated on timed tasks. When individual scores were examined, 50% or more of the subjects exhibited either unchanged or increased Vocabulary, Similarities, and DSF subtest scores between the mean ages of 63 and 73 years. During the next decade the percent of subjects with unchanged or increased scores declined, but Digit Symbol, highly weighted with a speed component, was the only subtest on which all persons showed a decline between the mean ages of 73 and 85 years.

As Lezak (1976) pointed out, the WAIS does have its share of methodological and diagnostic problems. However, the wide data base accumulated over decades argues powerfully in favor of its use. Since interpretation of scores on the basis of the verbal-performance discrepancy may be confounded by a number of variables other than age or organic deterioration, it is important to extract all the information one can from each test. In order to do that, individual patterns of performance should be observed. Further discussion of the analysis of intertest patterns and the issues of age-related scoring may be found in Lezak (1976) and Bromley (1966).

Primary Mental Abilities Test

The Primary Mental Abilities Test (PMA) consists of five subtests believed by their designers (Thurstone & Thurstone, 1949) to measure five independent functions. The subtests are Verbal Meaning (a vocabulary test in which the best synonym is selected from five possible choices), Verbal Fluency (a test of how many words beginning with a certain letter one can recall), Reasoning (a test of sequence patterns), Number Ability (a relatively simple test of addition), and Space (a figure matching and mental shifting test). All are timed.

Schaie and Strother (1968) have studied test performances in terms of both age differences and age changes. Their cross-sequential design has examined performance both cross-sectionally and longitudinally in the same subjects on the PMA test. Age was negatively related to performance, and all tests showed a decline with age when examined cross-sectionally. However, when examined longitudinally, only scores on those tests where speed of performance seemed critical (Reasoning and Fluency) declined with age, while scores on Verbal Meaning, Space, and Numerical Abilities were maintained between the ages of 20 and 70 years, and on a retest 7 years later. The authors concluded that changes over time within a given individual tended to be much smaller than differences between cohorts, not only on Number Ability, as mentioned earlier in this chapter, but in general on all the abilities measured by the PMA. These conclusions are in agreement with previous distinctions between age changes and age differences as stressed by Anastasi (1956), Bayley (1956), Birren (1960), Jarvik et al. (1963), Jones (1956), Lorge (1957), and Owens (1953). The greater cross-sectional decline may be due to environmental advantages of succeeding generations or genetic adaptations for the newer members of the species (Botwinick, 1977).

The PMA test is often criticized for its speed component, since all the subtests are timed. However, in one study, untimed administrations to subjects 53 to 78 years of age tended to exaggerate the deficits of the older subjects on the Space and Reasoning subtests (Schaie, Rosenthal, & Perlman, 1953).

In another study attempting to improve speed of performance through training (Hoyer, Labouvie, & Baltes, 1973), improvement was achieved by the subjects (ages 60–85) on a reinforced rote task but was not generalized to the PMA as measured on repeated testings. Like others before them (e.g., Jarvik et al., 1962), Hoyer et al. questioned the validity of single-occasion measures. Only through repeated testing can reversibility or rate of change of performance be detected.

Finally, the answer sheet of the PMA presents a problem in that the answer slots are small and closely packed. Marking them appropriately tends to be difficult for persons with impaired vision as well as for those unfamiliar with the mechanics of completing test forms, particularly in anxiety-provoking situations. Indeed the older person's possible difficulties in dealing with the answer sheet may reflect one aspect of cognitive impairment, but these difficulties should not be confused with an inability to answer the questions correctly, given that the testee understands and can follow the test format.

The Wechsler Memory Scale

The Wechsler Memory Scale (WMS) (Wechsler, 1945), perhaps the most widely used test of memory for older persons, attempts to span a wide range of memory functions. It has seven subtests: Personal and Current Information, Orientation, Mental Control, Logical Memory, Digit Span, Visual Reproduction, and Associate Learning. Norms are published for up to 64 years (Wechsler, 1945) and between 80 and 92 years (Klonoff & Kennedy, 1965, 1966; Meer & Baker, 1965). Unfortunately, it has been found to be ineffective in discriminating between various patient groups (Cohen, 1950; Howard, 1950; Ivinskis, Allen, & Shaw, 1971) and correlates poorly with other tests of memory (Hulicka, 1966). A factor-analytic study (Kear-Caldwell, 1973) suggested that certain subtests (such as Associate Learning and Logical Memory) measure specific memory aspects but, unlike the WAIS, there is no accepted system by which to compare the efficiency among the subtests, and thus one cannot establish a comprehensive picture of an individual's memory functions. The Scale may be most useful when scored on the basis of two or three factors, particularly Memory, and Attention and Concentration (Erickson & Scott, 1977).

Hulicka (1966) examined subjects 15 to 80 years of age (equated on WAIS Vocabulary) by first testing them on a name-and-picture-of-persons test that had both learning and recall components and then administering the WMS. Correlations between the WMS and the picture test showed that four of the six WMS subtests correlated more highly with learning than with recall scores (Logical Memory, Digit Span, Visual Reproduction, and Associate Learning). Based on these findings, Hulicka suggested that the performance of older persons on the WMS may be more a reflection of willingness to cooperate, ability to understand and follow directions, attention span, and willingness (or ability) to learn material of little intrinsic value than of ability to recall learned material. In numerous other studies as well, a relationship between intelligence and WMS performance has emerged (Dujovne & Levy, 1971; Fields, 1971; Hall & Toal, 1957; Ivinskis et al., 1971). Erickson and Scott (1977) raised the question of its utility in providing clearcut meaningful information about an individual's memory.

In a drug study (Salzman, Shader, Harmatz & Robertson, 1975) comparing diazepam (Valium) with placebo, the WMS was administered to 40 men who were over 60 years old. Upon retesting 2 weeks after drug administration, there was a significant difference in scores between the 2 groups, with a reduction in WMS performance in the diazepam group and improved performance in the placebo group. Diazepam, as a sedative, may have affected primarily the subjects' alertness; fatigue was, in fact, reported. The fact that unmedicated subjects showed improved scores on retesting stresses once again the value of testing more than once.

In other studies, no drug effects emerged on WMS performance for demented individuals prescribed deanol (Ferris, Sathananthan, Gershon, & Clark, 1977) or cyclandelate (Westreich, Alter, & Lundgren, 1975) or for moderately impaired persons given methylphenidate (Crook, Ferris, Sathananthan, Raskin, & Gershon, 1977).

To date, few drugs have demonstrated efficacy in improving memory or other cognitive functions. However, the WMS's dependence on attention and alertness may cloud true functional levels when it comes to testing memory of medicated patients.

A variant of the WMS has been developed called the Guild Memory Scale (Gilbert, Levee, & Catalano, 1968). It includes Recall of Paragraphs, Paired Associates, Numbered Designs, as well as Digit Span Forward and Backward. One advantage over other memory tests is its development of norms for each subtest with the supposition that there may be little relationship between different types of memory, and differential loss or gain may be missed in a composite score (Gilbert, 1941). Although developed a decade ago, considerable work still needs to be done on its validation. (For additional discussion of the WMS, as well as other memory tests, see Erickson & Scott, 1977.)

The Shipley-Hartford Institute of Living Scale

The Shipley-Hartford Institute of Living Scale (Shipley, 1940, 1946), often called the Shipley-Hartford, has both a vocabulary and a verbal abstraction section. As Lezak (1976) has pointed out, a number of studies reported the test to be far from adequate in separating organically impaired, psychiatrically disturbed patients, and normals (Aita, Armatage, Reitan, & Rabinowitz, 1947; Parker, 1957; Savage, 1970). Not surprisingly, scores in the organic range increase with age (Yates, 1954). When testing persons of known high premorbid intellectual functioning (Prado & Taub, 1966), examiners can detect significant changes in performance. However, if premorbid level of functioning is unknown, conclusions based on the test are hazardous.

Ganzler (1964) wondered if the poorer performance of old as compared to young subjects on this battery could be attributed to the fact that older persons were less motivated to do well. He tried to induce motivation experimentally but was unable to demonstrate differential improvement in score. It must be concluded, therefore, that either the attempt to increase motivation was unsuccessful or increase in motivation was insufficient to overcome decline in performance. Increasing motivation may serve primarily to increase speed of response, and since the Shipley-Hartford is not a timed test, no speed change would be detected. In support of this, another study noted no improvement on a test of vocabulary following experimental manipulation of motivation. However, scores on a test of verbal fluency, which is believed to be more affected by timing, did show an improvement (Kamin, 1957).

The Halstead-Reitan Battery

A neuropsychological battery originally developed to measure biological intelligence as a relationship between behavior and brain status, the Halstead-Reitan battery (Halstead, 1947; Reitan & Davison, 1974) has been used to discriminate a variety of organic disturbances as well as impaired and intact individuals (Goldstein, Deysack, & Kleinknecht, 1973; Reitan, 1955).

One study reported that measures on the battery that clearly separated old (over 60) from young subjects were similar to those previously found to be sensitive to brain damage (Reed & Reitan, 1963). However, older intact persons often score lower because of their tendency to proceed more slowly than their younger counterparts.

In a recent review of neuropsychological batteries, Luria and Majovski (1977) listed several strengths and limitations of the test. One strength is its history of reliably-based evaluations administered to and compared with many types of subjects. A severe limitation is the demanding length of administration (both for tester and testee) of 6–8 hours. In particular, the Categories Test and Tactual Performance Test (which are both considered to be highly associated with brain damage) take considerable time. In general, this approach concentrates on localization of lesions and is, therefore, most valuable in those conditions that respond to neurosurgical intervention. However, its utility diminishes in trying to explain cognitive impairment not attributable to distinct lesions. The Bender-Gestalt (Lacks, Harrow, Colbert, & Levine, 1970) and the WAIS (DeWolfe, Barrell, Becker, & Spaner, 1971; Watson, Thomas, Anderson, & Felling, 1968) both have been reported to show better discriminatory power than the Halstead-Reitan for comparing persons with brain damage and those with other psychiatric diagnoses.

Luria's Investigations

Luria's (1966) neuropsychological investigative approach, as spelled out in his book *Higher Cortical Functions of Man,* has provided useful guidelines for sequential testing. He has offered a logical progression for administration of tests, depending on individual symptoms and outcomes on prior tests, and he has related performance on them to specific cerebral areas. The clinician can hone in on the specific site of the disorder and also gain insight into the individual's intact abilities. Luria's approach differs from the psychometric position in that he focuses on qualitative observations about a deficit both for rehabilitative purposes and for an understanding of brain-behavior interactions.

Unlike Reitan, Luria emphasizes preliminary testing that includes a sufficiently extensive range to get a general overview of the patient's mental condition. Emphasis is on how a function suffers rather than which function is suffering (Luria & Majovski, 1977). These tests are in large measure unstandardized and the level of complexity depends on the patient's premorbid functioning, education, and cultural background. In the next stage of testing, individualization is the key to determining what areas of functioning are being underutilized by the patient and how, if at all, compensatory mechanisms are operating. Emphasis is placed on the extent of the persistence of a malfunction. In the final stage, a conclusion regarding the disturbance is reached by comparative analysis, linking the fundamental defect with related mental activity and psychophysiological processes. Unlike the aforementioned batteries, this approach stresses that

> Qualification of a symptom is never construed as the mechanistic application of a standardized test battery with formal quantitative interpretation of the results. In contradistinction, it is a clinically creative effort requiring from the neuropsychologist both critical thinking and readiness to reject initial hypotheses if they conflict with new data obtained or if there is confounding of the results. (Luria & Majovski, 1977, p. 964)

Gerontological studies utilizing Luria's approach are lacking but clearly deserve serious consideration in the areas of compensation and restoration of functions.

SINGLE TESTS OF COGNITIVE FUNCTIONING

In this section, single tests usually presumed to measure specific cognitive abilities are examined, whether originally administered in batteries or singly. We agree with Salzman et al. (1972) that:

> Memory assessment should be classified according to the mode of perception (e.g., visual, verbal, olfactory) and it should include not only the assessment of immediate recognition and recall but also the evaluation of memory for distant personal and impersonal events . . . and the capacity for learning new material. (p. 14)

Such a view is extended in this chapter to include a wide range of cognitive functions. The specific tests presented here are grouped by their primary modality of presentation: auditory-verbal, visual, auditory-nonverbal, and tactile. Tests of olfactory and gustatory sensations exist, but they have not been utilized in the assessment of cognitive performance and are not covered in this review. The tests presented here differ on such critical variables as the amount of research available, the levels of impairment of subjects, definitions of young and old (45-year-olds are old subjects in one study and young in another), and span of testing.

Auditory-Verbal Cognitive Ability

Auditory-verbal cognitive ability encompasses a wide variety of behaviors. The key element characterizing tests of verbal cognitive ability is dependence on verbal knowledge or on the processing of information in the verbal modality. Many of the studies examining age effects in this area have been confounded with extraneous variables such as education, motivation, speed, instructions, sex, and intellectual ability. In general, verbal ability is considered to be a relatively durable trait, regardless of personal or test characteristics, even in the profiles of persons with organic impairment. Verbal test scores are usually relied on as the best indicators of premorbid functioning level. Verbal cognitive ability can be divided as follows: vocabulary, verbal fluency, shifting, and verbal learning.

Vocabulary

There is widespread agreement that vocabulary test scores tend to remain stable and may even increase throughout the adult life span, including the period of old age. This finding, reported from cross-sectional (Botwinick, 1967; Garfield & Blek, 1952; Granick & Friedman, 1967; Jones & Conrad, 1933; Reed & Reitan, 1963; Strother, Schaie, & Horst, 1957; Sorenson, 1933; Thorndike & Gallup, 1944) as well as longitudinal studies (Blum, Fosshage, & Jarvik, 1972; Eisdorfer, 1968; Jarvik, 1973; Schaie & Strother, 1968), dates back to the earliest investigation of intellectual changes and is in accord with Cattell's (1963) postulate of the stability of crystallized intelligence.

A number of vocabulary tests are popular with gerontologists. Here are some brief descriptions of these tests.

Vocabulary subtest–WAIS or Wechsler-Bellevue. The overwhelming majority of studies, both longitudinal and cross-sectional, using the WAIS Vocabulary subtest have shown maintenance or rise of scores with increase in age for both intact and orgnically impaired persons (Blum et al., 1970; Goldstein & Shelly, 1975; Granick & Friedman, 1967; Reed & Reitan, 1963; Savage, Britton, George, O'Connor, & Hall, 1972; Traxler, 1972; Reitan, Note 6). One longitudinal study (Berkowitz & Green, 1963) showed a decline for all subjects, and the rate of decline was not related to subjects' original IQ scores. By contrast, another longitudinal study (Blum & Jarvik, 1974) showed that subjects who were initially more able (estimated by Vocabulary score) declined less on tests in a cognitive battery than did the initially less able, leading to the conclusion that age is kinder to those initially more able. While initial or pretested IQ scores may not reflect the degree to which one will change over time on the Vocabulary subtest, the evidence suggests that initial or pretested Vocabulary scores are sensitive to maintenance of cognitive capacity.

The effect of education on vocabulary has also been studied, but the results remain inconclusive. For example, in a study by Reed and Reitan (1963), 4 groups were compared: 2 young groups with a mean age of 28–brain damage versus intact, and 2 intact older groups–those with a mean age of 45 versus those with a mean age of 55. There was a significant difference in Vocabulary scores between the first two groups but not between the last two groups, indicating once more the stability of vocabulary from age decade to age decade in contrast to its sensitivity to brain damage. It must be pointed out, however, that the oldest group, the 50-year-olds, had significantly more education (mean = 16.7 years) than the group of 40-year-olds (mean = 13.9 years), which was not taken into account in the statistical analysis. The educational advantage of the older group may have masked age-related decline so that this study, like so many others, fails to clarify the issue of age-related decline.

Several studies have reported that brain damage affects Vocabulary performance less than it affects other WAIS subtests, especially in the case of diffuse or bilateral damage (Gonen & Brown, 1968) or dominant lesions (Parsons, Vega, & Burn, 1969). On the other hand, at least one study has reported that cognitively-impaired persons did worse on Vocabulary than on Comprehension, Arithmetic, and Picture Completion (Overall & Gorham, 1972). It is possible that many subjects of this study had left temporal lobe lesions that might have impaired vocabulary ability. The only information supplied by the authors about the cognitively-impaired group was that they had a clinical diagnosis of chronic brain syndrome.

A study was previously described that showed that differential Performance and Verbal scores for young and old subjects accounted for equivalent Full Scale scores (Harwood & Naylor, 1971). Botwinick and Storandt (1973) similarly analyzed overall scores as well as intratest patterns of response for young (ages 17–20) and old (ages 62–83) subjects on the Vocabulary subtest. They found that overall the scores did not differ significantly between the two age groups using the conventional scoring system. However, in an in-depth analysis of response quality, differences were noted. The younger subjects tended to give more concise, synonymous responses. By contrast, the older subjects knew more words and generally gave fuller explanations, which are considered less desirable than synonyms in the conventional scoring systems. Findings from both of these studies serve as reminders that even when scores of older persons appear to be quantitatively equivalent to those of younger persons, assumptions about intactness or stability of a particular function over the life span may be erroneous. There may be a redistribution of functional strengths and weaknesses. Care should be taken to consider both quantitative and qualitative aspects of performance.

Verbal Meaning Subtest (PMA). Although this test is timed, speed is not believed to contribute significantly to performance. Persons generally maintain or increase their original scores until about age 60. A decline is noted after that when the test scores are analyzed cross-sectionally, but, on longitudinal examination, individuals appear to retain this ability (Schaie & Strother, 1968). On this test, cohort differences outweigh individual changes over the life span.

Mill Hill Vocabulary Scale (MHVS). This multiple-choice, 80-word, long-term recall test has been found sensitive to dominant hemisphere damage (Costa & Vaughan, 1962; Lansdell, 1968). Using the MHVS, Foulds and Raven (1948) have noted that verbal recall ability increased with age for subjects considered above average in general functioning (based on their occupations) and decreased markedly for subjects considered below average. Although Eisdorfer (1963) used the WAIS and not the MHVS, findings of his relatively short-term (2.5–4.5 years) longitudinal study actually suggested a trend opposite to that found by Foulds and Raven (1948). In his study, both younger (ages 60–69) and older (ages 70 and older, mean of 75) subjects who initially had low IQs showed an increase on a retest of the WAIS. Subjects of both ages with middle-range IQs either maintained their scores or showed bidirectional variance. Subjects with initially high IQs maintained their scores if they were in the younger group and declined if they were in the older group. Eisdorfer attributed these findings to regression of subjects' scores to the mean. Regardless of age or intelligence scores, the rates of change of cognitive abilities were not significantly different.

The Peabody Picture Vocabulary Test. In this test, four pictures are presented at a time, and one word is either spoken by the tester or shown on a card that the subject must match with one of the four pictures (Dunn, 1965). Although norms are provided only for ages 2½–18, the Peabody has utility for testing older persons. Considering the high success rate on this test even among persons with some organic impairment, it may be a good test to include in a battery to alleviate anxiety stemming from fear of failure. Poor performance on the Peabody (in combination with poor performance on a battery of other tests) has been associated with cerebral atrophy (Kaszniak, Garron, Fox, Huckman, & Ramsey, Note 7).

Verbal Fluency

Tasks of verbal fluency require facility of word association as well as speed in the recognition and recall of words. Lezak's (1976) review reported that poor fluency may be due to aphasia or frontal (especially left) brain damage (Benton, 1968; Milner, 1967; Ramier & Hécaen, 1970).

Word fluency. The task on this test is to write as many words as possible beginning with the letter *S* during a 5-minute period. Left frontal lobe lesions have been related to impaired performance (Milner, 1967). Equivalence of verbal fluency was reported for young (17-year-olds) and old (ages 70-84) intact subjects (Strother et al., 1957).

When Kamin (1957) examined Word Fluency in younger and older subjects, he included two other variables of interest, residence and motivation. Subjects were not classified as brain damaged or intact. One result of the study was that older institutionalized individuals did far worse on Word Fluency (as well as on the other subtests) than did community elderly who in turn did less well than young subjects. However, without diagnostic confirmation, it is difficult to evaluate the results, although it is known that institutionalized groups in general are weighted more heavily with brain-damaged persons than are other subsamples. Motivation in this study (a cash prize) was reported effective in improving Word Fluency scores for the older subjects.

The Controlled Word Association Test. Another test of verbal functioning introduced to study speech fluency is the Controlled Word Association Test, requiring that on 3 1-minute trials subjects say as many words as possible that begin with F, A, and S, respectively (Benton, 1973). Scoring takes into account education, sex, and age (from 25 to 64). Scores are adjusted for age with higher scores given to older subjects, suggesting some decline on this skill as an accompaniment to the normal aging process. Because findings on similar tests have demonstrated poorer performance by persons with low intellectual ability but without brain damage than by bright persons who had suffered brain damage (Borkowski, Benton, & Spreen, 1967), premorbid level of functioning should be carefully considered if this test is to be utilized.

Reading ability. Reading ability may be regarded as a facet of verbal fluency. According to Nelson and McKenna (1975), it provides a good estimate of premorbid functioning in demented persons. The evidence supporting this view is based on the following observations: (a) word reading ability and general intellectual level on the WAIS showed high correlations for intact adults aged 16-69 (mean age of 47) and (b) IQ levels predicted on the basis of current reading levels closely approximated premorbid IQ levels estimated from other observations recorded for subjects aged 22-68 (mean age of 49) with suspected dementia. (All subjects had clinical evidence of organic cerebral disease and a history of generalized intellectual impairment.)

Verbal Shifting

Verbal shifting encompasses at least two important components, the ability to shift concepts and the ability to maintain steadfastness to the new concept. Performance on these tests consistently shows a relationship with brain damage. Age seems to be somewhat negatively related to performance, although external variables that often accompany aging (e.g., institutionalization and physical illness) can also cause suboptimal performance and need to be controlled to evaluate age effects per se.

Set Test. In the Set Test (Isaacs & Kennie, 1973), the subject's task is to name as many items as possible (up to 10) in each of 4 categories: colors, animals, fruits, and towns. The subject is given 1 point for each correct answer, up to a maximium of 40 points. This test is both short and portable. According to an early study by Isaacs & Kennie, a number of persons who scored under 15 points had been independently diagnosed as suffering from dementia, based on Roth's (1955) criteria of progressive or episodic intellectual decline and on an evaluation of current mental status. None of the subjects scoring 25 or more points had received a diagnosis of dementia. One caveat is that physical illness also was associated with low scores. The authors' interpretation that advanced physical disability and advanced brain disease may be related needs further documentation before it can be accepted.

Categories Test. Performance on the Categories Test, described as part of the Halstead-Reitan Battery (Halstead, 1947), was found to decline with age (Goldstein & Shelly, 1975; Reed & Reitan, 1963; Reitan, Note 6) and also with brain damage (DeWolfe et al., 1971; Goldstein & Shelly, 1975; Reed & Reitan, 1963; Shaw, 1966). The DeWolfe et al. study needs clarification, because young schizophrenics (mean age of 45) performed significantly worse than young brain-damaged persons (mean age of 44), whereas old brain-damaged persons (mean age of 70) and old schizophrenics (mean age of 73) performed similar to one another. Neither of these two latter groups performed as well as young brain-damaged persons nor as poorly as young schizophrenics. As is the case with most tests of brain damage, this test probably is more sensitive to long-standing deteriorative processes. This may explain why the younger brain-damaged persons, whose onsets of illness may have been more recent and less encompassing, were able to do better than their older counterparts.

Stroop Color-Word Test. The Stroop Color-Word Test (Stroop, 1935) requires verbal fluency as well as the ability to abstract and reintegrate material. On the first part, the subject must read four names of colors in black print; on the second part, the subject must name colors as printed in rectangles of colored ink; on the third and final part, the subject must name colors printed in ink different from that spelled by the letters. This test has been used to study a variety of psychological phenomena (for reviews, see Bettner, Jarvik, & Blum, 1971; Jensen & Rohwer, 1966). In regard to aging, Comalli and associates (Comalli, 1965; Comalli, Wapner, & Werner, 1962; Rand, Wapner, Werner, & McFarland, 1963) administered a modified version of the Stroop and found that subjects aged 7-13 (in grammar school) performed worst, subjects aged 17-44 (attending college) performed best and subjects aged 65-80 (community residents) performed in an intermediate range. Institutionalized elderly performed more like the grammar school children (Commalli, Krus, & Wapner, 1965). Bettner et al. (1971) also found poorer performance among their older subjects (aged 77-89) than is characteristic of younger persons. The group showing the poorest performance were subjects with organic brain syndrome, confirming the findings of Comalli et al. (1965) and suggesting that the Stroop may be useful in early detection of organic impairment.

Digit Span Backward. Digit Span Backward (DSB) is not as predictably stable as DSF. In several studies, no relationship between age and performance has been observed (Granick & Friedman, 1967; Zarit, Miller, & Kahn, Note 8). Some studies employing this test have observed the onset of decline before the age of 72 (Bromley, 1958; Gilbert, 1941), whereas other studies have shown decline occurring only after 80 years of age (Kral, 1959; Kubo, 1938). Kaszniak et al. (Note 2) have found no significant age or age-brain damage interaction, but brain damage alone was shown to affect scores significantly. Finally, Blum et al. (1970) have observed a decrease in scores over time in their longitudinal study, but the declines did not become increasingly larger as was the case for DSF.

The point has been made that attentional endurance alone cannot maintain normal performance on DSB, but rather performance on this test requires the ability to visually scan the verbally presented material before reciting it backwards.

Stability of performance on DSB, as well as on DSF, emerged from a study designed to assess the effects of a pipradrol-vitamin (Alertonic) elixir on intact older volunteers (age 65 and older) (Shader, Harmatz, Kochansky, & Cole, 1975). While one group of subjects received the elixir, a second group received a placebo, and a third group recieved no treatment for 1 week. No significant differences in pretest/posttest change scores on either DSF or DSB were found in the drug, placebo, or nontreatment groups. Consistency of performance on both these tests was not notably influenced by a placebo for older persons.

Lehmann (1971) reported on a psychopharmacological study of geriatric patients who received six different drugs, administered over separate time periods. Improved performance on DSB was associated with meprobamate (Miltown), a minor tranquilizer.

Verbal Learning

The rate of learning newly presented verbal material can also be taken as an indicator of skill in verbal processing. Comparing young and old almost inevitably reveals better performance of the young unless testing conditions are altered. Depending on the specifications of the experimental manipulations, such factors as varying time intervals, instructional sets, motivation, and relevance of material may significantly influence the learning of verbal material for older subjects.

Serial rote and associate learning tests. Serial rote and paired associates learning generally present greater difficulties to old than to young subjects (Arenberg, 1965; Canestrari, 1963; Eisdorfer, 1965, 1968; Eisdorfer, Axelrod, & Wilkie, 1963; Gilbert, 1935, 1941; Gladis & Braun, 1958; Hulicka, Sterne,

& Grossman, 1967; Hulicka & Weiss, 1965; Korchin & Basowitz, 1957; Monge & Hultsch, 1971; Ruch, 1934; Talland, 1966; Wimer, 1960; Witte, 1975; Witte & Freund, 1976).

Sex differences have been noted on these learning tasks with females generally scoring better than males. The relatively poor performance of males usually relates to failure to respond (omission errors) rather than to responding incorrectly (commission errors), particularly at fast pacing speeds. When presentation is slowed, significant improvement occurs in both sexes, and males no longer exhibit behavior markedly different from their female counterparts (Wilkie & Eisdorfer, 1977). The elimination of errors of omission and an increase in correct responses argues for a deficit of performance output rather than of inherent ability (Basowitz & Korchin, 1957; Botwinick, Brinley, & Robbins, 1958; Silverman, 1963).

Females tend to respond more frequently (Harkins, Nowlin, Ramm, & Schroeder, 1974), more quickly (Elias & Kinsbourne, 1974), and more correctly (Maccoby & Jacklin, 1974) on tests with high verbal loadings. However, when the initial level of verbal ability is high in both sexes, these sex differences are significantly diminished (Wilkie & Eisdorfer, 1977).

In 1963, Canestrari demonstrated the benefit for older people of extending the period of time to view and respond to lists of words on paired associates tests. Performance improved even more when the elderly had an unlimited amount of time and could pace their own learning, although they never did as well as younger subjects. When given unlimited time, the elderly increased the time for inspecting test items less than they increased the amount of time to respond (the anticipation interval). Similarly, when Monge and Hultsch (1971) manipulated both the inspection interval and the anticipation interval, they found that the anticipation interval interacted directly with age (increasing it benefited the old more than the young subjects), while increasing the inspection interval benefited all ages equally.

Arenberg (1965) reported that self-pacing on a paired associates test was of limited benefit to the less educated elderly subject, although differences between fast and slow pacing still held up. Since taking more time (the self-pacing condition) did not significantly raise their scores, Arenberg suggested that the errors made by the paced group, even at a fast pace, were not directly attributable to insufficient time to give a correctly learned response. Test-taking anxiety or unfamiliarity with the style of thinking required may have decreased the ability of the less educated to use self-pacing to advantage. Arenberg connected his findings with the search deficit theory in that the more information there is to be searched and choices and discriminations to be made, the more search time is required by older persons.

Arousal seems to play an important part in verbal learning. Eisdorfer, Nowlin, and Wilkie (1970) suggested that a state of heightened autonomic arousal is responsible for the decrement in learning performance so common in older persons. Evidence for their model is based on their study in which a group of intact volunteers (aged 60–78) did better on a serial rote learning task when given an arousal-suppressing drug (propranolol) than did a control group receiving a placebo. Their findings may be explained in part by their instruction to subjects to respond immediately. This instruction may have heightened their subjects' initial anxiety levels and aroused their autonomic nervous systems more than would be normal for them. Also, the 4-second exposure used in this study had previously been associated with greater performance deficit than had a longer exposure period (Eisdorfer et al., 1963), and thus anxiety may have been produced by the specific elements of the test situation.

Motivation may lead to improved scores, but it is not always clear whether the change reflects heightened capacity or an increase in rate of production. When Leech and Witte (1971) administered a paired associates task to older subjects (ages 59–85), they offered half of them cash for correct responses and the other half of them cash for both correct and incorrect responses. Subjects paid for both types of responses learned more quickly. However, it is possible that both groups learned the same amount; that is, motivation may have induced faster retrieval but without improving either storage or learning. Botwinick (1973) suggested that older people may be at least as motivated and involved in an experiment as younger people but may focus on inappropriate aspects of a test, implying that it may not be as critical to vary the amount of motivation for older persons as it is to help in the productive channeling of it.

Poor performance in paired associates tasks has been associated with organic problems in studies comparing older functionally and organically impaired individuals (Caird, Sanderson, & Inglis, 1962; Irving, Robinson, & McAdam, 1970). However, Kaszniak et al. (Note 2) showed a relationship between learning paired associates and age but not between learning paired associates and cerebral atrophy (as measured by computerized tomography). These authors suggested that further studies are needed to differentiate between age and cohort effects. Since cerebral atrophy, even postmortem, is not directly related to specific learning, Kaszniak and associates' results are not surprising.

Although the nature of the relationship between motivation and depression is unclear, the presence of either one usually implies the absence of the other. Specifically, what emerges from studies in this area is that the depressed do significantly less well than the nondepressed on rote or unfamiliar tasks, while the groups tend to be indistinguishable on serial learning tasks where there is a high degree of meaningfulness or familiarity.

Young depressives have been observed to show improved short-term memory after effective antidepressant medication (Sternberg & Jarvik, 1976). The better the remission rate of the affective disturbance, the greater was the improvement in short-term memory scores. In a study of older subjects, depression again affected short-term performance, this time on a serial learning task (Whitehead, 1974). The Whitehead study included 24 depressives, all over 60 years of age: 12 subjects were examined before they received treatment; the remainder were examined on remission of depressive symptoms. According to Whitehead, results indicated better performance by those tested after remission of depression than by those tested before treatment for depression. Because depressive disorder is often masked by memory complaints in older persons (Kahn et al., 1975), and because one treats memory disturbances and depressive disorders differently, the practitioner must be careful to distinguish memory loss associated with organic brain damage from memory problems related to depression.

The Synonyn Learning Test (SLT) was administered to persons (mean age of 68) classified as depressed, treated (formerly depressed), or demented both before and after treatment. The demented subjects received milieu therapy and the depressed patients were given electroconvulsive therapy (ECT) (Hemsi, Whitehead, & Post, 1968). The SLT did not significantly discriminate among the three groups. Although the depressives did significantly better than the demented subjects on the SLT before and after treatment, a considerable proportion of the depressives scored in the dementia range at both times of testing.

Performance on tests of new verbal learning may also be affected by the amount and type of instruction provided by the experimenter. For example, Hulicka and Grossman (1967) designed an experiment based on earlier findings that old subjects performed less well than young on a paired associates task and also reported less mediational relationships between paired associates items. Subjects in this study were placed in one of four conditions to learn paired associates: (1) no special instructions were given, (2) experimenter provided the images, (3) subjects were told to form their own images, and (4) experimenter gave standard instructions. Old subjects improved more than young did when told to increase usage of mediational devices, but still they did not perform as well as the young. They performed best when told to use their own mediational devices. Hulicka and Grossman concluded that old persons have the ability to improve their verbal learning when instructed to use their own images, but without instructions they do poorly, due either to the inappropriateness or lack of mediators.

Mason (Note 9) let young and old self-pace on a word-learning list and noted that both groups showed similar degrees of improvement and used similar amounts of inspection time. In another phase of the experiment, she found unexpectedly that only young subjects showed improvement with mnemonic devices and imagery instructions. The author suggested that the study may have exaggerated age differences on the basis of its particular combination of type of task (using peg words), type of instruction (imagery), and type of presentation (separate lists for abstract and concrete words). Mason also cited a comparative word-learning study by Rowe and Schnore (1971) that presented a paired associates task, standard word-pairing instructions, and lists of combinations of abstract and concrete words. In that study, older subjects recalled more of the concrete words that did younger subjects. Mason warned that exclusive use of concrete words in a mixed age sample may exaggerate age differences if the instructions encourage the use of imagery and may underestimate age differences if standard word-pairing instructions are given.

Other WAIS verbal tests. Some of the other verbal subtests on the WAIS have not been very helpful when used singly because of conflicting results. To mention but a handful of studies, Similarities, Comprehension, and Information have been shown to rise with age in one sample (Goldstein & Shelly, 1975), Information has been shown to remain stable in another study (Granick & Friedman, 1967), and Information, Comprehension, or Similarities have been shown to decline in other studies (Berkowitz & Green, 1963; Blum et al., 1970; Granick & Friedman, 1967; Overall & Gorham, 1972; Reed & Reitan, 1963). Brain damage is also associated with poor test performance on the Similarities and Information subtests (McFie, 1960; Newcombe, 1969; Reitan, 1955; Sheer, 1956; Smith, 1966; Spreen & Benton, 1965).

Rey's Auditory-Verbal Learning Test. A promising neuropsychological test that has been described in English (original in French) by Muriel Lezak (1976) is Rey's Auditory-Verbal Learning Test (Rey, 1964). One of its most attractive features is that it considers the meaningfulness of individual patterns of performance, rates of learning, age differences, and social class, rather than producing a single, composite memory score. A list of 15 words is read, 1 per second, with instructions for the subject to recite as many as he or she can remember in any order. The examiner records the order of the recalled words so that patterns of words may be ascertained and compared with later trials. On the next 4 trials the examiner reads the same list, and the subject is repeatedly asked to recite all words remembered, including those recited originally. On Trial 6, a new list of 15 words is read, with instructions to recite as many of those as the subject remembers. After recitation, the subject is asked to recite as many words as possible from List 1. Lezak has pointed out that most brain-damaged patients show a learning curve over the first 5 trials, albeit a small one. She has theorized that if the amount learned is maintained on the final delayed recall, it may demonstrate an ability to learn. Furthermore, it suggests that a brain-damaged person could benefit from psychotherapeutic guidance or from lessons tailored to the individual's rate of comprehension. She also has pointed out that a once bright subject who has experienced severe impairment may show a high score on Trial 1 and an insignificant increase after that.

Hebb's Digit-Sequences Test. Hebb's Digit-Sequences Test (Hebb, 1961) is a verbal learning task that helps differentiate left and right temporal lobe damage (Milner, 1971). The task is to recall strings of unrelated digits as they are presented sequentially. Although the subject is not so informed, the span exceeds by one digit the subject's pretested digit span recall. Every third span is identical although the two intervening ones are not repeated and serve as interference. Intact subjects perform increasingly well on the repeated sequences. However, a study by Corsi (cited in Milner, 1971) showed that persons with left (but not right) temporal lobectomies had a deficit in performance, and a direct correlation was observed between the amount of verbal learning impairment and the extent of hippocampal destruction. Nonetheless, the groups did not differ on the nonrepeated sequences or on the pretested Digit Span (another instance of the stability of Digit Span). The effect of age on test performance apparently was not assessed.

Dichotic listening. In dichotic listening studies, differing but similar stimuli are presented simultaneously to both ears. Stimuli in the form of digits, words, and consonants fall under the auditory-verbal dimension because they are better distinguished by the right ear, i.e., by the left hemisphere, which generally is associated with verbal functions (Darwin, 1971; Kimura, 1967; Milner, Taylor, & Sperry, 1968; Shankweiler & Studdert-Kennedy, 1967).

Milner et al. (1968) have presented digits dichotically to subjects who had previously undergone commissurotomy (their hemispheres were completely divided), and they were able to correctly repeat very few of the digits that had been presented to their left ears. However, when digits were presented monaurally, there were no left/right differences in reports of input to either ear for these subjects, indicating that both hemispheres were able to attend to simple digit spans when not in competition with one another. Their findings suggest that similar stimuli presented singly or dually appear to evoke different functions. This brings to mind the finding mentioned earlier (Thompson et al., 1963) that the same test administered at varying speeds may tap different functions.

In an examination of age effects, Inglis and Caird (1963) presented increasingly longer spans of different series of numbers to each of their subjects, who ranged in age from 11–70, and were considered physically and mentally intact. Results showed that with increasing age, subjects did not demonstrate an age-related deficit on recall of the first series. However, there was progressively greater difficulty with age in recalling the second series. The contention is that the first series does not need to enter memory storage and reflects the individual's attentional process while the second series must enter storage. Therefore, the results suggested that while intake and registration are as efficient in old as in young individuals, short-term memory is not. This finding was confirmed with different subjects by MacKay & Inglis (1963). However, neither motivational (Talland, 1968) nor attentional (Craik, 1965; Inglis & Ankus, 1965) differences between young and old subjects have adequately explained why one-half of the dichotic set is recalled better than the other by the old (Talland, 1968).

Visual Cognitive Abilities

According to Luria (1961), verbal processing is responsible for much orienting behavior and inhibition of impulsive actions early in life but later on is replaced by or integrated with visual analysis of a situation. The stereotypical picture of old age includes a waning of the cognitive abilities dependent on visual processing. However, experiments designed to tap visual processing often contain uncontrolled (confounding) factors, e.g., requiring verbal responses that encourage the use of verbal encoding strategies or demanding visuopractic coordination (McFie, 1975). Since visual tests that can be verbalized easily are poor discriminators of left and right hemispheric disturbances, McFie has suggested that the material should be either too simple, such as counting dots presented tachistoscopically, or too complex for verbalization.

In general, however, the literature on visual cognitive functioning appears to be less concerned with the effects of extraneous variables on performance than the literature on auditory-verbal functioning. Often such tests are administered to detect sites of brain lesions rather than as variations in experimental or environmental conditions. For example, on a visual test that is difficult to verbalize and easy to reproduce graphically, right parietal damage often is associated with disoriented reproduction and left parietal damage with oversimplified perseverative performance.

Visual tests are divided here on the basis of their presumed cognitive requirements, into recognition, recall, reproduction, and shifting.

Visual Recognition

Two studies using different tests reported impaired visual cognitive ability in intact older persons. On an Object Recognition Test (Granick & Friedman, 1967), older subjects checked for absence of organicity did less well than younger subjects in recognition of familiar objects. The degree of education did not seem to affect scores. On a neuropsychological test of Facial Recognition (unfamiliar faces) (Benton & Van Allen, 1968), intact controls showed slightly worse performance with increasing age, and education did not affect performance. Granick and Friedman's subjects may have done relatively worse than Benton and Van Allen's, because as 1 of 33 tests in their battery the Object Recognition Test may not have been administered under as fresh and challenging circumstances as was the Test of Facial Recognition, which was the only test administered to subjects in the Benton and Van Allen study.

Benton and Van Allen (1968) also tested brain-damaged subjects on the Facial Recognition test. Brain-damaged subjects (particularly right hemisphere) did significantly worse than normal controls. Other neuropsychological investigations have concurred in their findings of left-field superiority for Facial Recognition (Rizzolatti, Umilta, & Berlucchi, 1971) and greater impairment in Facial Recognition after right posterior cerebral lesions than left (DeRenzi, Faglioni, & Spinnler, 1968).

Visual Recall

The Paired Associates for Objects Test. The Paired Associates for Objects Test (Fowler, 1969) was devised as a visual analogue of the verbal paired associates test. Neither education nor age appeared to affect scores in intact subjects 30–70 years of age. If replication yielded similar results, and if cognitively impaired persons did significantly worse than intact persons, this test might prove useful in discriminating cognitive impairment. Useful data also might be derived by comparing an individual's performance on this test with performance on an auditory version of it, particularly in order to determine whether recall impairment is diffuse or modality-specific.

KIM Test. The KIM test, designed by Barbizet and Cany (1968), is a test of visual recall of 3-dimensional objects. It is a timed test of memory of 20 common objects presented on a tray. Subjects are tested immediately after viewing the items, as well as 1 hour, 1 day, and 1 week later. The authors have presented norms only for older controls aged 50–64. They have found 1-hour recall scores to be higher than immediate recall scores for all of the subjects. Scores at 1-week recall were higher than earlier scores only for the group over 64 years of age. The findings suggest improvement, or at least maintenance, of long-term recall in older adults. However, the test requires a verbal response that suggests possible reliance on verbal encoding of items.

Visual Reproduction

The Bender-Gestalt Visual Motor Test. The Bender-Gestalt consists of nine designs that are presented singly to the testee who is allowed unlimited time (within reason) to complete drawings (usually the total test runs 5–10 minutes).

The test has demonstrated effectiveness in distinguishing organic impairment from psychiatric disturbance, although an age-related decline between 17 and 84 has been noted (Brilliant & Gunther, 1963; Korman & Blumberg, 1963; Lacks et al., 1970). Parietal lobe lesions are associated with poor performance (Garron & Cheifetz, 1965), especially when right-sided (Diller, Ben-Yishay, Gerstman, Goodkin, Gordon, & Weinberg, 1974; Hirschenfang, 1960a). Right hemisphere damage is frequently manifested in rotational drawings (Billingslea, 1963; Diller et al., 1974). Biparietal damage is reflected by simplified, fragmented drawings with incorrect proportions and upward displacement (Horenstein, 1971). According to Horenstein, when dementia is secondary to a widespread process, such as Alzheimer's disease or hypertensive cerebrovascular disease, drawings appear abnormal, over- or undersized, displaced upward, with many corrections, and with simple, broken figures. Scores on the Bender-Gestalt Visual Motor Test have been found to vary on the basis of health, motor functioning, hospitalization, and marital status for older subjects (Klonoff & Kennedy, 1965, 1966). A test similar to the Bender-Gestalt showed no decline with age when the effect of education was separated out (Granick & Friedman, 1967).

A modification of this test, the Background Interference Procedure (BIP) screen (Canter & Straumanis, 1968), uses a mass of tangled lines to camouflage the design to be copied, and it has been reported to assess impairment with greater reliability than the original Bender-Gestalt. The BIP is also believed to be less influenced by such factors as intelligence, affective status, and age.

Benton Visual Retention Test. The Benton Visual Retention Test involves both visual recall and graphic reproduction requiring subjects to draw figures from memory after 10- and 5-second exposures, to copy the figures as accurately as they can, and to draw them after a 10-second exposure followed by a 15-second delay. Brain damage is negatively associated with performance (Benton, 1974; Brilliant & Gunther, 1963; Westreich et al., 1975).

External situations may affect Benton Visual Retention Test scores, as demonstrated by the studies done by Klonoff and Kennedy (1965, 1966) in which hospitalization related negatively to performance, while activeness and being married related positively. Their subjects were persons 80–90 years of age living in the community and persons of similar age and sex who were hospitalized for physical ailments. Within this narrow age range, there was no significant age-related decline on the test. Although the authors acknowledged the usual age sensitivity of the test with lower age ranges, they suggested that other variables overshadow the influence of age beyond the age of 80.

The Minnesota Percepto-Diagnostic Test. The Minnesota Percepto-Diagnostic Test (MP-DT) (Fuller & Laird, 1963), another visuomotor test, relies heavily on rotational errors in design copying as a measure of brain damage. Lezak (1976) summarized findings on this test; it has been reported to discriminate between brain-damaged and other patient and nonpatient groups (Fuller & Laird, 1963; Uyeno, 1963; Yates, 1966). Two questions that remain unanswered are whether the MP-DT measures variables related to normal aging beyond the seventh decade of life and whether and to what extent cohort differences influence the results of cross-sectional studies since the test has been reported sensitive to cultural background factors (Harrison & Chagnon, 1966). Further exploration of the usefulness of this test is needed.

Graham-Kendall Memory for Designs Test. The Graham Kendall Memory-for-Designs Test (G-K) (Graham & Kendall, 1960) requires that the subject reproduce designs of increasing complexity after viewing each for 5 seconds. Age-adjusted norms are provided; nonetheless, the data on age changes are conflicting. Kendall (1962) found that older persons suffering brain damage did significantly worse than intact subjects, but psychiatric disturbances confounded the scores to some degree. Jarvik and Kato (1969) reported a significant correlation between G-K scores and loss of chromosomes, the latter associated with the diagnosis of organic brain syndrome (Jarvik, Altshuler, Kato & Blumner, 1971).

According to Alexander (1970), the G-K is unreliable in discriminating brain damage (it misclassified 33% of older intact persons, 60–70 years of age) and fails to differentiate among patterns associated with various types of cerebral damage. Even in a study in which the experimenters were concerned only with the presence or absence of brain damage and not with the lateralization of it, the G-K contributed only minimally in discriminating organic impaired from intact subjects (Haglund & Shuckit, 1976). In younger samples as well, the validity of the G-K has been questioned (McIver, McLaren, & Philip, 1973; Turland & Steinhart, 1969) as has its reliability (Howard & Shoemaker, 1954).

Block Tapping. Block Tapping, developed by Corsi and described by Milner (1971), is the nonverbal analogue to Hebb's Digit-Sequences task (Hebb, 1961). Nine blocks, which are fixed to a board, are tapped by the experimenter in a specific order that the subject is asked to reproduce. The subject's initial "spatial span" of maximum number correct is recorded, and then 24 trials of tapped sequences are administered, all of which exceed the subject's spatial span by 1 block. As in the verbal test, intact subjects improve their recall of the repeated trial but not of the nonrepeated trials.

Left temporal lobectomy does not produce impairment on this task, but right temporal lobectomy produces difficulty in recalling the tapping pattern of the repeated sequence, even after a considerable number of trials. Furthermore, hippocampal damage affects performance in patients with right temporal damage but not in those with left temporal damage. Recalling that left temporal lobectomy is associated with lowered performance on Hebb's Digit Sequences task, Milner (1971) suggested that disorders of one temporal lobe may be material specific and merit close examination. Little is known regarding age effects on performance differences.

Visual Shifting Tests

Goldstein-Scheerer Test of Abstract and Concrete Thought. An extensively used battery of shifting ability is the Goldstein-Scheerer Test of Abstract and Concrete Thought (Goldstein & Scheerer, 1941, 1945). The five subtests are: (1) Goldstein-Scheerer Cube Test, a test somewhat similar to the WAIS Block Design subtest but with figures of increasing difficulty (to the extent that no hints are given for the number of blocks required to complete the arrangement); (2) Goldstein-Scheerer Object Sorting Test, a test that requires organizing commonplace objects based on categories of name, nature, and class; (3) Goldstein-Scheerer Stick Test, a test that requires reproduction of simple figures using sticks of varying lengths; (4) Gelb-Goldstein Wool Sorting Test, a test that requires sorting wool skeins according to various properties; and (5) Weigl-Goldstein-Scheerer Color-Form Sorting Test, a test in which 3-dimensional objects can be grouped by their shapes or colors.

Horenstein (1971) noted that poor performance on the Color-Form and Object Sorting tests may indicate bifrontal lobe disease, particularly if the WAIS score is little affected. If, however, performance is low on WAIS verbal tests (among other tests), left frontal damage is suspect. Poor performance on both the Object Sorting and Cube tests may reflect left parietal damage, especially if accompanied by better performance than verbal scores on the WAIS.

Poor performance on the Color-Form subtest was related to age (Thaler, 1956) in a study of subjects 60–101 years old (mean age of 73). The ability to abstract on the subtest was significantly related to higher Wechsler-Bellevue Scores, which in turn were significantly related to younger ages. The implication is that increasing age is associated with increasingly concrete thought.

Digit Symbol Substitution (DSS). The Digit Symbol Substitution (DSS) is one of the subtests of the WAIS. The task on this timed test is to match certain pairs of numbers and figures, by referring to a charted code. Poor performance on the DSS has been associated both with increasing age (Blum et al., 1970; Botwinick, 1967; Goldstein & Shelly, 1975; Granick & Friedman, 1967; Harwood & Naylor, 1971; Overall & Gorham, 1972; Reitan, Note 6) and with brain damage regardless of site. Deficits on the DSS have been noted for these groups even when there is minimal influence on performance on other subtests (Granick & Friedman, 1967; Hirschenfang, 1960b). Female superiority has been reported consistently for this subtest, both for middle-aged and for older samples (Blum et al., 1972; Doppelt & Wallace, 1955; Norman, 1953). The test also appears to have a heavy verbal component, as determined by factor analysis (Jarvik, Kallmann, Lorge, & Falek, 1962) and to depend more on perceptual, decisional or motoric factors than on memory (Salthouse, 1978).

Block Design Subtest (WAIS). The goal on this timed test is to reconstruct 10 2-dimensional designs using 3-dimensional blocks. Concepts that require shifting include color, shape, and angle.

Poor performance on Block Design generally is associated with increasing age (Blum et al., 1970; Goldstein & Shelly, 1975; Klodin, 1975; Reed & Reitan, 1963) and with organic impairment (Goldstein & Shelly, 1975; McFie, 1960; Milner, 1954; Smith, 1966). Ben-Yishay, Diller, Mendleberg, Gordon, and Gerstman (1971) examined numerous dimensions of individual performance on the test (style, speed, degree of activeness, and various types of errors). They reported that overall both left and right hemiplegic subjects (mean age = 63 years) scored significantly worse than controls (mean age = 70 years). Even though the brain-damaged subjects made more errors, their styles overlapped markedly with the controls to the degree that the researchers suggested a continuity of behavior between the performance of normal and brain-damaged persons on this task. However, right and left hemiplegics displayed enough stylistic differences to be distinguishable from one another. An examination of individual intratest performance for neuropsychological assessment would be valuable.

The Wisconsin Card Sorting Test. The Wisconsin Card Sorting Test (Berg, 1948; Grant & Berg, 1948), often part of a neuropsychological battery, requires visuomotor processing in order to demonstrate the ability to shift sets of organization (shape, color, number of items). In one study (Drewe, 1974), inability to conceptualize categories was associated with left frontal lobe damage, whereas preservation appeared regardless of the site of the brain damage. Frontal lobe damage was indicated in studies by Milner (1963, 1964) and Teuber, Pattersby, and Bender (1951) who also noted markedly deteriorated performance in persons with parieto-temporal lobe lesions. Another pattern on this test noted in brain-damaged persons was diminished ability for prolonged concentration, despite persisting ability to shift (Parsons, 1975).

Trail Making Test. The Trail Making Test, originally part of the Army Individual Test, 1944, and described as part of the Halstead-Reitan battery, is another neuropsychological measure that has been used with several samples but remains controversial. It provides a visuographic stimulus, is timed, and has subjects figure out how to proceed rather than simply reproduce or recognize the presented item. Intact older persons do worse than younger persons (Davies, 1968; Gordon, 1972; Goul & Brown, 1970; Lindsey & Coppinger, 1969; Reitan, Note 6) and tend to perform similarly to brain-damaged persons (Davies, 1968; Reitan, Note 6). Davies suggested a change in the standard cutoff scores for older people, implying that in his view visuomotor speed and coordination decrease with age without being symptomatic of the type of brain damage associated with senility. In a study where level of initial functioning was taken into account, TMT performance did not correlate with age (Lindsey & Coppinger, 1969). Goul and Brown (1970) similarly found TMT performance to be positively correlated with intelligence and negatively correlated with age. Age and IQ-corrected norms are therefore recommended.

Gordon (1972) tried to correct for age by using two different cutoff levels with a middle-aged sample of brain-damaged and non-brain-damaged patients. Finding numerous false positives among the older subjects and some false negatives among the younger subjects, he suggested a new approach for evaluating performance. Since the perfect test has not yet been developed, he felt a good test battery should include tests with complementary error rates of false positives and false negatives in order to keep checks on their over- and underdiagnostic powers.

Boll and Reitan (1973) reported that they found no significant differences with age on the TMT in their intact subjects, ranging in age from 15 to 65, while brain-damaged subjects performed significantly worse. The authors suggested that the regular cutoffs are valid for subjects of all ages. Yet, Reitan (Note 6) himself reported that subjects aged 30 to 65, all without brain damage, showed a sharp age-related decline on the TMT.

Studies conducted to assess the utility of the TMT for the detection of specific lesions have produced inconsistent findings (Lezak, 1976). The test is useful in obtaining behavioral observations of an individual's performance, relative to his or her other skills, but at this point it is not recommended for diagnostic purposes.

Auditory-Nonverbal Cognitive Functioning

Auditory-nonverbal tests are those that avoid the use of words or images that might be inherently more meaningful to some subjects than to others. The rationale for such test construction is to eliminate many extraneous variables that tend to affect persons differentially. Therefore, it is surprising that so little work has been done with older subjects, particularly since the older persons do not seem to function noticeably worse than younger ones in this area.

Seashore Rhythm Test

In the Reed and Reitan study (1963) of normal aging, the Seashore Rhythm Test was administered as part of their battery to all subjects: young intact and brain damaged (mean age = 28 years), old intact (mean age = 45 years), and older intact (mean age = 55 years). While young controls and young brain-damaged subjects performed significantly different from one another, the two older groups did not have differential scores. Raw scores are not provided so it is uncertain whether the young and old groups performed significantly differently. No explanation for the older groups' results is offered by the authors. However, since many of the other tests in this study (which showed similar results) contain abilities well maintained with age (e.g., Vocabulary and Arithmetic), the Seashore Rhythm test probably tests a similarly maintained ability. Further testing is warranted, because this area of functioning may have potential for rehabilitation or compensation.

Other Auditory-Nonverbal Tests

When presented with a variety of everyday sounds, defects in auditory-nonverbal cognitive functioning have been noted in younger subjects with right temporal lobe lesions (Bogen & Gordon, 1971; Milner, 1962, 1971). Lezak (1976) has suggested several other tests for right temporal lobe lesions, e.g., recognition of popular tunes that the tester hums, discriminating the relative pitch of two notes, and distinguishing between or mimicking tapping patterns (without allowing visual access to the tester's tapping). Again, it must be stressed that if a deficit is noted, tests that are similar in concept but constructed in other modalities should be administered to assess whether the paradigm is modality-specific or conceptual. The effect of age remains to be studied.

Tactile Cognitive Functioning

Tactile cognitive ability is processing that is done primarily on the basis of tactile stimulation and involves bodily sensation or stereognostic recall. The response is often nonverbal (usually a gesture). While it is true that persons are less likely to demonstrate impaired performance on such tests, it is also true that impaired tactile cognitive functioning is more likely to be related to organic factors, uncontaminated by intervening variables, e.g., education, cohort, socioeconomic status, than impaired performance on verbal or visual cognitive tests.

The Face-Hand Test

The Face-Hand Test (FHT) (Fink, Green, & Bender, 1952), a test of double simultaneous tactile stimulation, is widely used as a gross measure of organic impairment. While it may miss mild brain damage, it is not likely to yield false positives.

Haglund and Shuckit (1976) compared the diagnostic power of the FHT with several other measures: the Mental Status Questionnaire (MSQ), the Pfeiffer Short Portable MSQ, and the G-K. None of the tests confirmed brain damage in even half of the subjects (aged 65–97, mean age of 76), who had been diagnosed clinically as brain damaged. Since the FHT contributed less than 5% to the diagnostic power of the battery, the authors suggested it be used only as an adjunct to other tests. In another study, however, the FHT, when administered with the MSQ to subjects aged 50 to 91 (mean age of 65), showed significant discrimination between subjects who performed at varying levels on other intellectual measures (Zarit et al., Note 8).

One of the advantages of the FHT is its insensitivity to education or intelligence. Also, normally dull persons or adults anxious about the experiment are allowed an opportunity to get accustomed to the format of the test and their expected role in it, without a scoring penalty, by being given more than one trial to perform the requested task. There are four testing trials and two orientation trials. Once oriented, most people, regardless of affective state, perform normally. On the other hand, brain-damaged persons often respond correctly to the two orientation trials, but they cannot seem to retain their sense of bodily orientation when stimulated on two nonsymmetrical parts of their bodies simultaneously (Pollack & Fink, 1962).

On the basis of the FHT, Bender and Fink (1952) were able to discriminate adult psychiatric patients from those with massive brain lesions and accompanying behavior deficit. The psychiatric patients performed like normal intact adults. Fink and Bender (1952) found patterns of errors in children under 6 years of age similar to those in brain-damaged adults. A commonly noted error in brain-damaged adults is face dominance, in which response to stimulation of the face is displaced, often external to the body.

Tactual Performance Test

An apparently valuable neuropsychological test is the Tactual Performance Test (TPT) (Arthur, 1947; Halstead, 1947). Its three trials not only measure discrete cognitive abilities but also can be examined in relation to one another. When the trial with the nondominant hand (Trial II) takes longer or as long as the trial with the dominant hand (Trial I), but the trial with both hands (Trial III) is done relatively quickly, signs of a lesion in the non-dominant hemisphere should be further investigated using tactile and other modalities. If the first trial takes much longer than the second one, the intactness of the dominant hemisphere should be examined further. Brain-damaged persons have performed significantly less well than non-brain-damaged persons (Reed & Reitan, 1962) and old intact persons have performed significantly less well than young (Goldstein & Shelly, 1975; Reed & Reitan, 1962, 1963). Equally interesting was the finding that young and old non-brain-damaged persons improved with practice, while young and old brain-damaged persons did worse with practice, suggesting a discrepancy over time between brain damage and intactness, regardless of age (Reed & Reitan, 1962).

In one study of performance on the TPT with intact older persons, Reed and Reitan (1963) noted significantly poorer performance of dominant hand and both hands sections by older (mean age of 55) as opposed to younger subjects (mean age of 45). Poorer performance on this test also has characterized young brain-damaged persons compared to young intact persons. The authors believe that differences in TPT performance associated with aging may be explained partially on the basis of changes in the organic condition of the brain.

The type of organicity detected by the TPT is not clearly delineated, although brain-damaged persons in general show difficulty doing the task. Patients with left-hemisphere lesions tend to do better than those with right-sided lesions (Teuber & Weinstein, 1954), although patients with right-hemisphere lesions have exhibited superior performance to left-hemisphere-damaged patients on the drawing recall section of the test (DeRenzi et al., 1968). One explanation is that there is possibly greater access to verbal encoding in persons with right-hemisphere lesions. Lack of agreement among several studies (discussed by Lezak, 1976) suggests that the test may not be as clear a discriminator of frontal versus nonfrontal lesions as had been believed originally.

Tactile Nonsense Figures

Brenda Milner (1971) offered a test designed to assess intactness of the right hemisphere. The task involves what she calls "matching-to-sample" of tactile nonsense figures. The subject is first given a figure to examine tactilely (screened from view) and then is asked to pick it out of a large collection of objects. The number of objects, their similarities, and the delay between the tactile examination and the choosing are all factors that can be altered to make the test more or less difficult. Because the figures in this test are composed of variously twisted pieces of wire, they do not lend themselves easily to verbal encoding. All seven subjects in Milner's study had undergone commissurotomy prior to the experiment, and, therefore, the functions assumed by each hemisphere could be observed separately. At first, the subjects were taught to perform the experiment without any delay, and gradually a delay was introduced, increasing to a maximum of 2 minutes. With the left hand tested first (i.e., the right hemisphere), 4 patients performed successfully to 2 minutes. With the right hand (left hemisphere), none of them did. It appears that encoding (which is associated with left hemisphere functions) is not always the most effective strategy by which to perceive and remember complex information. This task is most useful for assessment of right hemispheric intactness and is particularly useful for deaf, blind, or mute patients.

Cognitive Potential and Compensatory Functioning

A small number of studies have gone beyond descriptive analyses of older persons' typical performance. These studies have attempted to disclose latent capabilities; they have either experimentally manipulated factors believed to influence test performance in the elderly (e.g., time allotments, modalities, motivation, instructions) or they have attempted to enhance compensatory functioning in cases of irreversible deterioration of particular brain-behavior mechanisms.

In his investigation of the role of speech as a regulator of normal and abnormal behavior, Luria (1961) provided a fascinating example of the restoration of a behavioral function through compensation. He noted in some cases of cerebral degeneration that only the subcortical levels of the nervous system were affected (such as in Parkinson's disease) leaving the complex cortical connections (including those of the verbal system) relatively intact and able to compensate for damaged systems. He cited an experiment conducted with persons suffering from cerebral asthenia, a subcortical disorder in which unusually heightened impulsiveness and excitement leads to premature weakness or exhaustion. In the first phase, subjects with this disorder were told to press a key in response to a red but not a green light. Although often consciously aware of erring, subjects were unable to refrain from responding incorrectly. In the second phase, when Luria told the subjects to say "press" or "don't press" instead of pressing the key when the appropriate lights came on, performance was unimpaired. In the third phase, subjects were to respond to the lights both by saying the correct word and by simultaneously either pressing or not pressing the correct key; motor behavior improved significantly compared to Phase I. When the speech response was excluded, the original impulsive excitable behavior returned. Finally, when subjects were given a phrase to say that was unrelated to the motor task in response to the light and were to simultaneously press or not press the key, they performed as poorly as they had in Phase I, illustrating the particular value of appropriate speech to compensate for deficits and to produce desired motor behavior.

Another example of performance potential was observed on a test of visual retention of geometric shapes (Arenberg, 1977). After initial testing of retention, half of the subjects of each age group (17-20 and 59-77) included auditory augmentation in their strategies to retain the images, and the other half did not. The old committed significantly more errors than the young both with and without augmentation. Augmentation reduced errors for all who used it, but the older auditorily augmented group improved relatively more than the respective younger group. To some degree the older control group also improved on retest, increasing their scores relatively but not absolutely more than the younger control group. Auditory cues and verbal coding clearly are helpful strategies for older persons on this visual memory task. Arenberg (1976) has reported similar findings on a word-reading test.

In another example where instructions showed differential effects (Labouvie-Vief & Gonda, 1976), four possible conditions of training were offered to the older subjects (ages 63-95): Two conditions focused on differing but specific structured cognitive strategy training (cognitive training and anxiety training), one condition offered nonspecific training, and one control condition provided no training. The most effective training was found to be in the unstructured condition. Subjects were instructed to generate their own strategies to improve on certain cognitive tasks (a training task, the Letter Sets Test, and a transfer test, Raven's Standard Progressive Matrices), and they were not given corrective feedback. The authors suggested that the elderly are not deficient in initiating task-relevant behaviors but are relatively ineffective in using experimenter-imposed strategies (Goulet, 1973). In attempting to resolve the discrepancy between their findings and those of others (Hulicka & Grossman, 1967; Mason, Note 9) who noted better performance when mediators were offered to older persons, Labouvie-Vief & Gonda (1976) contended that the elderly often conveniently fall into the role of helplessness and dependency expected of them and, in a self-fulfilling manner, exhibit lowered competence levels.

Another variable that clearly interacts with age is test timing, but as pointed out earlier, the precise nature of the relationship remains to be determined. On the one hand, the assumption is implicit that reduced time constraints will induce improved performance. Yet, Kinsbourne and Berryhill (1972) found that the slowest of three inspection rates on a paired associates task tended to be the least favorable learning condition for subjects between the ages of 60 and 85 (mean age of 70) and suggested that such a pattern may reflect boredom or lapsed attention.

Storandt (1977) also manipulated time in her study by comparing scoring systems for the WAIS: timed with credit provided for speed, timed but without bonus for speed, and untimed. Older subjects were matched on verbal intelligence with younger subjects. In general, elimination of bonuses for rapid performance differentially improved the scores of older subjects (community members, ages 65-76) but still did not raise them to the level of the scores of younger subjects (students, ages 20-30). The untimed test was not of special benefit to the old who had higher initial ability. When allowed to go beyond the standard time, older subjects improved significantly on Picture Arrangement only, although they benefited more than the younger subjects on the bonus questions on the Arithmetic and Block Design subtests. Overall, Storandt recommended retaining the standard cutoff times but warned that the time-dependent nature of the bonus questions can underestimate performance levels of older persons. Older subjects did not take significantly longer to complete the main body of the test, but they were able to reach the bonus questions more often when time constraints were removed. Storandt suggested letting older persons work on the bonus questions after the main time is up. It remains to be seen whether older persons devote more concentration and processing time to each question than do younger persons and therefore take longer overall, or whether their attention gets diverted more easily.

Eisdorfer and Stotsky (1977) reviewed some other interventions that have been used to improve cognitive performance in psychiatrically disturbed older persons (including laboratory and environmental manipulations and psychotherapies). They stressed the importance of accurate diagnosis and evaluation of resources in developing a treatment plan. In particular, they advised "controlled experimental studies using reliable well-standardized measures to evaluate the efficiency of a particular modality against a standard procedure on the relative efficiency of one modality versus another" (p. 740).

RECOMMENDATIONS

In spite of the heterogeneity of results derived from many of the cited studies, certain general recommendations can be made. Clearly, the examiner must establish the existence of an adequate level of attention before proceeding with tasks that demand higher level cognitive functioning. Test batteries are useful when the locus of malfunctioning is unknown so that a broad spectrum of functions may be examined; since no battery is totally comprehensive, testing of specific functions should often follow. Performance tends to approach an optimal level if the subject is able to achieve a reasonable degree of success and derive a sense of accomplishment and challenge from the testing situation. The levels of test difficulty must be considered in conjunction with the person's background. Intertest comparisons may identify specific areas of cognitive deficit that can be examined further on the basis of in-depth analyses of performance on carefully selected single tests.

There is no way to eliminate all extraneous influences upon test performance, but awareness of the probable contributing variables (such as testing conditions, individual personality, and background factors) permits a more realistic, accurate interpretation of test results than is possible without taking these factors into consideration.

The clinician should also evaluate the patient's potential. Luria (1961) described Vigotsky's approach to what he calls the investigation of the child's zone of potential development, an approach worth exploring in regard to the elderly. Not only are intellectual abilities assessed on the basis of repeated performance on a task (to check for initial situational anxiety or distraction), but subjects also are given test trials with and without the aid of another person. If a patient performs poorly alone but improves markedly when assisted, such information about the subjects' learning ability and independence enhances that information provided by test scores alone and has prognostic as well as therapeutic implications. To ask at what level of cognitive functioning an older person is performing is only part of the evaluative task. It is more important to determine the mechanisms underlying less than optimal performance. Will performance spontaneously reverse (as is the case in some situationally reactive conditions)? If not, can it be reversed or slowed down with clinical guidance? Or, can one learn to compensate for performance deficits? In order to answer these questions, a combination of cognitive assessments drawn from neuropsychodiagnostic, psychometrics, and clinical observations is desirable.

REFERENCES

Aita, J. A., Armitage, S. G., Reitan, R. M., & Rabinowitz, A. The use of certain psychological tests in the evaluation of brain injury. *Journal of General Psychology,* 1947, *37,* 25–44.

Alexander, D. A. The application of the Graham-Kendall Memory-for-Designs to elderly normal and psychiatric groups. *British Journal of Social and Clinical Psychology,* 1970, *9,* 85–89.

Anastasi, A. Age changes in adult test performance. *Psychological Reports,* 1956, *2,* 509.

Arenberg, D. Anticipation interval and age differences in verbal learning. *Journal of Abnormal Psychology,* 1965, *70,* 419–425.

Arenberg, D. The effects of input conditions on free recall in young and old adults. *Journal of Gerontology,* 1976, *31,* 551–555.

Arenberg, D. The effects of auditory augmentation on visual retention for young and old adults. *Journal of Gerontology,* 1977, *32,* 192–195.

Arenberg, D., & Robertson-Tchado, F. Learning and aging. In J. E. Birren & K. W. Schaie (Eds.), *Handbook of the psychology of aging.* New York: Van Nostrand Reinhold, 1977.

Arthur, G. *A point scale of performance tests. Revised form II.* New York: Psychological Corporation, 1947.

Barbizet, J., & Cany, E. Clinical and psychometric study of a patient with memory disturbance. *International Journal of Neurology,* 1968, *7,* 44–54.

Basowitz, H., & Korchin, S. J. Age differences in the perception of closure. *Journal of Abnormal and Social Psychology,* 1957, *54,* 93–97.

Bayley, N. The place of longitudinal studies in research on intellectual factors in aging. In J. E. Anderson (Ed.), *Psychological aspects of aging.* Washington, D.C.: American Psychological Association, 1956.

Bender, M. B., & Fink, M. Tactile perceptual tests in the differential diagnosis of psychiatric disorders. *Journal of Hillside Hospital,* 1952, *1,* 21.

Benton, A. L. Differential behavioral effects in frontal lobe disease. *Neuropsychologia,* 1968, *6,* 53–60.

Benton, A. L. The measurement of aphasic disorders. In A. Caceres Velasques (Ed.), *Aspectos patologicas del lengage.* Lima: Centro Neuropsicologica, 1973.

Benton, A. L. *The Revised Visual Retention Test* (4th Ed.). New York: Psychological Corporation, 1974.

Benton, A. L., & Van Allen, M. W. Impairment in facial recognition in patients with cerebral disease. *Cortex,* 1968, *4,* 344–358.

Ben-Yishay, Diller, L., Mendleberg, I., Gordon, W., & Gerstman, L. J. Similarities and differences in block design performance between older normal and brain injured persons: A task analysis. *Journal of Abnormal Psychology,* 1971, *78,* 17–25.

Berg, E. A. A simple objective technique for measuring flexibility in thinking. *Journal of General Psychology,* 1948, *39,* 15–22.

Berkowitz, B., & Green, R. F. Changes in intellect with age: Longitudinal study of Wechsler-Bellevue scores. *Journal of Genetic Psychology,* 1963, *103,* 3–21.

Bettner, L. G., Jarvik, L. F., & Blum, J. E. Stroop color-word test, non-psychotic organic brain syndrome and chromosome loss in aged twins. *Journal of Gerontology,* 1971, *26,* 458–469.

Billingslea, F. The Bender-Gestalt: A review and a perspective. *Psychological Bulletin,* 1963, *60,* 233–251.

Birkhill, W. R., & Schaie, K. W. The effect of differential reinforcement of cautiousness in intellectual performance among the elderly. *Journal of Gerontology,* 1975, *30,* 578–583.

Birren, J. E. Psychological aspects of aging. *Annual Review of Psychology,* 1960, *11,* 161–198.

Birren, J. E., Butler, R. N., Greenhouse, S. W., Sokoloff, L., & Yarrow, M. R. *Human aging* (U.S. Public Health Service Publication No. 986). Washington, D.C.: U.S. Government Printing Office, 1963.

Birren, J. E., & Morrison, D. F. Analyses of the WAIS scores relative to age and education. *Journal of Gerontology,* 1961, *16,* 363–369.

Birren, J. E., & Spieth, W. Age, response speed, and cardiovascular functions. *Journal of Gerontology,* 1962, *17,* 390–391.

Blessed, G., Tomlinson, B. E., & Roth, M. The association between quantitative measures of dementia and of senile change in the cerebral gray matter of elderly subjects. *British Journal of Psychiatry,* 1968, *114,* 797–811.

Blum, J. E., Fosshage, J. L., & Jarvik, L. F. Intellectual changes and sex differences in octogenarians: A twenty-year longitudinal study of aging. *Developmental Psychology,* 1972, *7,* 178–187.

Blum, J. E., & Jarvik, L. F. Intellectual performance of octogenarians as a function of education and initial ability. *Human Development,* 1974, *17,* 364–375.

Blum, J. E., Jarvik, L. F., & Clark, E. T. Rate of change on selective tests of intelligence: A twenty-year longitudinal study of aging. *Journal of Gerontology,* 1970, *25,* 171–176.

Bogen, J. E., & Gordon, H. W. Musical tests for functional lateralization with intracarotid/amobarbitol. *Nature,* 1971, *230,* 524.

Boll, T. J., & Reitan, R. M. Effect of age on performance of the Trail Making Test. *Perceptual Motor Skills,* 1973, *36,* 691–694.

Borkowski, J. G., Benton, A. L., & Spreen, O. Word fluency and brain damage. *Neuropsychologia,* 1967, *5,* 135–140.

Botwinick, J. Cautiousness in advanced age. *Journal of Gerontology,* 1966, *21,* 347–351.

Botwinick, J. *Cognitive processes in maturity and old age.* New York: Springer, 1967.

Botwinick, J. Disinclination to venture response versus cautiousness in responding: Age differences. *Journal of Genetic Psychology,* 1969, *115,* 55–62.

Botwinick, J. *Aging and behavior.* New York: Springer, 1973.

Botwinick, J. Intellectual abilities. In J. E. Birren & K. W. Schaie (Eds.), *Handbook of the psychology of aging.* New York: Van Nostrand Reinhold, 1977.

Botwinick, J., Brinley, J. F., & Robbins, J. S. The interaction effects of perceptual difficulty and stimulus exposure time on age differences in speed and accuracy of response. *Gerontologia,* 1958, *2,* 1–10.

Botwinick, J., & Storandt, M. Speed functions, vocabulary ability and age. *Perceptual Motor Skills,* 1973, *36,* 1123–1128.

Brilliant, P. J., & Gunther, M. D. Relationships between performance on three tests for organicity and selected patient variables. *Journal of Consulting Psychology,* 1963, *27,* 474–479.

Bromley, D. B. Some effects of age on short-term learning and remembering. *Journal of Gerontology,* 1958, *13,* 398–406.

Bromley, D. B. *The psychology of human aging.* Baltimore: Penguin, 1966.

Caird, W. K., Sanderson, R. F., & Inglis, J. Cross-validation of a learning test for use with elderly patients. *Journal of Mental Science,* 1962, *108,* 368–370.

Canestrari, R. E. Paced and self-paced learning in young and elderly adults. *Journal of Gerontology,* 1963, *18,* 165–180.

Canter, A., & Straumanis, J. J. Performance of senile and healthy older persons on the BIP Bender test. *Perceptual Motor Skills,* 1968, *28,* 695–698.

Cattell, R. B. Theory of crystallized and fluid intelligence: A critical experiment. *Journal of Educational Psychology,* 1963, *54,* 1–22.

Cohen, J. Wechsler Memory Scale performance of psychoneurotic, organic and schizophrenic groups. *Journal of Consulting Psychology,* 1950, *14,* 371–375.

Cohen, J. The factorial structure of the WAIS between early adulthood and old age. *Journal of Consulting Psychology,* 1957, *21,* 283–290.

Comalli, P. E., Jr. Cognitive functioning in a group of 80–90 year-old men. *Journal of Gerontology,* 1965, *20,* 14–17.

Comalli, P. E., Jr., Krus, D. M., & Wapner, S. Cognitive functioning in two groups of aged; one institutionalized, the other living in the community. *Journal of Gerontology,* 1965, *20,* 9–13.

Comalli, P. E., Jr., Wapner, S., & Werner, H. Interference effects of Stroop Color-Word Test in childhood, adulthood and aging. *Journal of Genetic Psychology,* 1962, *100,* 47–53.

Corsini, R. J., & Fassett, K. K. Intelligence and aging. *Journal of Genetic Psychology,* 1953, *83,* 249–264.

Costa, L. D., & Vaughan, H. G., Jr. Performance of patients with lateralized cerebral lesions: I. Verbal and perceptual tests. *Journal of Nervous and Mental Disease,* 1962, *134,* 162–168.

Craik, F. I. M. The nature of the age decrement in performance on dichotic listening tasks. *Quarterly Journal of Experimental Psychology,* 1965, *17,* 227–240.

Crook, T., Ferris, S., Sathananthan, G., Raskin, A., & Gershon, S. The effect of methylphenidate in test performance in the cognitively impaired aged. *Psychopharmacology,* 1977, *52,* 251–255.

Crookes, T. G. Indices of early dementia on WAIS. *Psychological Reports,* 1974, *34,* 734.

Darwin, D. J. Ear differences in the recall of fricatives and vowels. *Quarterly Journal of Experimental Psychology,* 1971, *23,* 46–62.

Davies, A. D. M. The influence of age on Trail-Making Test Performance. *Journal of Clinical Psychology,* 1968, *24,* 96–98.

Davies, A. D. M., & Davies, D. R. The effects of noise and time of day upon age differences in performance at two checking tasks. *Ergonomics,* 1975, *18,* 321–326.

DeRenzi, E., Faglioni, P., & Spinnler, H. The performance of patients with unilateral brain damage on face recognition tasks. *Cortex,* 1968, *4,* 17.

DeWolfe, A. S., Barrell, R. P., Becker, B. C., & Spaner, F. E. Intellectual deficit in chronic schizophrenia and brain damage. *Journal of Consulting Psychology*, 1971, *36*, 197–204.

Diller, L., Ben-Yishay, Y., Gerstman, L. J., Goodkin, R., Gordon, W., & Weinberg, J. *Studies in cognition and rehabilitation in hemiplegia (Rehabilitation Monograph No. 50)*. New York: New York University Medical Center Institute of Rehabilitation Medicine, 1974.

Doppelt, J. E., & Wallace, W. L. Standardization of the Wechsler Adult Intelligence Scale for older persons. *Journal of Abnormal and Social Psychology*, 1955, *51*, 312–330.

Drewe, E. A. The effect of type and area of brain lesion on Wisconsin Card Sorting Test Performance. *Cortex*, 1974, *10*, 159–170.

Dujovne, B. E., & Levy, B. I. The psychometric structure of the Wechsler Memory Scale. *Journal of Clinical Psychology*, 1971, *27*, 351–354.

Dunn, L. M. *Expanded manual for the Peabody Picture Vocabulary Test*. Circle Pines, Minn.: American Guidance Service, 1965.

Eisdorfer, C. The WAIS performance of the aged: A retest evaluation. *Journal of Gerontology*, 1963, *18*, 169–172.

Eisdorfer, C. Verbal learning and response time in the aged. *Journal of Genetic Psychology*, 1965, *107*, 15–22.

Eisdorfer, C. Arousal and performance: Experiments in verbal learning and a tentative theory. In G. Talland (Ed.), *Human behavior and aging*. New York: Academic Press, 1968.

Eisdorfer, C., Axelrod, S., & Wilkie, F. L. Stimulus exposure time as a factor in serial learning in an aged sample. *Journal of Abnormal and Social Psychology*, 1963, *67*, 594–600.

Eisdorfer, C., Busse, E. W., & Cohen, L. D. The WAIS performance of an aged sample: The relationship between verbal and performance IQ. *Journal of Gerontology*, 1959, *14*, 197–201.

Eisdorfer, C., & Cohen, L. D. The generality of the WAIS standardization for the aged. *Journal of Abnormal and Social Psychology*, 1961, *62*, 520–527.

Eisdorfer, C., Nowlin, J., & Wilkie, F. L. Improvement in the aged by modification of autonomic nervous system activity. *Science*, 1970, *170*, 1327–1329.

Eisdorfer, C., & Stotsky, B. Intervention, treatment, and rehabilitation of psychiatric disorders. In J. E. Birren & K. W. Schaie (Eds.), *Handbook of the psychology of aging*. New York: Van Nostrand Reinhold, 1977.

Eisdorfer, C., & Wilkie, F. L. Changes with advancing age. In L. F. Jarvik, C. Eisdorfer, & J. E. Blum (Eds.), *Intellectual functioning in adults*. New York: Springer, 1973.

Elias, M. F., & Kinsbourne, M. Age and sex differences in the processing of verbal and nonverbal stimuli. *Journal of Gerontology*, 1974, *29*, 162–171.

Erickson, R. C., & Scott, M. L. Clinical memory testing: A review. *Psychological Bulletin*, 1977, *84*, 1130–1149.

Ferris, S., Sathananthan, G., Gershon, S., & Clark, C. Senile dementia: Treatment with deanol. *Journal of the American Geriatrics Society*, 1977, *35*, 240–244.

Fields, F. Relative effects of brain damage on the Wechsler memory and intelligence quotients. *Diseases of the Nervous System*, 1971, *32*, 673–675.

Fink, M., & Bender, M. B. Perception of simultaneous tactile stimuli in normal children. *Neurology*, 1952, *3*, 27.

Fink, M., Green, A., & Bender, M. B. The Face-Hand Test as a diagnostic sign of organic mental syndrome. *Neurology*, 1952, *2*, 48–56.

Foulds, G. A., & Raven, J. C. Normal changes in the mental ability of adults as age advances. *Journal of Mental Science*, 1948, *94*, 133–142.

Fowler, R. S. A simple non-language test of new learning. *Perceptual Motor Skills*, 1969, *29*, 895–901.

Fuller, G. B., & Laird, J. T. The Minnesota Percepto-Diagnostic Test. *Journal of Clinical Psychology Monograph,* 1963, *16.*

Ganzler, H. Motivation as a factor in the psychological deficit of aging. *Journal of Gerontology,* 1964, *19,* 425–429.

Garfield, S. L., & Blek, L. Age, vocabulary level, and impairment. *Journal of Consulting Psychology,* 1952, *16,* 395–398.

Garron, D. C., & Cheifetz, D. I. Comment on Bender-Gestalt discernment of organic pathology. *Psychological Bulletin,* 1965, *63,* 197–200.

Gilbert, J. G. Mental efficiency in senescence. *Archives of Psychology,* 1935, *27,* 188.

Gilbert, J. G. Memory loss in senescence. *Journal of Abnormal and Social Psychology,* 1941, *36,* 73–86.

Gilbert, J. G., Levee, R. F., & Catalano, F. L. A preliminary report on a new memory scale. *Perceptual Motor Skills,* 1968, *27,* 277–278.

Gladis, M., & Braun, H. W. Age differences in transfer and retroaction as a function of intertask response similarity. *Journal of Experimental Psychology,* 1958, *55,* 25–30.

Goldstein, K., & Scheerer, M. Abstract and concrete behavior: An experimental study with special tests. *Psychological Monographs,* 1941, *53.*

Goldstein, K., & Scheerer, M. *Goldstein-Scheerer Test of Abstract and Concrete Thinking.* New York: Psychological Corporation, 1945.

Goldstein, S. G., Deysack, R. E., & Kleinknecht, R. A. Effect of experience and amount of information on identification of cerebral impairment. *Journal of Consulting and Clinical Psychology,* 1973, *41,* 30–34.

Goldstein, S. G., & Shelly, C. H. Similarities and differences between psychological deficits in aging and brain damage. *Journal of Gerontology,* 1975, *30,* 448–455.

Gonen, J. Y., & Brown, L. Role of vocabulary in deterioration and restitution of mental functioning. *Proceedings of the 76th Annual Convention of the American Psychiatric Association,* 1968, *3,* 469–470. (Summary)

Gordon, N. G. The Trail-Making Test in neuropsychological diagnosis. *Journal of Clinical Psychology,* 1972, *28,* 167–169.

Goul, W. R., & Brown, M. Effects of age and intelligence on Trail Making Test performance and validity. *Perceptual Motor Skills,* 1970, *30,* 319–326.

Goulet, L. R. The interfaces of acquisition: Models and methods for studying the active, developing organism. In J. R. Nesselroade & R. W. Reese (Eds.), *Life-Span Developmental Psychology.* New York: Academic Press, 1973.

Graham, F. K., & Kendall, B. S. Memory-for-Designs Test: Revised general manual. *Perceptual Motor Skills,* 1960, *11,* 147–188.

Granick, S., & Friedman, A. L. The effect of education on the decline of psychomotor test performance with age. *Journal of Gerontology,* 1967, *22,* 191–195.

Grant, D. A., & Berg, F. A. A behavioral analysis of degree of reinforcement and ease of shifting to new responses in a Weigl-type card-sorting problem. *Journal of Experimental Psychology,* 1948, *38,* 404–411.

Green, R. F. Age-intelligence relationships between ages sixteen and sixty-four: A rising trend. *Developmental Psychology,* 1969, *1,* 618–627.

Griew, S., & Davies, D. R. The effects of aging on auditory vigilance performance. *Journal of Gerontology,* 1962, *17,* 88–90.

Haglund, R. M. J., & Shuckit, M. A. A clinical comparison of tests of organicity in elderly patients. *Journal of Gerontology,* 1976, *6,* 654–659.

Hall, J. C., & Toal, R. Reliability (internal consistency) of the Wechsler Memory Scale and correlation with the Wechsler-Bellevue Intelligence Scale. *Journal of Consulting Psychology,* 1957, *21,* 131–135.

Halstead, W. C. *Brain and intelligence.* Chicago: University of Chicago Press, 1947.

Harkins, S. W., Nowlin, J. B., Ramm, D., & Schroeder, S. Effects of age, sex, and time-on-watch on a brief continuous performance task. In E. Palmore (Ed.), *Normal Aging II.* Durham, N.C.: Duke University Press, 1974.

Harrison, D. M., & Chagnon, J. G. The effect of age, sex and language on the Minnesota Percepto-Diagnostic Test. *Journal of Clinical Psychology,* 1966, *22,* 302–303.

Harwood, E., & Naylor, G. Changes in the constitution of the WAIS intelligence pattern with advancing age. *Journal of Psychology,* 1971, *23,* 297–303.

Hayman, M. Two minute clinical test for measurement of intellectual improvement in psychiatric disorders. *Archives of Neurology and Psychiatry,* 1942, *47,* 454–464.

Hemsi, L. K., Whitehead, A., & Post, F. Cognitive functioning and cerebral arousal in elderly depressives and dements. *Journal of Psychosomatic Research,* 1968, *12,* 145–156.

Hine, W. D. The abilities of partially hearing children. *British Journal of Educational Psychology,* 1970, *40,* 171–178.

Hirschenfang, S. A comparison of Bender Gestalt reproductions of right and left hemiplegic patients. *Journal of Clinical Psychology,* 1960, *16,* 439. (a)

Hirschenfang, S. A comparison of WAIS scores of hemiplegic patients with and without aphasia. *Journal of Clinical Psychology,* 1960, *16,* 351. (b)

Horenstein, S. The clinical use of psychological testing. In C. E. Wells (Ed.), *Dementia.* Philadelphia: F. A. Davis, 1971.

Howard, A. R. Diagnostic value of the Wechsler Memory Scale with selected groups of institutionalized patients. *Journal of Consulting Psychology,* 1950, *14,* 376–380.

Howard, A. R., & Shoemaker, D. J. An evaluation of the Memory-for-Designs test. *Journal of Consulting Psychology,* 1954, *18,* 266.

Hoyer, W. J., Labouvie, G. V., & Baltes, P. B. Modification of response speed and intellectual performance in the elderly. *Human Development,* 1973, *16,* 233–242.

Hulicka, I. M. Age differences in Wechsler Memory Scale scores. *Journal of Genetic Psychology,* 1966, *109,* 135–145.

Hulicka, I. M., & Grossman, J. L. Age-group comparisons for the use of mediators in paired-associate learning. *Journal of Gerontology,* 1967, *22,* 46–51.

Hulicka, I. M., Sterne, H., & Grossman, J. Age-group comparisons of paired-associate learning as a function of paced and self-paced association and response time. *Journal of Gerontology,* 1967, *22,* 274–280.

Hulicka, I. M., & Weiss, R. L. Age differences in retention as a function of learning. *Journal of Consulting Psychology,* 1965, *29,* 125–129.

Inglis, J., & Ankus, M. Effects of age on short-term storage and serial rote learning. *British Journal of Psychology,* 1965, *56,* 183–195.

Inglis, J., & Caird, W. K. Age differences in successive responses to simultaneous stimulation. *Canadian Journal of Psychology,* 1963, *17,* 98–105.

Irving, G., Robinson, R. A., & McAdam, W. The validity of some cognitive tests in the diagnosis of dementia. *British Journal of Psychiatry,* 1970, *117,* 149–156.

Isaacs, B., & Kennie, A. T. The Set Test as an aid to the detection of dementia in old people. *British Journal of Psychiatry,* 1973, *123,* 467–470.

Ivinskis, A., Allen, S., & Shaw, E. An extension of Wechsler Memory Scale norms to lower age groups. *Journal of Clinical Psychology,* 1971, *27,* 384–387.

Jarvik, L. F. Survival and psychological aspects of aging in men. *Symposium for the Society for Experimental Biology,* 1967, *21,* 463–482.

Jarvik, L. F. Discussion: Patterns of intellectual functioning in the later years. In L. F. Jarvik, C. Eisdorfer, & J. Blum (Eds.), *Intellectual functioning in adults.* New York: Springer, 1973.

Jarvik, L. F., Altshuler, K. Z., Kato, T., & Blumner, B. Organic brain syndrome and chromosome loss in aged twins. *Diseases of the Nervous System,* 1971, *32,* 159–170.

Jarvik, L. F., & Blum, J. E. Cognitive declines as predictors of mortality in twin pairs: A twenty-year longitudinal study of aging. In E. Palmore & F. C. Jeffers (Eds.), *Prediction of life span.* Washington, D.C.: Health and Company, 1971.

Jarvik, L. F., & Falek, A. Intellectual stability and survival in the aged. *Journal of Gerontology,* 1963, *18,* 173–176.

Jarvik, L. F., Kallmann, F. J., & Falek, A. Intellectual changes in aging twins. *Journal of Gerontology,* 1962, *17,* 289–294.

Jarvik, L. F., Kallmann, F. J., Falek, A., & Klaber, M. M. Changing intellectual functions in senescent twins. *Acta Genetic et Statistica Medica,* 1957, *7,* 421–430.

Jarvik, L. F., Kallmann, F. J., Lorge, I., & Falek, A. Longitudinal study of intellectual changes in senescent twins. In C. Tibbits & W. Donahue (Eds.), *Social and psychological aspects of aging.* New York: Columbia University Press, 1962.

Jarvik, L. F., & Kato, T. Chromosome and mental changes in octogenarians: Preliminary findings. *British Journal of Psychiatry,* 1969, *115,* 1193–1194.

Jensen, A. R., & Rohwer, W. D. The Stroop Color-Word Test: A review. *Acta Psychologica,* 1966, *25,* 36–93.

Jones, H. Problems of aging in perceptual and intellectual functioning. In J. E. Anderson (Ed.), *Psychological aspects of aging.* Washington, D.C.: American Psychiatric Association, 1956.

Jones, H. E., & Conrad, H. S. The growth and decline of intelligence: A study of a homogenous group between the ages of ten and sixty. *Genetic Psychology Monographs,* 1933, *13,* 223–298.

Kahn, R. L., Zarit, S. H., Hilbert, N. M., & Niederehe, G. Memory complaints and impairment in the aged. *Archives of General Psychiatry,* 1975, *32,* 1569–1573.

Kallmann, F. J., & Jarvik, L. F. Individual differences in constitution and genetic background. In J. E. Birren (Ed.), *Handbook of aging and the individual: Psychological and biological aspects.* Chicago: University of Chicago Press, 1959.

Kamin, L. J. Differential changes in mental abilities in old age. *Journal of Gerontology,* 1957, *12,* 66–70.

Kear-Caldwell, J. J. The structure of the Wechsler Memory Scale and its relationship to brain damage. *British Journal of Social and Clinical Psychology,* 1973, *12,* 394–392.

Kendall, B. S. Memory-for-Designs performance in the seventh and eighth decades of life. *Perceptual Motor Skills,* 1962, *14,* 399–405.

Kimura, D. Functional asymmetry of the brain in dichotic listening. *Cortex,* 1967, *3,* 163–178.

Kinsbourne, M., & Berryhill, J. L. The nature of the interaction between pacing and the age decrement in learning. *Journal of Gerontology,* 1972, *27,* 471–477.

Kleemeier, R. W. Intellectual changes in the senium. *Proceedings of the Social Statistics Section of the American Statistical Association,* 1962, 290–295.

Klodin, V. M. The relationship of scoring treatment and age in perceptual integrative performance. *Experimental Aging Research,* 1975, *2,* 303–313.

Klonoff, H., & Kennedy, M. Memory and perceptual functioning in octogenarians and nonagenarians in the community. *Journal of Gerontology,* 1965, *20,* 328–333.

Klonoff, H., & Kennedy, M. A. A comparative study of cognitive functioning in old age. *Journal of Gerontology,* 1966, *21,* 239–243.

Korchin, S. H., & Basowitz, H. Age differences in verbal learning. *Journal of Abnormal Psychology,* 1957, *54,* 64–69.

Korman, M., & Blumberg, S. Comparative efficiency of some tests of cerebral damage. *Journal of Consulting Psychology,* 1963, *27,* 303–309.

Kral, V. A. Types of memory dysfunction in senescence. In D. E. Cameron & M. Greenblatt (Eds.), *Recent advances in new physiological research. Psychiatric Research Reports,* 1959, *11,* 30–40.

Kubo, Y. Mental and physical changes in old age. *Journal of Genetic Psychology,* 1938, *53,* 101–108.

Labouvie-Vief, G., & Gonda, J. Cognitive strategy training and intellectual performance in the elderly. *Journal of Gerontology,* 1976, *31,* 327–332.

Lacks, P. B., Harrow, M., Colbert, J., & Levine, J. Further evidence concerning the diagnostic accuracy of the Halstead organic test battery. *Journal of Clinical Psychology,* 1970, *26,* 480–481.

Lansdell, A. C. Effects of temporal lobe ablations on two lateralized deficits. *Physiology and Behavior,* 1968, *3,* 271–273.

Leech, S., & Witte, K. L. Paired-associate learning in elderly adults as related to pacing and incentive conditions. *Developmental Psychology,* 1971, *5,* 180.

Lehmann, H. E. Psychopharmacological aspects of geriatric medicine. In C. M. Gaitz (Ed.), *Aging and the brain.* New York: Plenum Press, 1971.

Lezak, M. D. *Neuropsychological Assessment.* New York: Oxford Press, 1976.

Lieberman, M. A. Psychological correlates of impending death: Some preliminary observations. *Journal of Gerontology,* 1965, *20,* 181–190.

Lindsey, B. A., & Coppinger, N. W. Age-related deficits in simple capabilities and their consequences for Trail-Making performance. *Journal of Clinical Psychology,* 1969, *25,* 156–159.

Lorge, I. Methodology of the study of intelligence and emotion in aging. In G. E. W. Wolstenholme & C. M. O'Connor (Eds.), *Ciba Foundation Colloquia on Aging (Vol. 3).* London: J and A Churchill, 1957.

Luria, A. R. *The role of speech in the regulation of normal and abnormal behavior.* New York: Liveright, 1961.

Luria, A. R. *Higher cortical functions in man.* New York: Basic Books, 1966.

Luria, A. R., & Majovski, L. V. Basic approaches used in American and Soviet clinical neuropsychology. *American Psychologist,* 1977, *32,* 959–968.

Maccoby, E. E., & Jacklin, C. N. *The psychology of sex differences.* Stanford, Calif.: Stanford University Press, 1974.

MacKay, H. A., & Inglis, J. The effect of age on a short-term auditory storage process. *Gerontologia,* 1963, *8,* 193–200.

Maxwell, A. F. Obtaining factor scores on the WAIS. *Journal of Mental Science,* 1960, *106,* 1060–1062.

McFie, J. Psychological testing in clinical neurology. *Journal of Nervous and Mental Diseases,* 1960, *131,* 383–393.

McFie, J. Recent advances in phrenology. *Lancet,* 1961, *2,* 360–363.

McFie, J. Preliminary results with an intelligence test. *West African Journal of Education,* 1966, *11,* 5–7.

McFie, J. *Assessment of organic intellectual impairment.* New York: Academic Press, 1975.

McGhie, A., Chapman, J., & Lawson, J. S. Changes in immediate memory with age. *British Journal of Psychology,* 1965, *56,* 69–75.

McIver, W. F., McLaren, S. A., & Philip, A. E. Inter-rater agreement on the Memory-for-Designs Test. *British Journal of Social and Clinical Psychology,* 1973, *12,* 194–198.

Meer, B., & Baker, J. A. Reliability of measurements of intellectual functioning of geriatric patients. *Journal of Gerontology,* 1965, *20,* 110–114.

Milner, B. Intellectual function of the temporal lobes. *Psychological Bulletin,* 1954, *51,* 42–62.

Milner, B. Laterality effects in audition. In V. B. Mountcastle (Ed.), *Interhemispheric relations and cerebral dominance.* Baltimore: Johns Hopkins University Press, 1962.

Milner, B. Effects of different brain lesions on card sorting. *Archives of Neurology,* 1963, *9,* 90–100.

Milner, B. Some effects of frontal lobectomy in men. In J. M. Warren & K. Akert (Eds.), *The frontal granular cortex and behavior.* New York: McGraw-Hill, 1964.

Milner, B. Brain mechanisms suggested by studies of frontal lobes. In C. H. Millikan & F. L. Darley (Eds.), *Brain mechanisms underlying speech and language.* New York: Grune & Stratton, 1967.

Milner, B. Interhemispheric differences in the localization of psychological processes in man. *British Medical Journal,* 1971, *27,* 272–274.

Milner, B., Taylor, L., & Sperry, R. W. Lateralized suppression of dichotically presented digits after commissural section in man. *Science,* 1968, *161,* 184–186.

Monge, R. H., & Hultsch, D. F. Paired associate learning as a function of adult age and the length of the anticipation and inspection intervals. *Journal of Gerontology,* 1971, *26,* 157–162.

Murdoch, B. B. Visual and auditory stores in short term memory. *Quarterly Journal of Experimental Psychology,* 1966, *18,* 206–211.

Nelson, H. E., & McKenna, P. The use of current reading ability in the assessment of dementia. *British Journal of Social and Clinical Psychology,* 1975, *14,* 259–267.

Newcombe, F. *Missile wounds of the brain.* London: Oxford University Press, 1969.

Norman, R. D. Sex differences and other aspects of young superior adult performance on the Wechsler-Bellevue. *Journal of Counselling Psychology,* 1953, *17,* 411–418.

Overall, J. E., & Gorham, D. R. Organicity versus old age in objective and projective test performance. *Journal of Consulting and Clinical Psychology,* 1972, *39,* 98–105.

Owens, W. A., Jr. Age and mental abilities. *Genetic Psychology Monographs,* 1953, *48,* 3–54.

Palmore, E. B. Physical, mental and social factors in predicting longevity. *The Gerontologist,* 1969, *9,* 103–108.

Parker, J. W. The validity of some current tests for organicity. *Journal of Consulting Psychology,* 1957, *21,* 425–438.

Parsons, O. A. Brain damage in alcoholics: Altered states of unconsciousness. In M. M. Gross (Ed.), *Alcohol intoxication and withdrawal.* New York: Plenum Press, 1975.

Parsons, O. A., Vega, A., Jr., & Burn, J. Different psychological effects of lateralized brain damage. *Journal of Consulting and Clinical Psychology,* 1969, *33,* 551–557.

Perez, F. I., Rivera, V. M., Meyer, J. S., Gay, J. R. A., Taylor, R. L., & Mathew, N. T. Analysis of intellectual and cognitive performance in patients with multi-infarct dementia, vertebro-basilar insufficiency with dementia and Alzheimer's disease. *Journal of Neurology, Neurosurgery and Psychiatry,* 1975, *38,* 533–540.

Pollack, M., & Fink, M. Disordered perception of simultaneous stimulation of face and hand: A review and theory. *Recent advances in biology and psychiatry* (Vol. 4). New York: Plenum Press, 1962.

Prado, W. M., & Taub, D. V. Accurate prediction of individual intellectual functioning by the Shipley-Hartford. *Journal of Clinical Psychology,* 1966, *22,* 294–296.

Ramier, A. M., & Hecaen, H. Role respectif des atteintes frontales et de la lateralisation lesionnelle drasles deficits de la "fluence verbale". *Revue Neurologique,* 1970, *123,* 17–22.

Rand, G., Wapner, S., Werner, H., & McFarland, J. M. Age differences in performance on the Stroop Color-Word Test. *Journal of Personality,* 1963, *31,* 534–558.

Reed, H. B. C., & Reitan, R. M. The significance of age in the performance of a complex psychomotor task by brain-damaged and non-brain-damaged subjects. *Journal of Gerontology,* 1962, *17,* 193–196.

Reed, H. B. C., & Reitan, R. M. A comparison of the effects of the normal aging process with the effects of organic brain damage on adaptive abilities. *Journal of Gerontology,* 1963, *18,* 177–179.

Reitan, R. M. Investigation of the validity of Halstead's measures of biological intelligence. *American Medical Association Archives of Neurology and Psychiatry,* 1955, *73,* 28–35.

Reitan, R. M., & Davison, L. A. *Clinical neuropsychology: Current status and applications.* Washington: Hemisphere, 1974.

Rey, A. *L'Examen clinique en psychologie.* Paris: Presses Universitaires de France, 1964.

Riegel, K. F. History as a nomothetic science: Some generalizations from theories and research in developmental psychology. *Journal of Social Issues,* 1969, *25,* 99–127.

Riegel, K. F., Riegel, R. M., & Meyer, G. A study of the drop-out rates in longitudinal research on aging and the prediction of death. *Journal of Personality and Social Psychology,* 1967, *4,* 342–348.

Rizzolatti, G., Umilta, C. A., & Berlucchi, G. Opposite superiorities of the right and left cerebral hemispheres in discriminative reaction time to physiognomical and alphabetical material. *Brain,* 1971, *94,* 431–442.

Rosvold, H. E., Mirsky, A. F., Sarason, I., Bransome, E. D., Jr., & Beck, L. H. A continuous performance test of brain damage. *Journal of Consulting Psychology,* 1956, *20,* 343–350.

Roth, M. The natural history of mental disorder in old age. *Journal of Mental Science,* 1955, *101,* 281–301.

Rowe, E. J., & Schnore, M. M. Item concreteness and reported strategies in paired associate learning as a function of age. *Journal of Gerontology,* 1971, *26,* 470–475.

Ruch, F. L. The differentiation effects of age upon human learning. *Journal of Genetic Psychology,* 1934, *11,* 261–286.

Russell, E. W. WAIS factor analysis with brain-damaged subjects using criterion measures. *Journal of Consulting and Clinical Psychology,* 1972, *39,* 133–139.

Salzman, C., Kochansky, G. E., & Shader, R. I. Rating scales for geriatric psychopharmacology—A review. *Psychopharmacology Bulletin,* 1972, *8,* 3–50.

Salzman, C., Shader, R. I., Harmatz, J., & Robertson, L. Psychopharmacological investigations in elderly volunteers: Effect of diazepam in males. *Journal of the American Geriatric Society,* 1975, *23,* 451–455.

Satthouse, T. A. The role of memory in the age decline in digit-symbol substitution. *Journal of Gerontology,* 1978, *2,* 232–238.

Savage, R. D. Intellectual assessment. In P. Mittler (Ed.), *The psychological assessment of mental and physical handicaps.* London: Methuen, 1970.

Savage, R. D., Britton, P. G., George, S., O'Connor, D., & Hall, E. H. A developmental investigation of intellectual functioning in the community aged. *Journal of Genetic Psychology,* 1972, *121,* 163–164.

Schaie, K. W., & Labouvie-Vief, G. Generational vs. ontogenetic components of change in adult cognitive behavior: A fourteen year cross-sequential study. *Developmental Psychology,* 1974, *10,* 305–320.

Schaie, K. W., Rosenthal, F., & Perlman, P. M. Differential mental deterioration of factorially pure functions in later maturity. *Journal of Gerontology,* 1953, *8,* 191–196.

Schaie, K. W., & Strother, C. R. A cross-sequential study of age changes in cognitive behavior. *Psychological Bulletin,* 1968, *70,* 671–680.

Shader, R. I., Harmatz, J. S., Kochansky, G. E., & Cole, J. O. Psychopharmacological investigations in healthy older volunteers: Effect of pipradol-vitamin (Alertonic) elixir and placebo in relation to research design. *Journal of the American Geriatric Society,* 1975, *23,* 277–279.

Shankweiler, D., & Studdert-Kennedy, M. Identification of consonants and vowels presented to left and right ears. *Quarterly Journal of Experimental Psychology,* 1967, *18,* 59–63.

Shaw, D. J. The reliability and validity of the Halstead Category Test. *Journal of Clinical Psychology,* 1966, *22,* 176–180.

Sheer, D. E. Psychometric studies. In N. D. C. Lewis, C. Landis, & H. E. King (Eds.), *Studies in topectomy.* New York: Grune & Stratton, 1956.

Shipley, W. C. A self-administering scale for measuring intellectual impairment and deterioration. *Journal of Psychology,* 1940, *9,* 371–377.

Shipley, W. C. *Institute of Living Scale.* Los Angeles: Western Psychology Services, 1946.

Siegler, I. Terminal drop hypothesis: Factor artifact. *Experimental Aging Research,* 1975, *1,* 169–185.

Silverman, I. Age and the tendency to withhold response. *Journal of Gerontology,* 1963, *18,* 372–375.

Smith, A. Intellectual functions in patients with lateralized frontal tumors. *Journal of Neurology, Neurosurgery and Psychiatry,* 1966, *29,* 52–59.

Smith, A. The Serial Sevens Subtraction Test. *Archives of Neurology,* 1967, *17,* 78–80.

Sorenson, H. Mental abilities over a wide range of adult ages. *Journal of Applied Psychology,* 1933, *17,* 729–741.

Spieth, W. Cardiovascular health status, age and psychological performance. *Journal of Gerontology,* 1964, *19,* 277–284.

Spieth, W. Slowness of task performance and cardiovascular diseases. In A. T. Welford and J. E. Birren (Eds.), *Behavior, aging and the nervous system.* Springfield, Ill.: Charles C Thomas, 1965.

Spreen, O., & Benton, A. L. Comparative studies of some psychological tests for cerebral damage. *Journal of Nervous and Mental Disease,* 1965, *140,* 323–333.

Sternberg, D. E., & Jarvik, M. E. Memory functions in depression. *Archives of General Psychiatry,* 1976, *33,* 219–224.

Sterne, D. M. The Benton, Porteus and WAIS digit span tests with normals and brain injured subjects. *Journal of Clinical Psychology,* 1969, *25,* 173–175.

Storandt, M. Age ability level and methods of administering and scoring the WAIS. *Journal of Gerontology,* 1977, *32,* 175–178.

Stroop, J. R. Studies of interference in serial verbal reactions. *Journal of Experimental Psychology,* 1935, *18,* 643-662.

Strother, C. R., Schaie, K. W., & Horst, P. The relationship between advanced age and mental abilities. *Journal of Abnormal and Social Psychology,* 1957, *55,* 166–176.

Talland, G. A. Performance studies in human aging and their theoretical significance. *Psychiatric Digest,* 1966, *27,* 37–53.

Talland, G. A. (Ed.). *Human Aging and Behavior.* New York: Academic Press, 1968.

Taub, H. Mode of presentation, age and short-term memory. *Journal of Gerontology,* 1975, *30,* 56–59.

Teuber, H.-L., Pattersby, W. S., & Bender, M. B. Performance of complex visual tasks after cerebral lesions. *Journal of Nervous and Mental Disease,* 1951, *114,* 413–429.

Teuber, H.-L., & Weinstein, S. Performance on a formboard-task after penetrating brain injury. *Journal of Psychology,* 1954, *38,* 177–190.

Thaler, M. Relationships among Wechsler, Weigl, Rorschach, EEG findings and abstract concrete behavior in a group of normal aged. *Journal of Gerontology,* 1956, *11,* 404–409.

Thompson, L. W., Eisdorfer, C., & Estes, E. H. Cardiovascular disease and behavioral changes in the elderly. *Proceedings of the 7th International Congress of Gerontology,* 1966, 387–390.

Thompson, L. W., Optin, E., & Cohen, L. D. Effects of age, presentation speed, and sensory modality on performance of a vigilance task. *Journal of Gerontology,* 1963, *18,* 366–369.

Thorndike, R. L., & Gallup, G. H. Verbal intelligence of the American adult. *Journal of General Psychiatry,* 1944, *30,* 75–85.

Thurstone, L. L., & Thurstone, T. C. *SRA Primary Mental Abilities.* Chicago: Science Research Associates, 1949.

Traxler, A. J. Negative transfer effects in paired associates learning in young and elderly adults. *Proceedings of the 80th Annual Convention of the American Psychological Association,* 1972, *7,* 655–666. (Summary)

Turland, D. N., & Steinhart, M. The efficiency of the Memory-for-Designs Test. *British Journal of Social and Clinical Psychology,* 1969, *8,* 44–49.

Uyeno, E. Differentiating psychotics from organics on the Minnesota Percepto-Diagnostic Test. *Journal of Consulting Psychology,* 1963, *27,* 462.

Wallach, M. A., & Kogan, N. Aspects of judgment and decision-making interrelationships and change with age. *Behavioral Science,* 1961, *6,* 23–36.

Wang, H. S., & Busse, E. W. Heart disease and brain impairment among aged persons. In E. Palmore (Ed.), *Normal aging II.* Durham, N.C.: Duke University Press, 1974.

Watson, C. G., Thomas, R. W., Anderson, D., & Felling, J. Differentiation of organics from schizophrenics at two chronicity levels by use of the Haldtead-Reitan organic test battery. *Journal of Consulting and Clinical Psychology,* 1968, *32,* 679–684.

Wechsler, D. A standardized memory scale for clinical use. *Journal of Psychology,* 1945, *19,* 87–95.

Wechsler, D. *Manual for the Wechsler Adult Intelligence Scale.* New York: The Psychology Corporation, 1955.

Wechsler, D. *The management and appraisal of adult intelligence.* Baltimore: Williams & Wilkins, 1958.

Westreich, G., Alter, M., & Lundgren, S. The effect of cyclandelate on dementia. *Stroke,* 1975, *6,* 535–538.

Whitehead, A. Verbal learning and memory for elderly depressives. *British Journal of Psychiatry,* 1973, *123,* 203–208.

Whitehead, A. Factors in the learning deficit of elderly depressives. *British Journal of Social and Clinical Psychology,* 1974, *13,* 201–208.

Wilkie, F., & Eisdorfer, C. Intelligence and blood pressure in the aged. *Science,* 1971, *172,* 959–962.

Wilkie, F., & Eisdorfer, C. Sex, verbal ability and pacing differences in serial learning. *Journal of Gerontology,* 1977, *32,* 63–67.

Wimer, R. E. Age differences in incidental and intentional learning. *Journal of Gerontology,* 1960, *15,* 79–82.

Witte, K. L. Paired associate learning in young and elderly adults as related to presentation rate. *Psychological Bulletin,* 1975, *82,* 975–985.

Witte, K. L., & Freund, J. S. Paired associate learning in young and old adults as related to stimulus concreteness and presentation method. *Journal of Gerontology,* 1976, *31,* 186–192.

Yates, A. J. The validity of some psychological tests for brain damage. *Psychological Bulletin,* 1954, *51,* 359–379.

Yates, A. J. Psychological deficit. *Annual Review of Psychology,* 1966, *17,* 111–144.

REFERENCE NOTES

1. Teuber, H.-L. Personal communication, 1974.
2. Kaszniak, A. W., Garron, D. C., & Fox, J. H. *Differential effects of age and cerebral atrophy upon span of immediate recall and paired-associate learning.* Paper presented at the Fourth Annual Meeting of the International Neuropsychology Society, Toronto, 1976.
3. Canestrari, R. E. *The effects of aging on vigilance performance.* Paper presented at the meeting of the Gerontological Society, Miami, 1962.
4. Kleemeier, R. W. *Intellectual changes in the senium or death and the I.Q.* Presidential address, Division on Maturity and Old Age, American Psychiatric Association, New York, 1961.
5. Granick, S., & Birren, J. E. *Cognitive functioning of survivors and nonsurvivors: A twelve-year follow-up of healthy aged.* Paper presented at the Eighth International

Congress of Gerontology, Washington, D.C., August 1969.
6. Reitan, R. M. *Behavioral manifestations of impaired brain function in aging.* Paper presented at the 81st Annual Convention of the American Psychiatric Association, 1973.
7. Kaszniak, A. W., Garron, D. C., Fox, J. H., Huckman, M. S., & Ramsey, R. G. *Relation between psychometric assessment of dementia and computerized tomography measures of cerebral atrophy.* Paper presented at the 27th Annual Meeting of the American Academy of Neurology, Bal Harbour, Fla., May 1975.
8. Zarit, S. H., Miller, N., & Kahn, R. L. *Brain function, intellectual improvement and education in the aged.* Paper presented at the 29th Gerontological Society, New York, 1976.
9. Mason, S. *The use of mnemonic devices by subjects of different ages.* Paper presented at the annual meeting of the Southeastern Psychiatric Association, New Orleans, 1976.

11

Cognitive Theory and the Assessment of Change in the Elderly

Donna Cohen and Carl Eisdorfer
University of Washington

INTRODUCTION

The assessment of cognitive performance in the aged has become an issue of more than theoretical significance. There is a growing recognition that it is difficult, if not impossible, to evaluate the efficacy of management and therapy in the older patient without an appropriate set of behavioral constructs. This problem is particularly salient when there is significant cognitive deficit or dysfunction, e.g., senile dementia of the Alzheimer type, the cerebrovascular variant of senile dementia, or the depressions. In a practical sense, research on outcome of drug or behavioral therapies is only as good as the measures of change, and the assessment instruments that define and measure cognitive change in the impaired elderly are severely limited (Eisdorfer, 1975; Erickson & Scott, 1977; Schaie & Schaie, 1977).

Current laboratory studies of attention, learning, and memory may give us a better basis from which to evaluate clinical change. It has become popular to conceptualize the individual as an information processing system, and the disoriented behavior of the impaired older adult can be analyzed as a disruption somewhere along the line in this information handling system. For the purpose of analysis and measurement, we propose to think of cognition as a continuous system of processes or structures with a flexible working space, e.g., a working memory and attention. Figure 1 presents a simple version of information processing that combines the common elements of many cognitive models in the current literature.

Information arrives at the sense organs, passes through a series of sensory stages of analysis, and a short-term or primary memory system. Information

Working Attention		
Information and Sensory buffers	Short-term memory store STS Primary memory Secondary memory	Long-term memory structure LTS
Working Memory		

FIGURE 1 Information handling system outlining the cognitive working space to be measured in the assessment of the impaired elderly.

held in short-term memory appears to be already coded and categorized to some extent. This process of encoding is thought to occur with little input from the memory system and has been called automatic processing by some theorists (Keele, Note 1).

Active use of control processes or cognitive strategies can be measured in short-term memory. Rehearsal is one way to maintain information in short-term memory, but there are other control or integrative processes that can be performed with short-term memory to organize information in a way that it can be found again when needed. Furthermore, there may be another level of cognitive control, executive functions, that is concerned with choosing what strategy will be performed at a point in time. Long-term memory processes are poorly understood, but several control processes are presumed to encode information in memory units or schemata (Norman, Note 2).

The problem for the cognitive theorist has been to chart the flow of information from input to output, and the problem for the experimentalist has been to develop appropriate techniques to measure the information flow at various points along its course (Craik, 1977; Rumelhart, 1977). The aim of this chapter is to identify key theoretical concepts and methods in the current psychological literature that may improve our understanding of cognitive dysfunction. These may be useful in the development of a framework to assess mental functioning in the aged that is (a) practical, (b) appropriate for the aged, and (c) sensitive to rapid change in a person's cognitive functioning, e.g., positive or negative changes induced by drug therapy. This chapter will consider five cognitive components: (1) sensory processing, (2) pattern recognition, (3) language, (4) memory, and (5) attention. They represent five points at which cognitive processing could be assessed in the older (impaired) patient. Furthermore, specific experimental paradigms are described that may be used to assess the efficiency of these cognitive components. Knowledge of component processes of behaviors operative during specific tasks provides a more precise idea about what a particular somatic or nonsomatic treatment can really do.

SENSORY PROCESSING

Cognitive processing begins with presentation of a stimulus to one or more sensory modalities. These sensory stores provide the input to perceptual processors that detect the presence of a stimulus and recognize it by interacting with a short-term store (STS) and a long-term store (LTS). It is interesting that, in essentially every stimulus modality a very short-term memory (VSTM) has been identified that continues to provide information after the stimulus is no longer present (Sperling, 1963). Neisser (1967) has described the existence of a visual iconic store and an auditory echoic store, and other researchers have explored the nature of these VSTMs with some success (Rumelhart, 1977). However, the processes leading to pattern detection and recognition are less well understood. It is generally accepted that recognition processes involve feature extraction and analysis guided by expectancies developed over time.

The information processing approach to perception provides a useful framework for evaluating the cognitively impaired elderly. Masking techniques permit measurement of the duration of VSTM and the duration of recognition processes. The ability to access information in VSTM along various physical dimensions can be tapped with partial report or whole report techniques (Darwin, Turvey, & Crowder, 1972; Sperling, 1960, 1963).

In a partial report experiment, a subject might be asked to view a matrix of letters for a specified time interval. Then, either before or after the stimulus matrix is turned off, the subject is cued to report a portion of the matrix. The closer in time the cue is presented to the stimulus presentation, the greater the number of cued items reported correctly. If the cue is delayed sufficiently, the subjects will respond with the same number of correct items as if they simply reported all the stimuli they could remember, i.e., whole report technique. A whole report technique might be an appropriate starting point to evaluate the cognitively impaired elderly before advancing to a partial report technique. The patient is presented with a series of target matrices, asked to observe each matrix, and after its removal asked to report verbally as many targets as possible.

PATTERN RECOGNITION

The iconic or echoic memory is a transient sensory memory where information is stored for further processing. Feature extraction is carried out at this level, and this may be a critical locus of cognitive dysfunction.

Impaired older adults often report becoming disoriented in familiar as well as new environments. Such confusion may be due to a deficit in visual scanning, a process people engage in when they enter a room or new environment and search for something or someone.

Paradigms developed by Rabbit (1967) and Neisser (1974) that measure the ability to test features in the environment during visual scanning, i.e., transfer from sensory store to STS, offer a useful beginning. A model task requires the subject to sort several decks of 48 cards on which strings of 9 letters appear. On each card 8 of the letters belong to an irrelevant background set, and the ninth determines in which of the 2 piles the card is to be sorted. The subject is asked to sort several card decks as quickly as possible, and total sorting time per deck is the dependent variable. Total sorting time is viewed as the sum of the times required for processing and handling the 48 individual pieces of information. The paradigm just described is only a starting point for assessment. The experimental exploration of a pattern recognition system requires careful research regarding how features are extracted and synthesized, how expectancies are formed, and how attention mediates information processing.

LANGUAGE

Language is one of the most important complex tasks performed by the information processing system, and it is strikingly impaired in cognitive disorders. Language disorder in dementia must be distinguished from specific aphasic syndromes that occur in dementia. Although there may be qualitatively different types of dementia, and the language deficits may vary with the type of dementia, there are certain characteristics of impaired language performance found in all cognitive diseases. These include a breakdown in logical association, naming deficits, simplified syntax, perseveration, echolalia, introduction of improbable phrases, and impaired ability to receive and interpret the language of others (Albert, Note 3). However, these language disorders in patients with dementia (but without significant aphasia) are heavily influenced by nonlinguistic cognitive factors, e.g., attention and memory impairment.

A linguistic verification task developed by Clark and Chase (1972) may be adapted for use with the cognitively impaired elderly. It involves the presentation of sentences such as "plus above star" or "star below plus" or "plus isn't above star." The patient is presented with a figure display such as $\overset{+}{*}$ and asked to identify whether the sentence and the figural representation are the same or different. The variable of interest is the time taken to verify whether the sentence is true or false with respect to the picture.

Several other paradigms may be used and adapted to evaluate syntactic knowledge, the form of language (Kaplan, 1972; Stevens & Rumelhart, 1975), and content (Bransford & Johnson, 1973). The conclusions of Irigaray (1967,

1973) and Albert (Note 3) suggesting that the content rather than the form of language may be impaired in cognitive disorders deserves further evaluation.

Specific aphasic syndromes may occur in the cognitive disorder, and can be evaluated using a variety of examinations (Goodglass & Kaplan, 1972; Reitan & Davison, 1974; Schuell, 1965). In senile dementia of the vascular type, infarction of the zone of language may provoke an aphasic syndrome that may occur in three ways: (1) it may appear abruptly in a patient who already has significant cognitive dysfunction; (2) the aphasia may precede the general impairment, or (3) a slowly evolving aphasia beginning as anomic aphasia may occur in connection with a series of multi-infarcts in the left hemisphere.

In senile dementia of the Alzheimer type, aphasias are common (Delay & Brion, 1962; Sjogren, Sjogren, & Lindgren, 1952). Anomic aphasia is the most common and sensory aphasia the next most common type; both agraphia and alexia are frequent (Albert, Note 3). The primary clinical features observed are word finding difficulties and the inability to comprehend spoken or written language. In a person with impaired learning, attention, and memory, the additional impact of aphasia may give the appearance of a more severe cognitive deficit than really exists.

What we know about language and aging may have a direct influence on our clinical evaluation of the elderly. The history of aphasia research has clearly shown that once the neurological basis of language disturbance was elaborated, effective therapy programs could be developed. Some of these, constructed by Albert and his colleagues (Albert, Sparkes, & Helm, 1973; Gardner, Zurif, Berry, & Baker, 1976), are based upon knowledge of what the damaged brain can do. The extent of reversibility of language dysfunction in dementia remains to be determined.

MEMORY

Memory impairment is one of the hallmark symptoms of the cognitively impaired elderly. Numerous theories abound in the literature to guide research to determine which cognitive components are most affected during the course of the cognitive disease and which components may respond to treatment strategies. Despite the controversy regarding theories of memory, there remains some agreement on basic issues. Perceptual processing can activate information stored in long-term memory (LTM) that becomes available in short-term memory (STM), and this information can be maintained in STM by processes such as verbal rehearsal. Information may also be organized to form a new, larger conceptual structure in LTM.

Despite the controversies regarding theories of memory, several test paradigms can be usefully adapted to measure different cognitive processes. A memory search experiment modeled after the original Sternberg paradigm (Sternberg, 1969) measures retrieval from STS. Subjects receive a memory set followed by a series of test trials. Each test trial consists of the presentation of a single item and the subject is told to indicate as rapidly as possible whether the item was or was not present in the memory set. Size of the memory set is the independent variable and reaction time the dependent variable. The general finding is that reaction time is a linear function of the size of the memory set. The slope of this function can be used as a measure of memory search, and the intercept represents a combination of response and decision times. Changes in the intercepts and slopes offer a potentially useful scale for the objective assessment of cognitive change over time (Parkinson, Note 4).

Another task adapted from Peterson and Peterson (1959) measures retrieval from STS by presenting a 3-consonant set followed by a 3-digit number. The subject's task is to count backwards from the number and after a delay of 3 or 9 seconds, to repeat the syllable. In general, unrehearsed information is forgotten from STS quite rapidly. Hellyer (1962), therefore, adapted the previous task to measure the retrieval of information from STS using rehearsal. A consonant trigram is presented for the subject to study. However, on some trials the subject rehearses the trigram several times, while on others, presentation and rehearsal of the trigram are followed by a variable interval of another task to prevent rehearsal.

A letter identification task adapted from a procedure by Posner and his colleagues (Posner & Mitchell, 1967; Posner, 1969) measures access to overlearned information in LTM. The impaired elderly often report difficulties recognizing objects, and an operational definition of "I recognize something," is to say that a stimulus activates information in LTM. Patients are shown two letters simultaneously and told to respond "same" if the letters share the same name (e.g., Aa, AA) and "different" if the names are not the same (e.g., AB). Response latency varies with the physical similarity of the letters. Same responses to letters that are physically identical (e.g., AA) are made 70–80 milliseconds faster than responses to letters similar in name only (e.g., Aa).

Posner has suggested that information is first stored in a form that retains the physical properties of the letter stimulus. If an identity match is made, a "same" response is given. If there is no physical identity, two possibilities remain: the same name or a different name, both of which require the matching of name codes. The advantage of physical identity over name identity is thought to represent the time required to generate a name code from long term memory store.

In a model task, the stimuli could be a series of trials with the upper and lower case letters A, F, H, and T. An equal number of same name and different name trials would be administered, and of the same name trials half would be physically identical and half identical in name only. Median reaction time would be calculated for physical identity (PI), name identity (NI), and different name trials. The PI time is another variable of interest. Parkinson (Note 4) has reported that older individuals have large NI-PI measures than the young, and we might predict even larger NI-PI measures in the cognitively impaired.

ATTENTION

Senile dementias are traditionally defined in terms of learning and memory impairment, and attentional difficulties are largely ignored. A systematic evaluation of attention as well as memory in the cognitively impaired elderly would be useful not only to assess change but also to document behavioral heterogeneity in dementias. The confused behavior of the elderly person could be described in terms of selective attention deficit, which could be further analyzed as a divided attention deficit or a focused attention deficit. In the early stages of cognitive dysfunction we might be able to influence or manipulate the individual's ability to focus attention, e.g., follow a conversation and not be distracted, as well as regulate the person's ability to divide attention, e.g., attend to more than one task. In later stages we might not be able to manipulate either focused or divided attention.

A test of what happens to attended and nonattended information is a dichotic listening task. The stimuli are lists of three digits presented at a set rate, and the task is conducted in three phases. In Phase 1 each subject receives digits in the right ear and the left ear for identification. In Phase 2, the subjects are given dichotic presentations with instructions to ignore one list and report the other. And, in Phase 3 the trials are dichotic and the subjects are instructed to report both lists as accurately as possible.

Recently, a process-oriented framework for the study of attention (Kahneman, 1973; Posner & Snyder, 1975) has emerged that has important implications for the assessment of the impaired elderly. Keele's theory of attention (Keele, 1973; Keele, Note 1) assumes two kinds of processes, automatic and control processes (Schneider & Shiffrin, 1977; Shiffrin & Schneider, 1977). Automatic processes require no attention and many of them can be done simultaneously. A control process requires all available attention; thus, only one control process can operate at an instant in time. In order to perform two tasks concurrently, two or more control processes must be time shared. That is, only one process occurs at an instant in time, but attention is rapidly shifted between processes so that each receives some attention. According to this theory, codes in memory are activated by automatic perceptual processes, but the conscious perceptions are determined by a control process that selects from among all those that are activated. Thus, the "bottleneck" occurs at the level of the control processes that determine which stimuli receive further processing.

Keele (Note 1) has suggested that age-related deficits reflect changes in control processes, while automatic processes remain stable with increasing age. Thus, the study of control and automatic processes may reveal different patterns of change with increasing age or with progressive deficits in cognitive ability that are related to age.

There are four aspects of control processes amenable to study and assessment (Poltrock, Note 5). These four aspects are: (1) whether the control process is available as a strategy for that individual, (2) whether the individual can maintain the strategy, (3) whether the control process is effective, and (4) whether the control process takes differential processing capacity or effort at different points in time. There are two aspects of automatic processing that deserve study over time: (1) speed of learning of automatic processes and (2) efficiency of automatic processes. The study of automatic processes may have important implications in accounting for deficits of the impaired elderly on tasks involving complex skills. In particular, deficits in the development of automatic processes may account for difficulty in learning new skills.

Control processes play an important part in a wide range of cognitive activities. For example, control processes influence the use of memory, perceptual speed and ability, and ability at processing verbal and spatial material. Control processes influencing memory performance include rehearsal of information in STS and LTS and organization of material presented for a later memory test. Control processes also influence the ability to mentally rotate spatial representations of objects and to perceive figures hidden among other distracting lines. In the realm of perception, control processes influence comparative judgments such as the determination of which object is bigger or which duration is longer. Furthermore, control processes limit the speed of a visual search for a target item among a group of distractors. The aspect of control processes most appropriate for study depends on the degree of impairment of the individual to be tested. For very impaired individuals it is appropriate to first ask whether the subject will make use of the control process, and if not, whether the process be maintained if the subject is instructed to use the strategy. For the less impaired, the efficiency and attention-demanding characteristics of the task deserve study.

One useful experimental paradigm involves variations on a basic visual and auditory search procedure (Schneider & Shiffrin, 1977) that requires the person to search for the presence of one or more of a set of X targets that have previously been memorized from among a set of Y visual stimuli (distractors). If the targets and the distractors are dissimilar, then across trials learning performance should steadily increase. This change is interpreted as evidence for the development of automatic processing. On the other hand, if targets and distractors are mixed across trials, then the subject must use a serial search of the stimuli presented. This is a slow deliberate process requiring attention by the individual, and the results are ascribed to the use of controlled search. The tasks range in design from those with a small number of simultaneous inputs (with reaction time as the measure) to tasks in which successive inputs are presented and performance accuracy is measured.

The visual and auditory search paradigms can also be adapted to examine perceptual learning, learning in general, categorization, and the ability to focus attention. In each case the variability in utilization and efficiency of processing can be evaluated. The complexity of tasks can be manipulated by varying (a) the time for which information is presented, (b) the amount of information (number of characters) presented at any one time, and (c) the number of characters held in STM.

CONCLUSION

An important problem challenging psychologists is the accurate analysis and measurement of cognition in the cognitively and emotionally impaired elderly. Subsidiary subproblems include identification of the component processes of cognition, establishment of specific measures of the efficiency of each, and analysis of biologically and clinically relevant processes. Although new tests and procedures need to be designed, some paradigms in the literature should be considered in the development of a cognitive assessment system to improve our understanding of performance limitations in terms of the rate, accuracy, and quality of information processing as well as the available repertoire of cognitive strategies. Adequate cognitive scales coupled with sophisticated psychophysiological techniques may provide a key to better understanding of brain/behavior relationships.

REFERENCES

Albert, M. L., Sparkes, R., & Helm, N. Melodic intonation therapy for aphasia. *Archives of Neurology,* 1973, *29,* 130–131.

Bransford, J. D., & Johnson, M. K. Considerations of some problems of comprehension. In W. G. Chase (Ed.), *Visual information processing.* New York: Academic Press, 1973.

Clark, H. H., & Chase, W. G. On the process of comparing sentences against pictures. *Cognitive Psychology,* 1972, *3,* 472–515.

Craik, F. I. M. Age differences in human memory. In J. E. Birren & K. W. Schaie (Eds.), *Handbook of the psychology of aging.* New York: Van Nostrand Reinhold, 1977.

Darwin, C. J., Turvey, M. T., & Crowder, R. G. An auditory analogue of the Sperling partial report procedure: Evidence for brief auditory storage. *Cognitive Psychology,* 1972, *3,* 255–267.

Delay, J., & Brion, E. *Les démences tardives.* Paris: Masson, 1962.

Eisdorfer, C. Intelligence and cognition in the aged. In E. Busse & E. Pfeiffer (Eds.), *Behavior and adaptation in later life* (2nd ed.). Boston: Little Brown, 1975.

Erickson, R., & Scott, M. L. Clinical memory testing: A review. *Psychological Bulletin,* 1977, *84,* 1130–1149.

Gardner, H., Zurif, E., Berry, T., & Baker, E. Visual communications in aphasia. *Neuropsychologia,* 1976, *14,* 275–292.

Goodglass, H., & Kaplan, E. *The assessment of aphasia and related disorders.* Philadelphia: Lea and Fehiger, 1972.

Hellyer, S. Frequency of stimulus presentation and short-term decrement in recall. *Journal of Experimental Psychology,* 1962, *64,* 650.

Irigaray, L. Approaches psycholinguistique du language des dements. *Neuropsychologia,* 1967, *5,* 25–52.

Irigaray, L. *Le language des dements.* The Hague: Mouton, 1973.

Kahneman, D. *Attention and effort.* New Jersey: Prentice-Hall, 1973.

Kaplan, R. M. Augmented transition networks as psychological models of sentence comprehension. *Artificial Intelligence,* 1972, *3,* 77–100.

Keele, S. *Attention and human performance.* Pacific Palisades, Calif.: Goodyear, 1973.

Neisser, U. *Cognitive psychology.* New York: Appleton-Century-Crofts, 1967.

Neisser, U. Practiced card-sorting for multiple targets. *Memory and Cognition,* 1974, *2,* 781–785.

Peterson, L. R., & Peterson, M. J. Short-term retention of individual verbal items. *Journal of Experimental Psychology,* 1959, *58,* 193–198.

Posner, M., Boies, S., Eichelman, W., & Taylor, R. Retention of visual and name codes of single letters. *Journal of Experimental Psychology,* 1969, *79,* 1–16.

Posner, M., & Mitchell, R. Chronometric analysis of classification. *Psychological Review,* 1967, *74,* 392–409.

Posner, M. I., & Snyder, C. R. R. Attention and cognition control. In P. L. Solo (Ed.), *Information-processing and cognition.* New Jersey: LEA, 1975.

Rabbit, P. M. A. Learning to ignore irrelevant information. *American Journal of Psychology,* 1967, *80,* 1–13.

Reitan, R., & Davison, L. A. *Clinical neuropsychology: Current status and applications.* New York: Wiley, 1974.

Rumelhart, D. E. *Introduction to human information processing.* New York: Wiley, 1977.

Schaie, K. W., & Schaie, J. Psychological evaluation of the cognitively impaired elderly. In C. Eisdorfer & R. O. Friedel (Eds.), *The cognitively and emotionally impaired elderly.* Chicago: Year Book Medical, 1977.

Schneider, W., & Shiffrin, R. M. Controlled and automatic human information processing: I. Detection, search, and attention. *Psychological Review,* 1977, *84,* 1–126.

Schuell, H. *Differential diagnosis of aphasia with the Minnesota test.* Minneapolis: University of Minnesota Press, 1965.

Shiffrin, R. M., & Schneider, W. Controlled and automatic human information processing: II. Perceptual learning, automatic attending, and a general theory. *Psychological Review,* 1977, *84,* 127–177.

Sjogren, T., Sjogren, H., & Lindgren, A. G. H. Morbus Alzheimer and morbus Pick. A genetic, clinical, and patho-anatomical study. *Acta Psychiatrica Neurologica Scandinavica,* 1952, *82* (Suppl.).

Sperling, G. The information available in brief visual presentations. *Psychological Monographs,* 1960, *74,* 1–29.

Sperling, G. A model for visual memory tasks. *Human Factors,* 1963, *5,* 19–39.

Sternberg, S. The discovery of processing stages: Extension of Donder's method. *Acta Psychologia,* 1969, *30,* 276–315.

Stevens, A. L., & Rumelhart, D. E. Errors in reaching: Analysis using an augmental network model grammar. In D. A. Norman, D. E. Rumelhart, and LNR Research Group (Eds.), *Explorations in cognition.* San Francisco: Freeman, 1975.

REFERENCE NOTES

1. Keele, S. *Theories of attention and skill: Implications for the study of aging.* Paper presented at the Conference on Cognition and Aging, Seattle, January 1977.
2. Norman, D. *Cognitive psychology and the process of aging.* Paper presented at the Conference on Cognition and Aging, Seattle, January 1977.
3. Albert, M. *Language in the aging brain.* Paper presented at the Conference on Cognition and Aging, Seattle, January 1977.
4. Parkinson, S. *Aging: An information processing analysis.* Paper presented at the Conference on Cognition and Aging, Seattle, January 1977.
5. Poltrock, S. Personal Communication, February 1977.

Appendix

GLOSSARY OF FREQUENTLY USED ACRONYMS AND ABBREVIATIONS

AEP	Auditory Evoked Potential
AER	Auditory Evoked Response
BDI	Beck Depression Inventory
BPRS	Brief Psychiatric Rating Scale
CNS	Central Nervous System
CNV	Contingent Negative Variation
CPS	Cycles Per Second
CPT	Continuous Performance Test
DQ	Deterioration Quotient
ECDEU	Early Clinical Drug Evaluation Unit
ECT	Electroconvulsive Therapy
EEG	Electroencephalogram
EMG	Electromyograph
EP	Evoked Potential
GRS	Geriatric Rating Scale
HAMA	Hamilton Anxiety Scale
HAMD	Hamilton Psychiatric Rating Scale for Depression
HSCL	Hopkins Symptom Checklist
K-scale	Correction Scale (MMPI)
L-scale	Lie Scale (MMPI)
MAS	Manifest Anxiety Scale
MMPI	Minnesota Multiphasic Personality Inventory
MMPI-D	Minnesota Multiphasic Personality Inventory Depression Scale
MSQ	Mental Status Questionnaire
NIMH	National Institute of Mental Health
NOSIE	Nurse's Observation Scale for Inpatient Evaluation
OBD	Organic Brain Disease
PAMIE	Physical and Mental Impairment of Function Evaluation
POMS	Profile of Mood Scales
RDC	Research Diagnostic Criteria
REM	Rapid Eye Movement
SAS	Social Adjustment Scale
SCAG	Sandoz Clinical Assessment–Geriatric
SDRS	Social Dysfunction Rating Scale
SDS	Self-rating Depression Scale (Zung)
SSIAM	Structured and Scaled Interview to Assess Maladjustment
WAIS	Weschler Adult Intelligence Scale
W–B	Wechsler Bellevue
WMS	Wechsler Memory Scale

Author Index

Subject Index